Tooth Whitening in Esthetic Dentistry

So-Ran Kwon
Seok-Hoon Ko
Linda H. Greenwall

Tooth Whitening in Esthetic Dentistry

Tooth Whitening Communication Tool

So-Ran Kwon
Seok-Hoon Ko
Linda H. Greenwall

With contributions from
Ronald E. Goldstein, DDS
Van B. Haywood, DMD
Hisashi Hisamitsu, DDS, PhD
Stephen J. Chu, DMD, MSD, CDT

quintessence books

Quintessence Publishing Co, Ltd
London, Berlin, Chicago, Tokyo, Barcelona, Beijing, Istanbul, Milan,
Moscow, Mumbai, Paris, Prague, São Paulo, and Warsaw

British Library Cataloguing in Publication Data
Kwon, So-Ran
Tooth Whitening in Esthetic Dentistry : principles and techniques
1. Teeth – Bleching 2. Dentistry – Aesthetic aspects
I. Title II. Ko, Seok-Hoon III. Greenwall, Linda
617.6
ISBN-13: 978-1-85097-177-1

Quintessence Publishing Co, Ltd
Grafton Road
New Malden
Surrey KT3 3AB
United Kingdom
www.quintpub.co.uk

Editor: Suzyon O'Neal Wandrey

ISBN-13: 978-1-85097-177-1
Printed in Singapore

Contents

Tooth whitening communication tool

■ How does whitening work?

The tooth is a semi-permeable membrane, and the tooth whitening materials – carbamide peroxide and hydrogen peroxide – penetrate into the tooth, thus removing extrinsic and intrinsic stains.

■ How white will my teeth look like after whitening?

There are individual variations since the color improvement depends on the cause of discoloration, tooth characteristics and your cooperation. In very rare, cases there may be no visible color change after whitening but, if you follow the instructions of your dentist, your teeth will definitely become whiter and brighter so that you should be happy with your smile.

■ How long will it take?

The duration of treatment depends on the degree of discoloration and your cooperation. Generally, tooth whitening takes 2 to 6 weeks. For severe discolorations, extended treatment times ranging from 3 to 6 months may be required.

■ What kind of discomfort may I experience during whitening?

Sensitivity to cold is a common discomfort during tooth whitening. It usually disappears in a few hours, but if it continues, please consult your dentist or dental staff for immediate relief. A burning sensation of the gums and, occasionally, a transient change of taste may occur.

■ How do I maintain the shade after completion of tooth whitening?

To maintain your white and bright smile for a long time, avoid food that contains strong colorants that cause rediscoloration of your teeth. A proper prophylaxis every 6 months is recommended, and a simple touch-up whitening procedure may be repeated every 1 to 2 years.

1. Single dark tooth

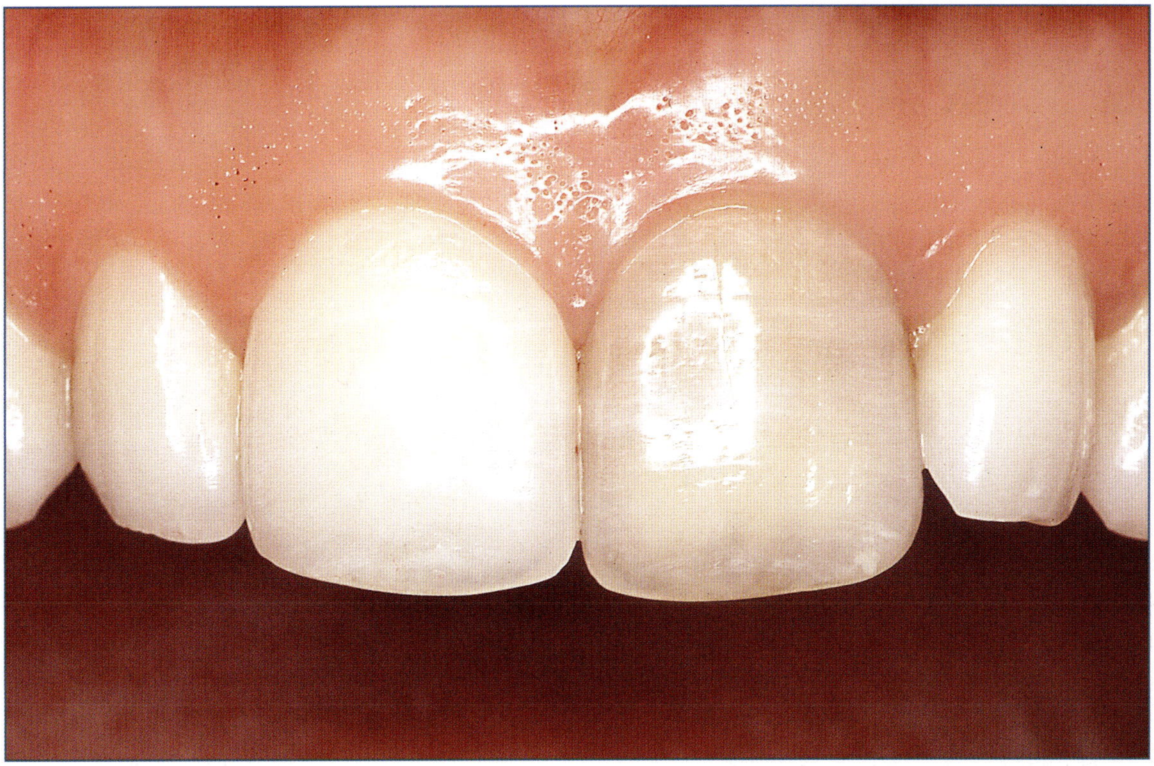

before whitening

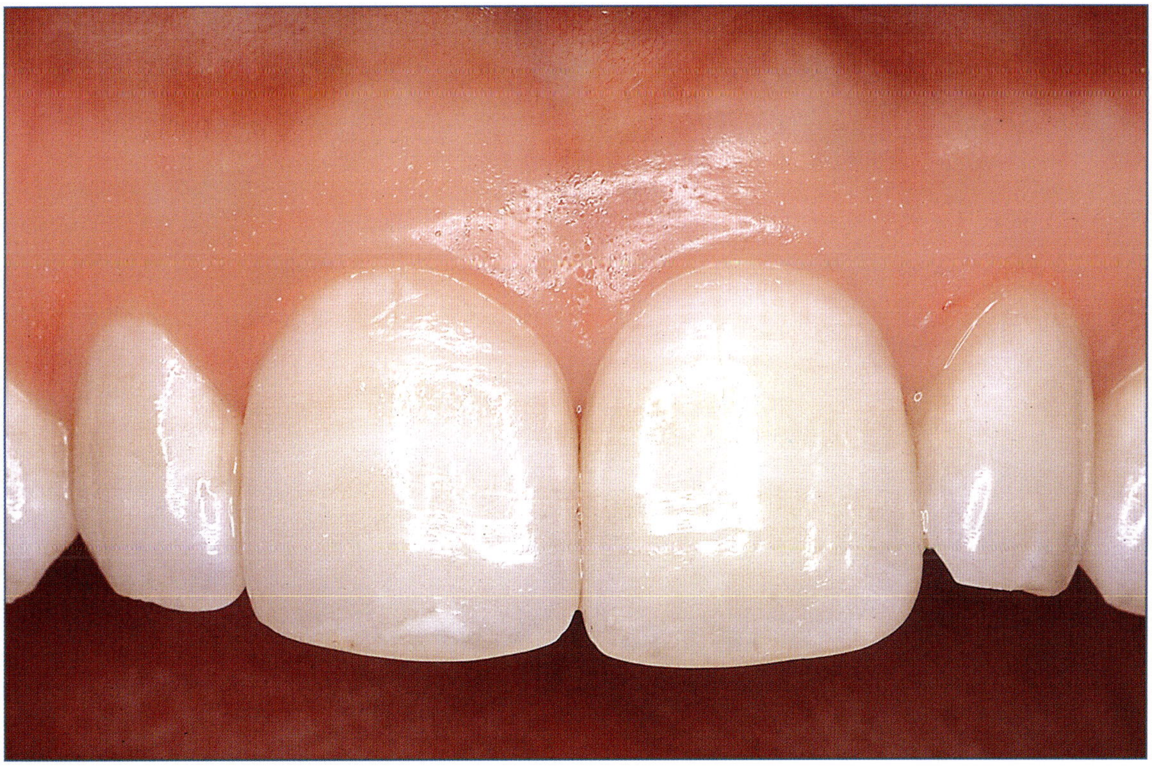

after whitening

2. Generalized yellow teeth with a single dark tooth

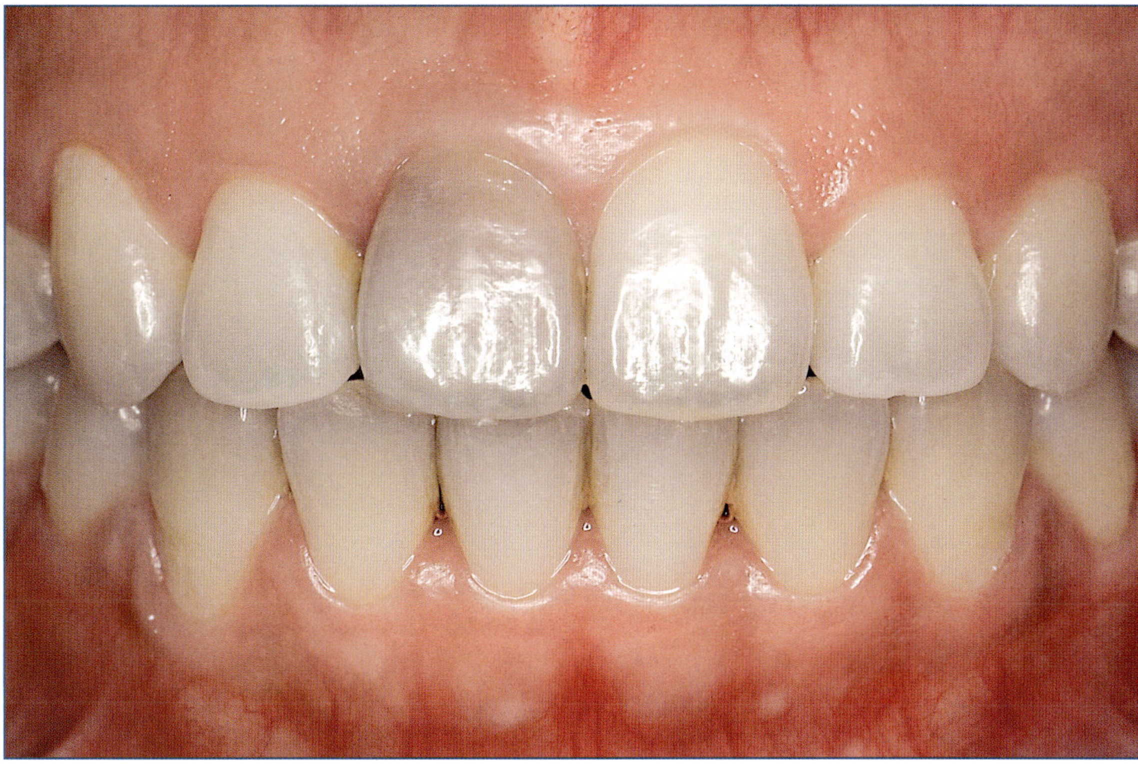

before whitening

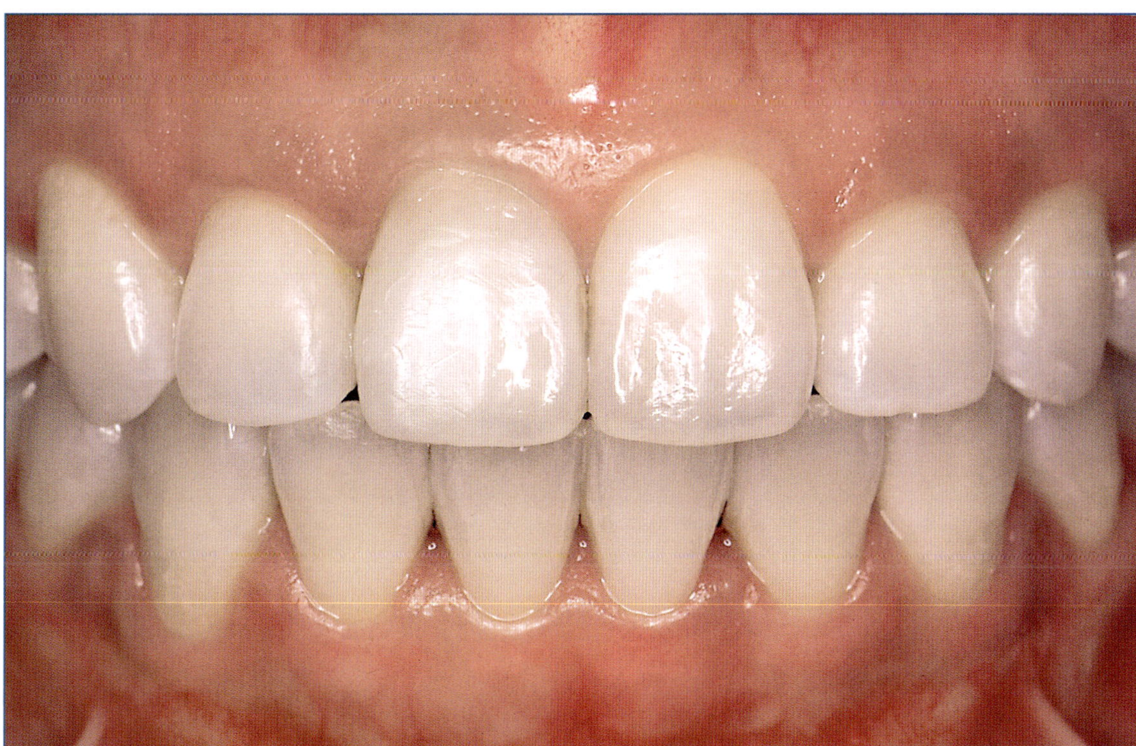

after whitening

3. Congenital yellow teeth

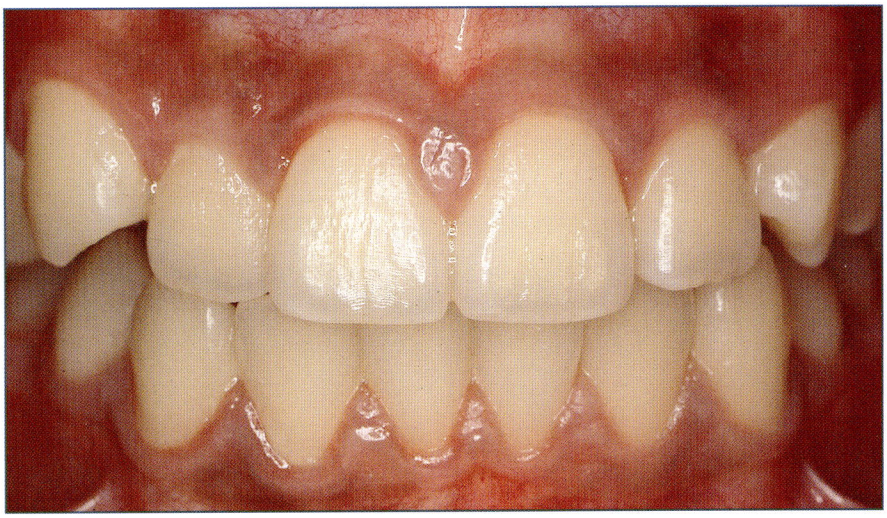

before whitening

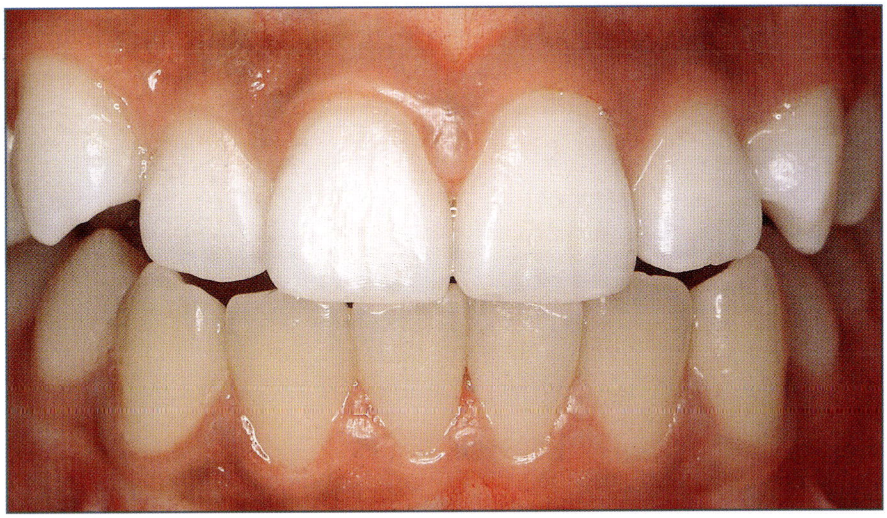

during whitening

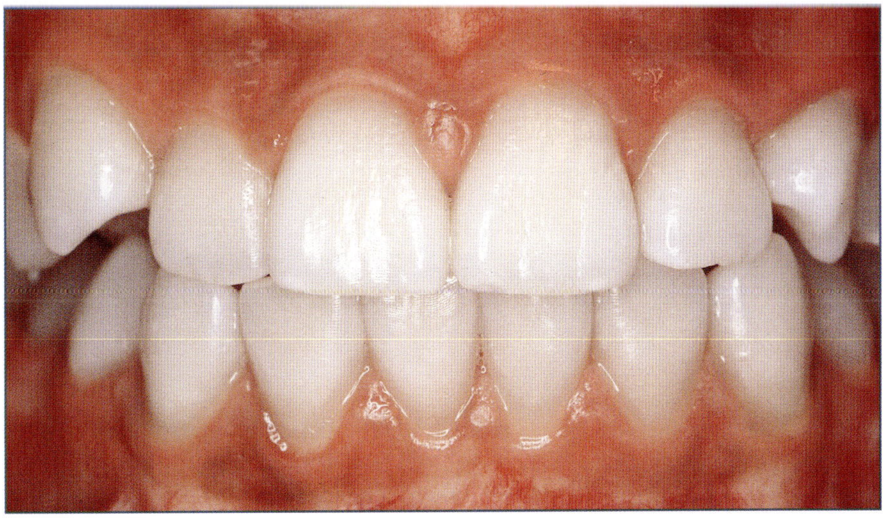

after whitening

4. Generalized yellow teeth with superficial brown stains

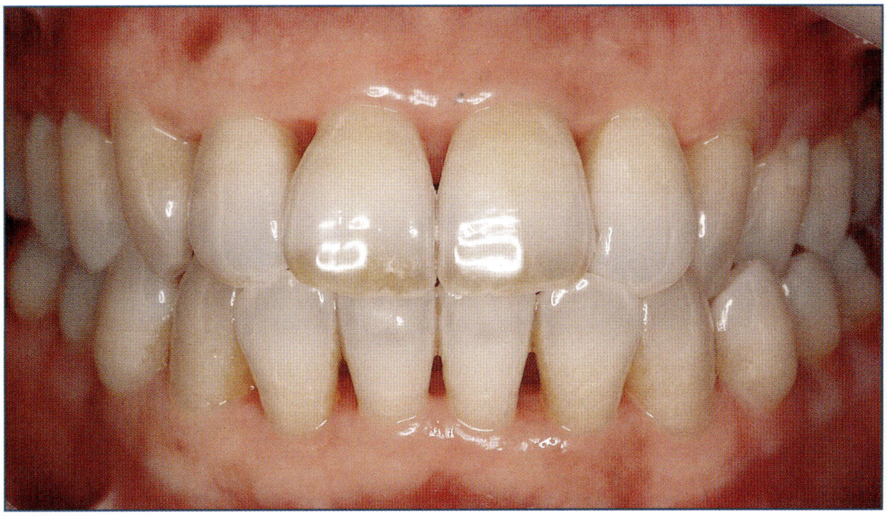

before whitening

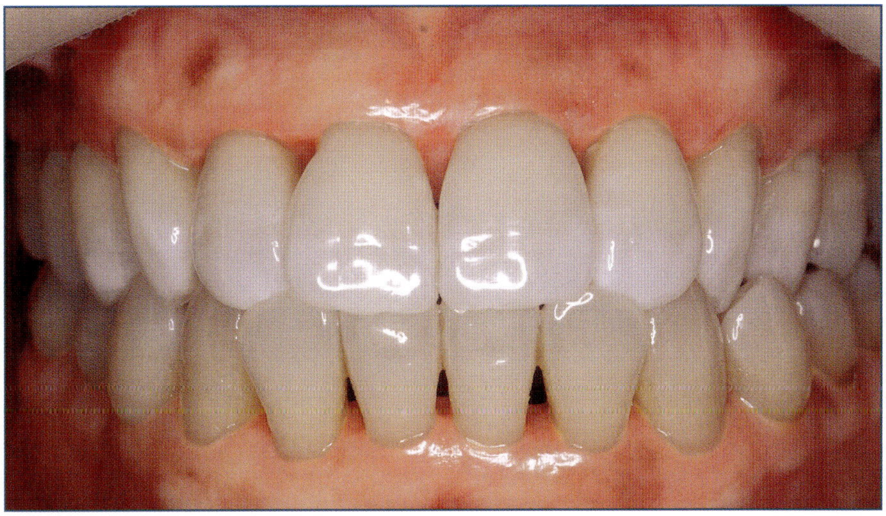

during whitening

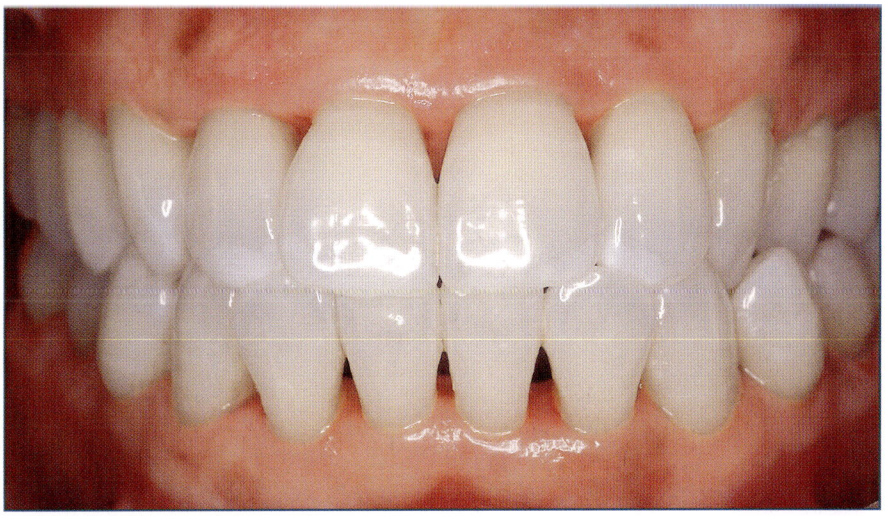

after whitening

5. Whitening for a natural smile

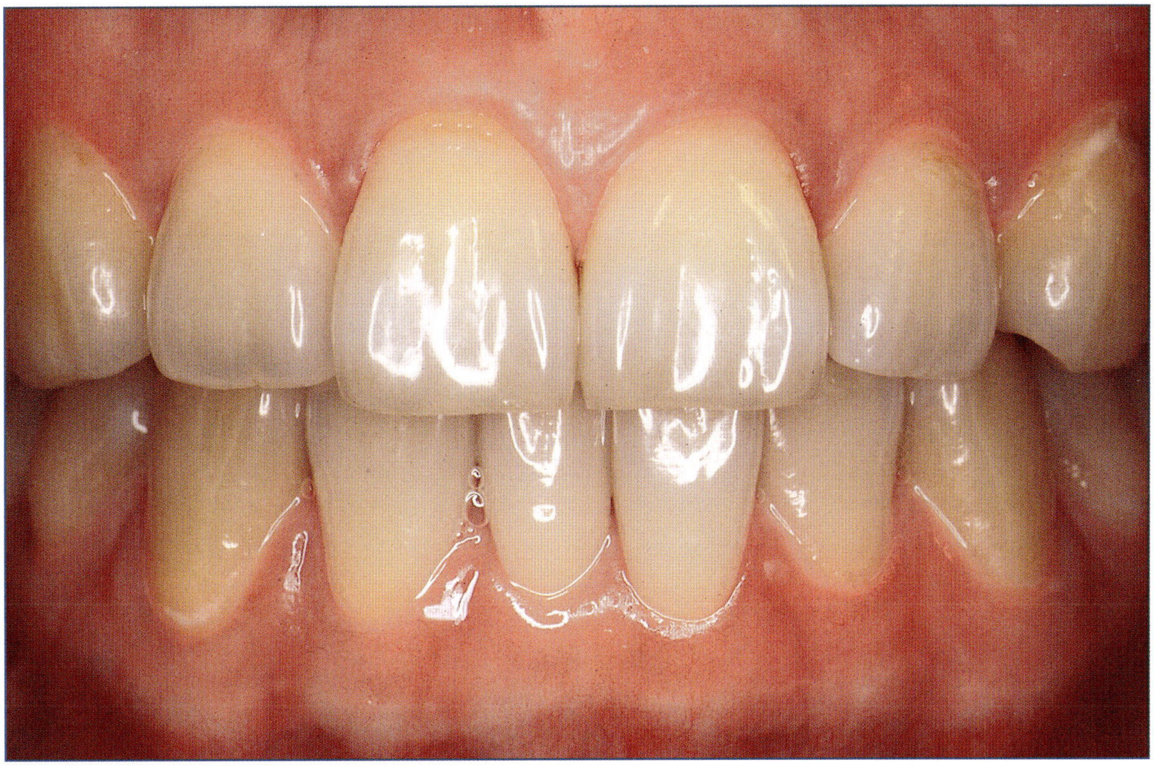

before whitening

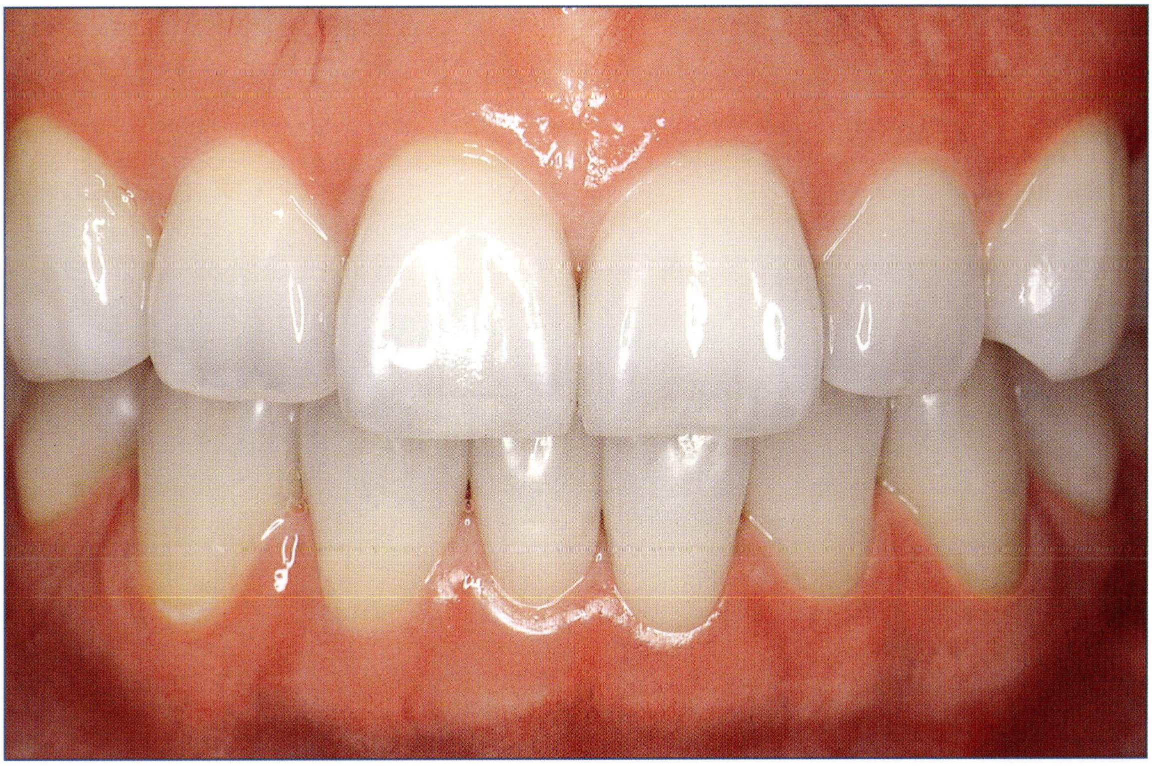

after whitening

6. Whitening after orthodontic treatment

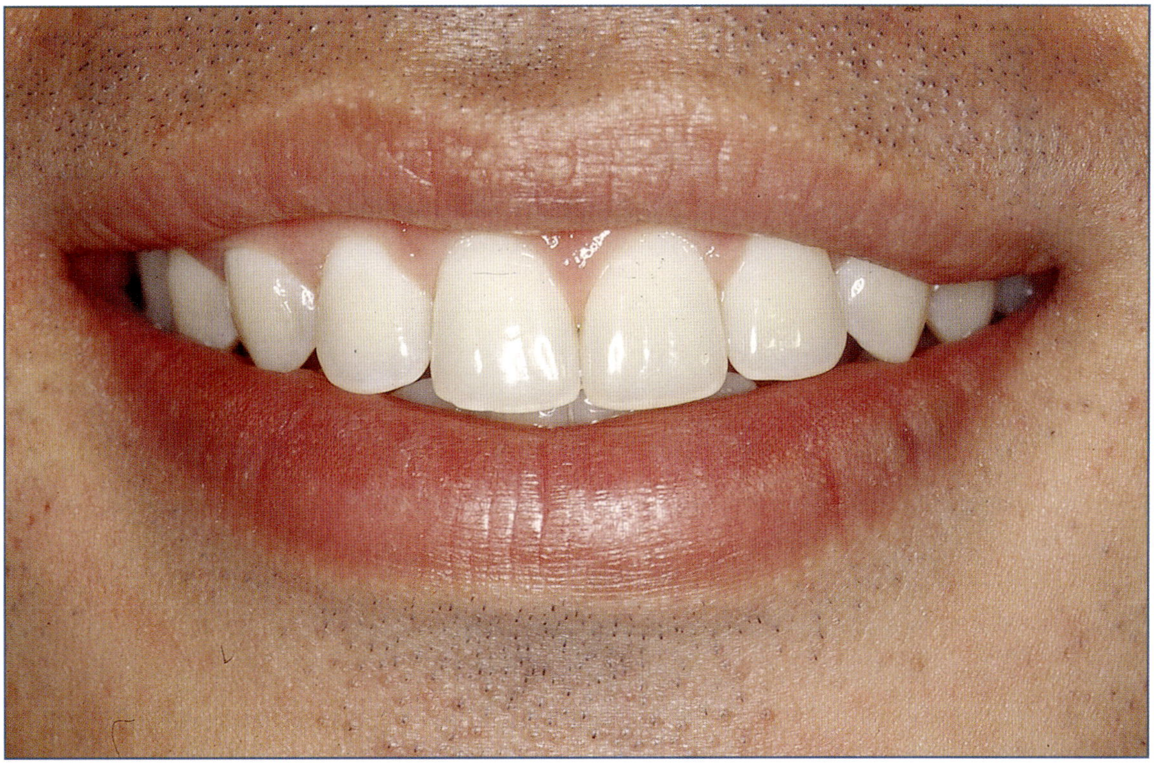

before whitening

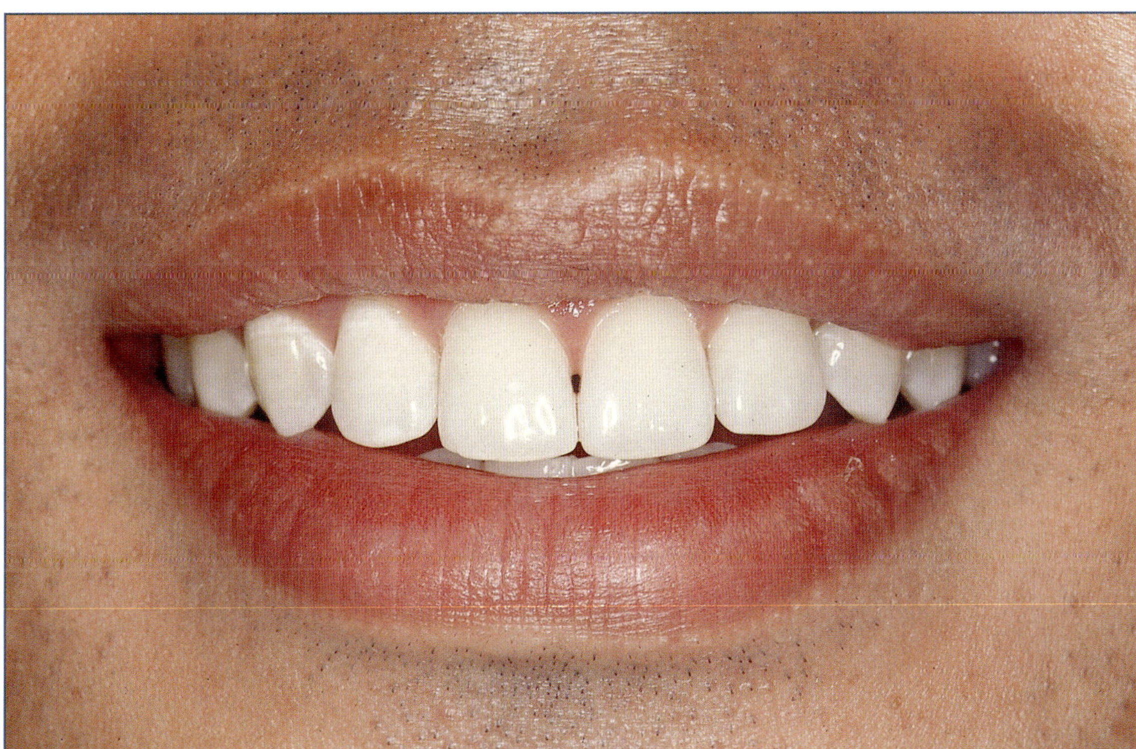

after whitening

7. Whitening in heavy smokers

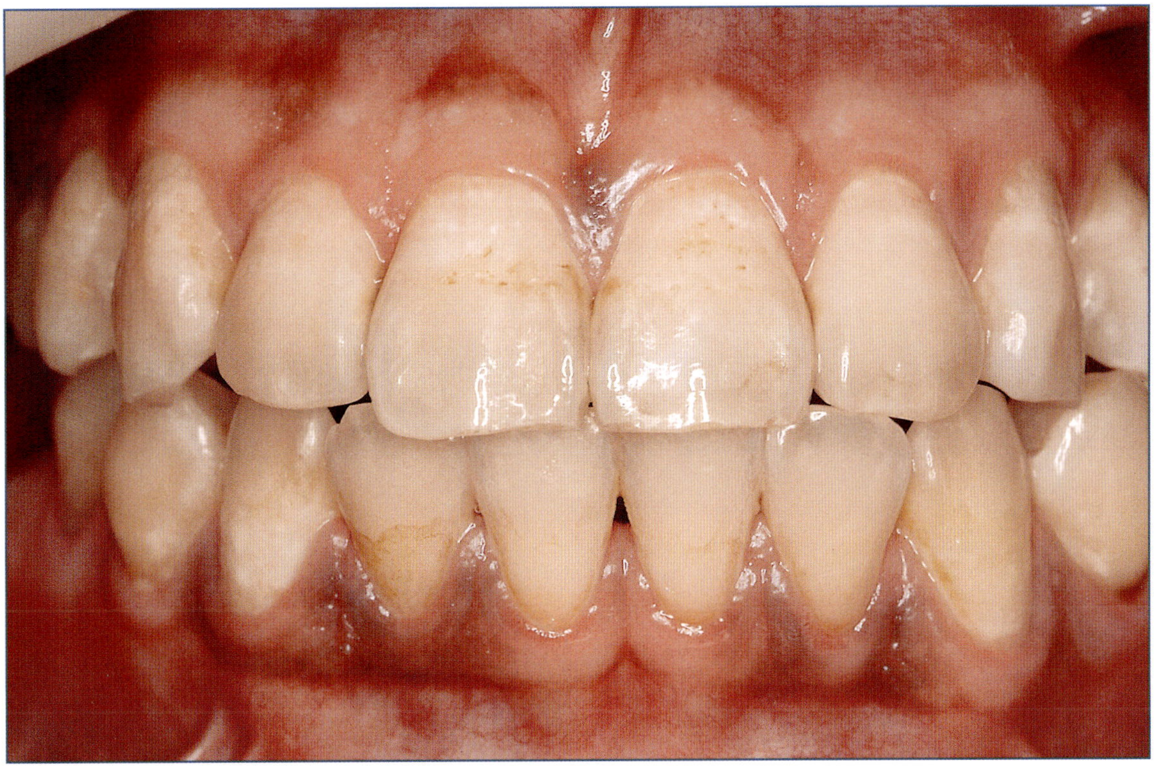

before whitening

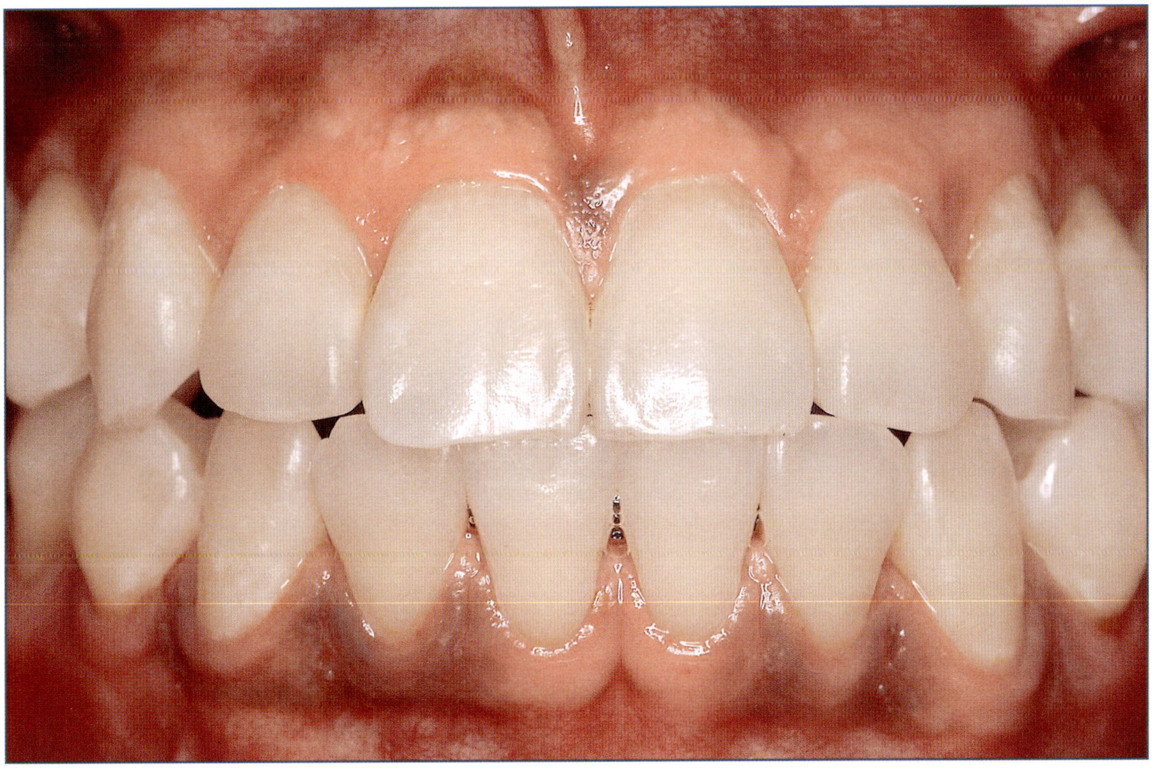

after whitening

8. Whitening to look 10 years younger

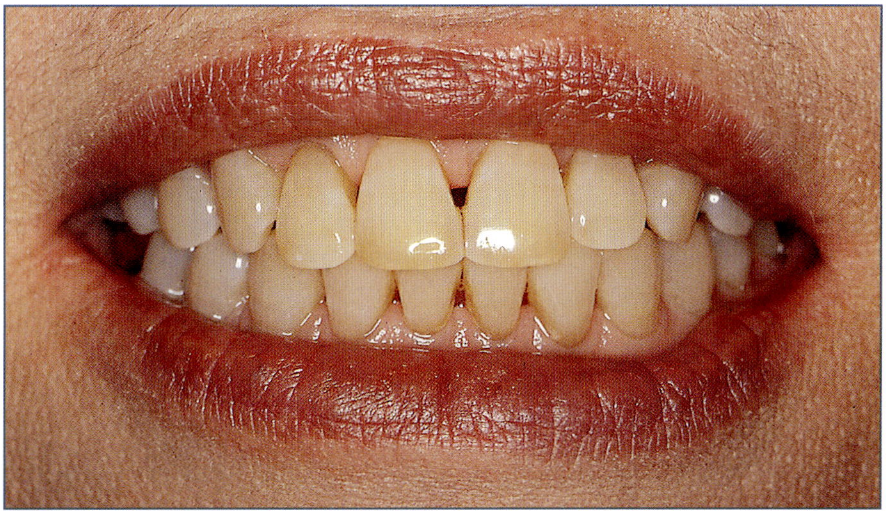

before whitening

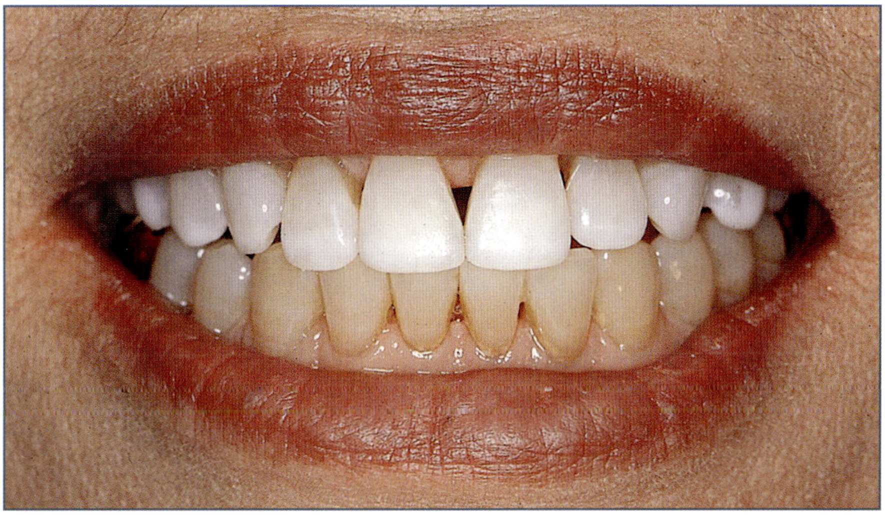

during whitening

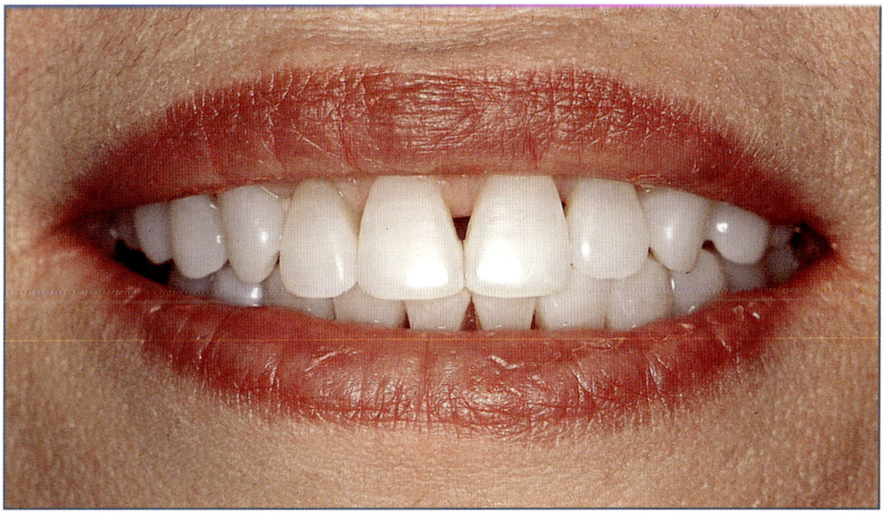

after whitening

9. Whitening combined with esthetic bonded restorations

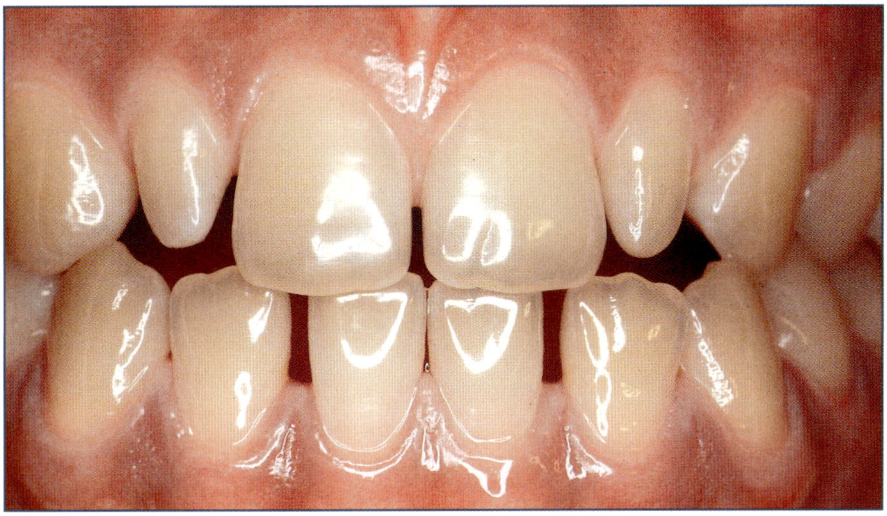

before whitening

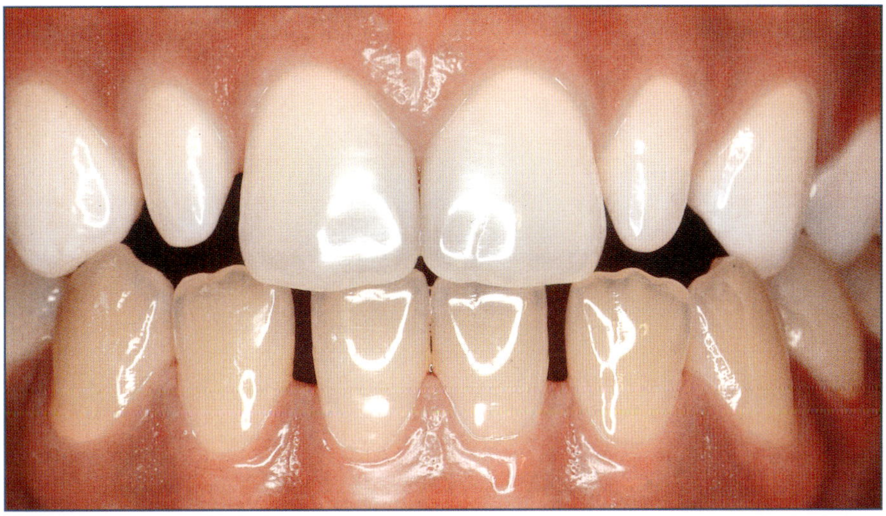

during whitening

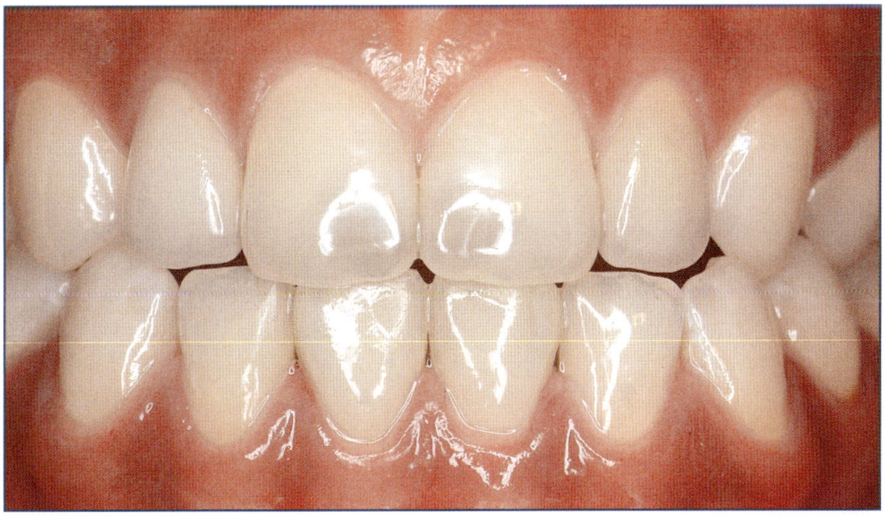

after whitening and esthetic bonded restorations

10. Whitening combined with porcelain laminate veneers

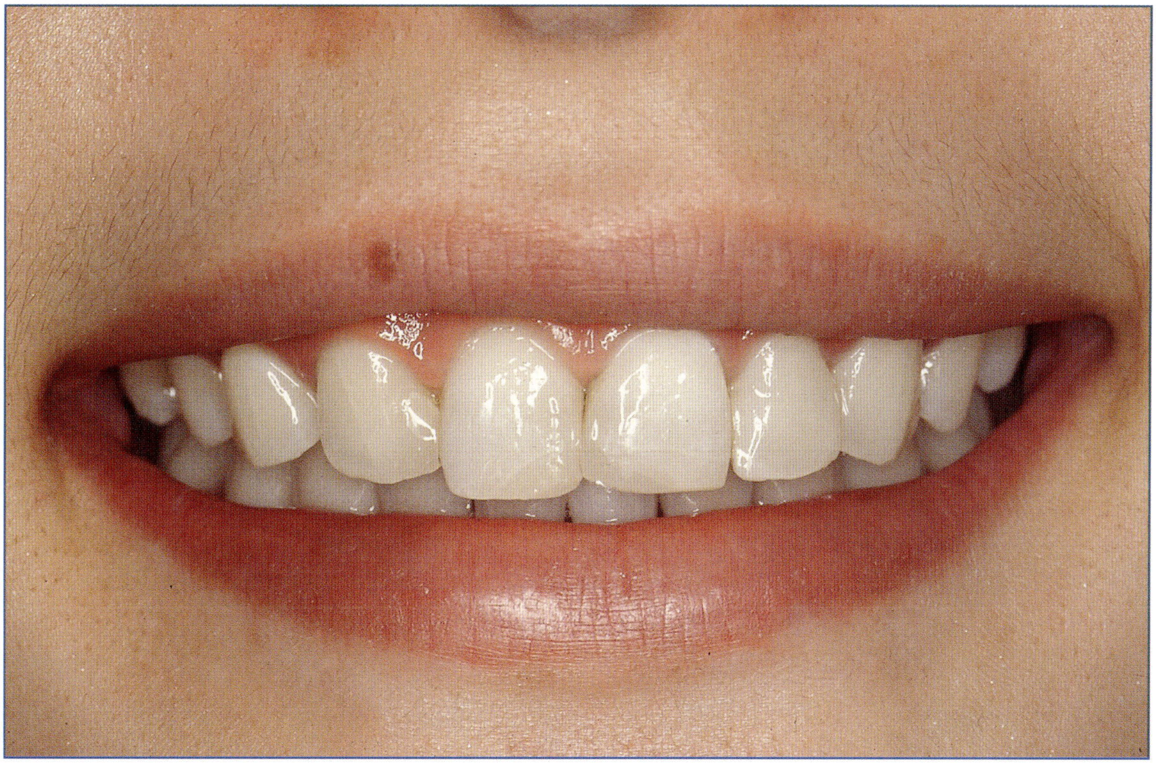

before whitening

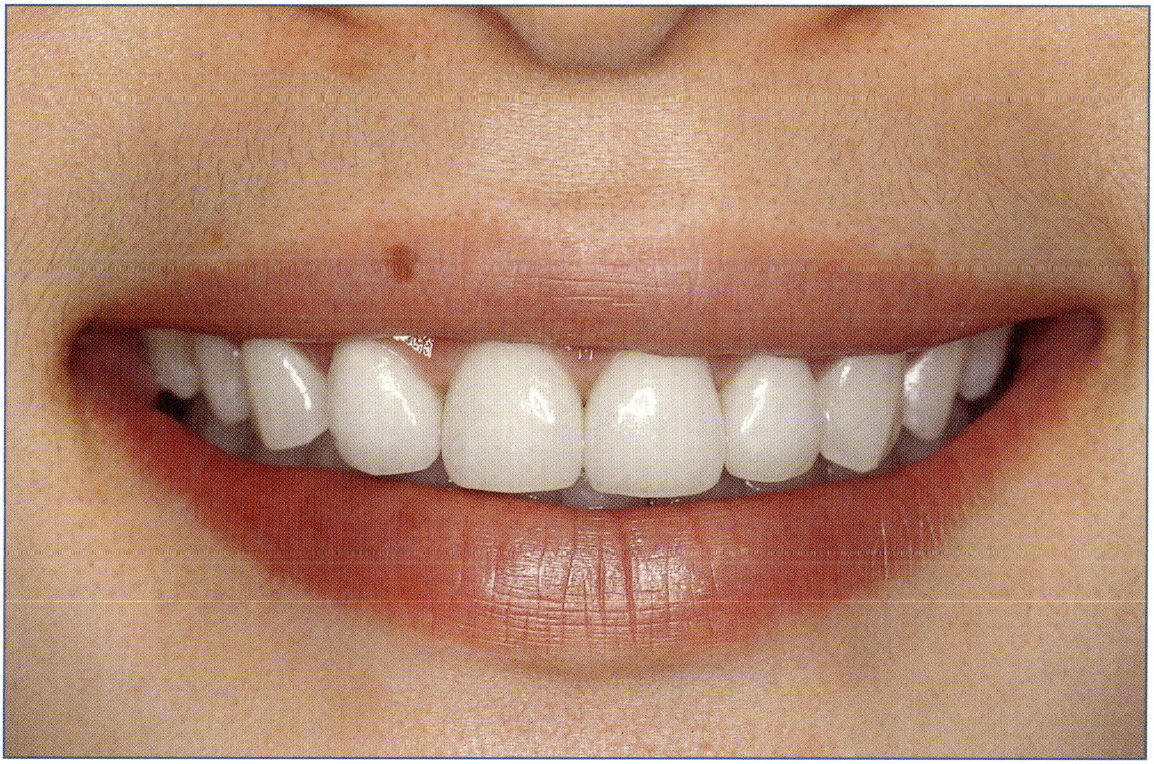

after whitening and four upper porcelain laminate veneers

11. Whitening in short teeth

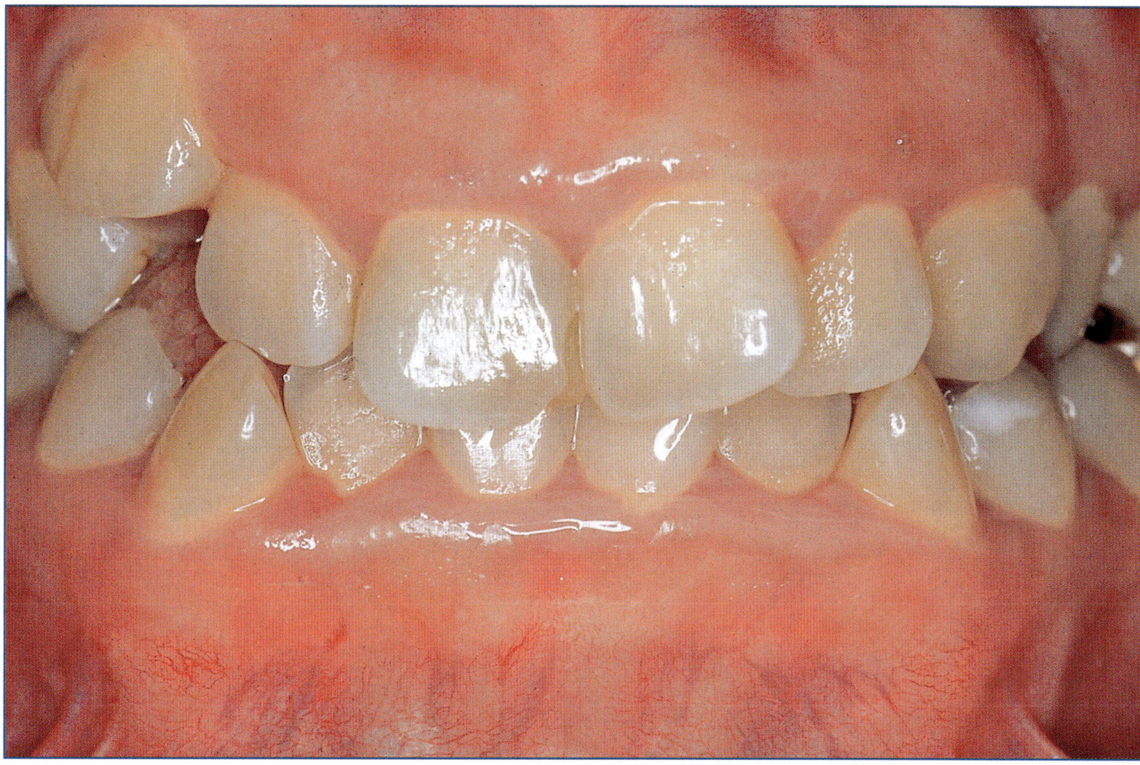

before whitening

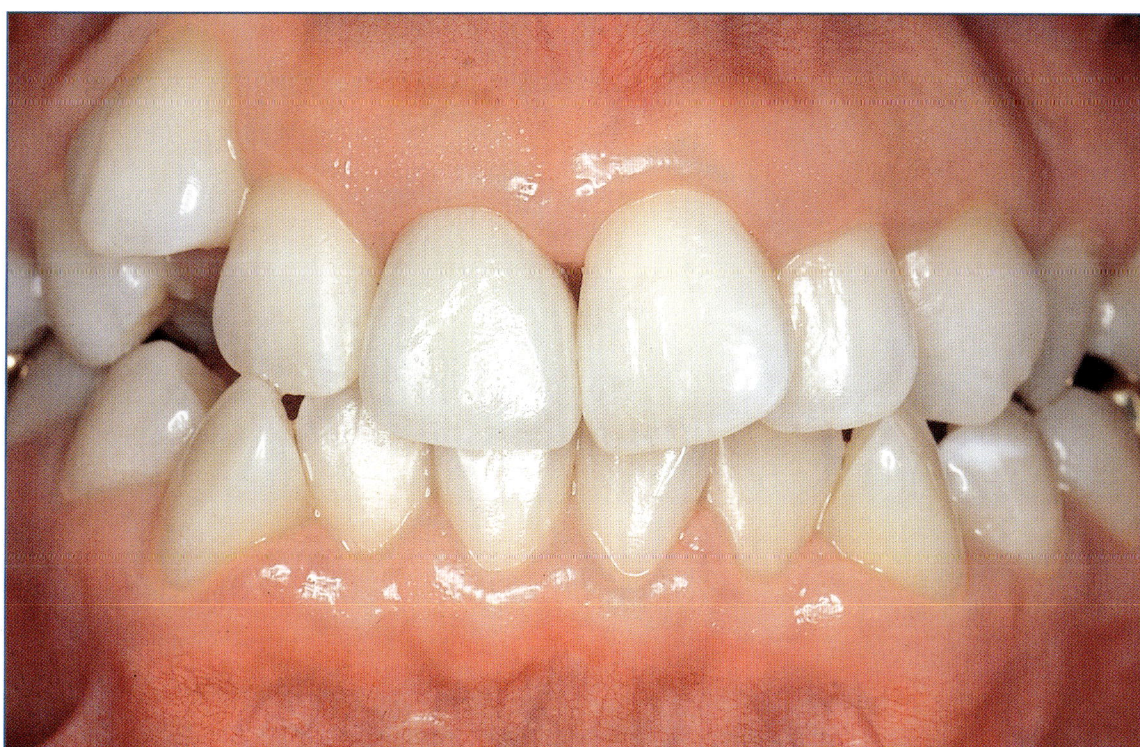

after crown lengthening and whitening

12. Whitening for children

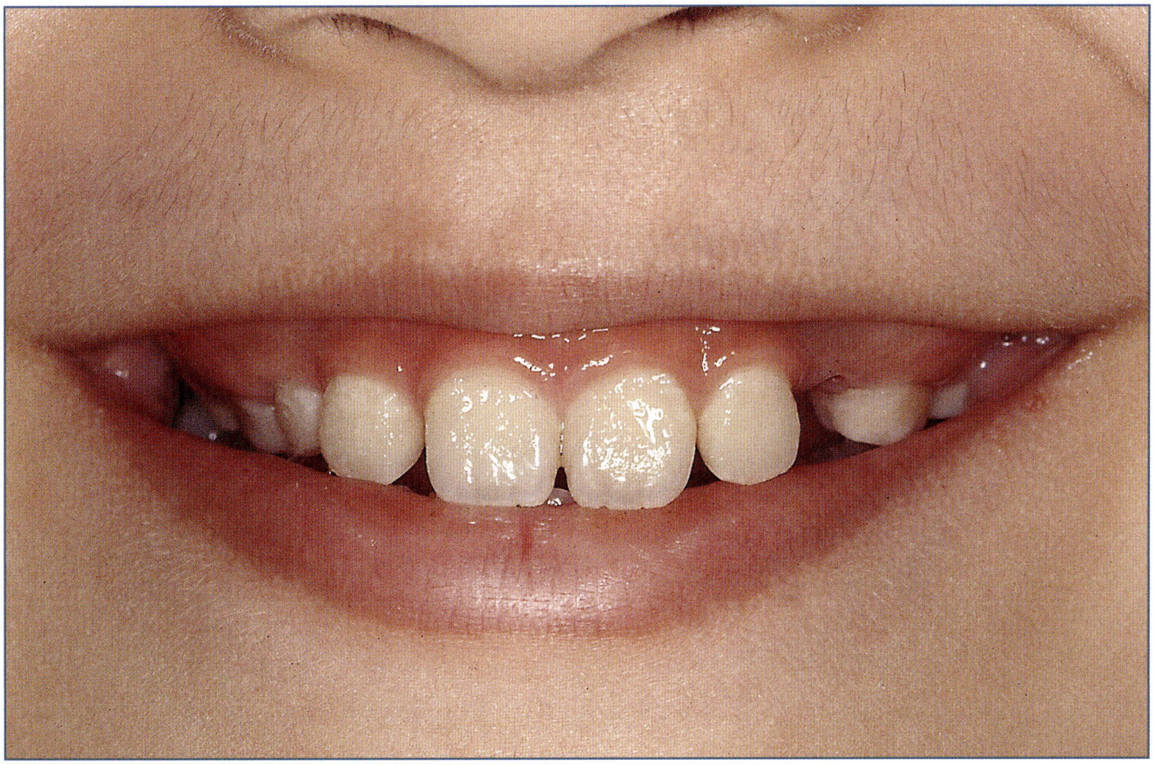

before whitening

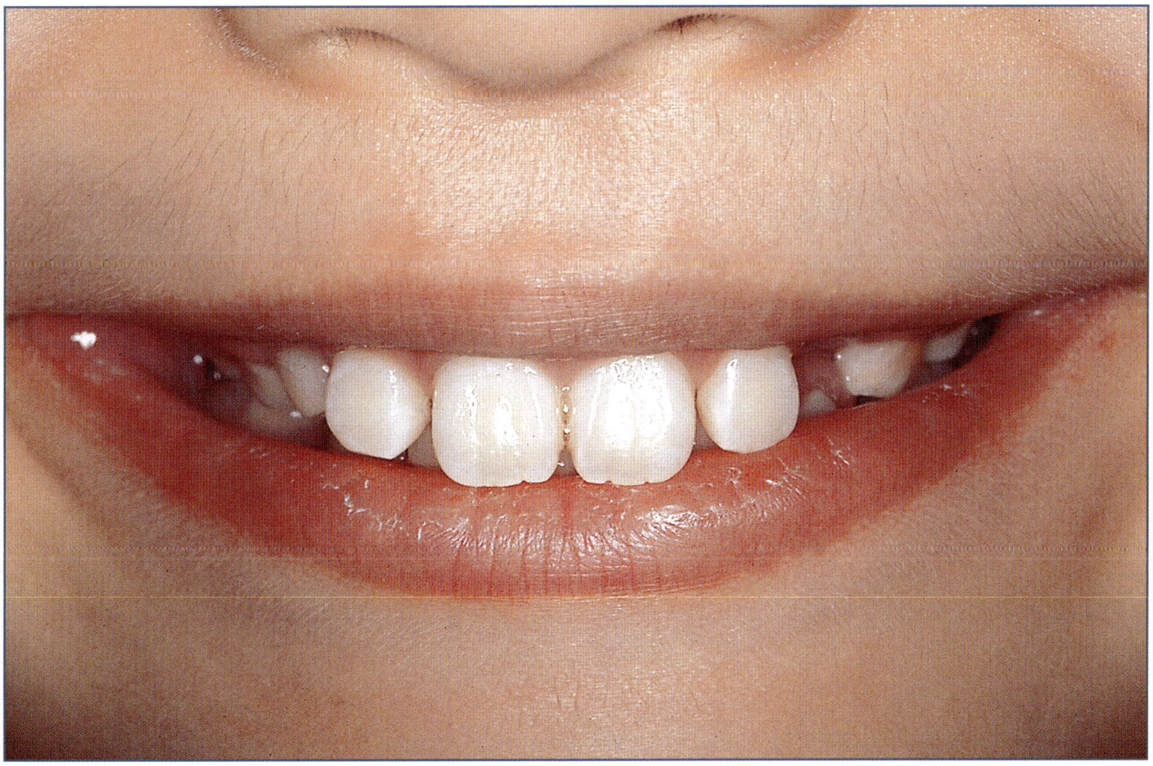

after whitening

13. White spots

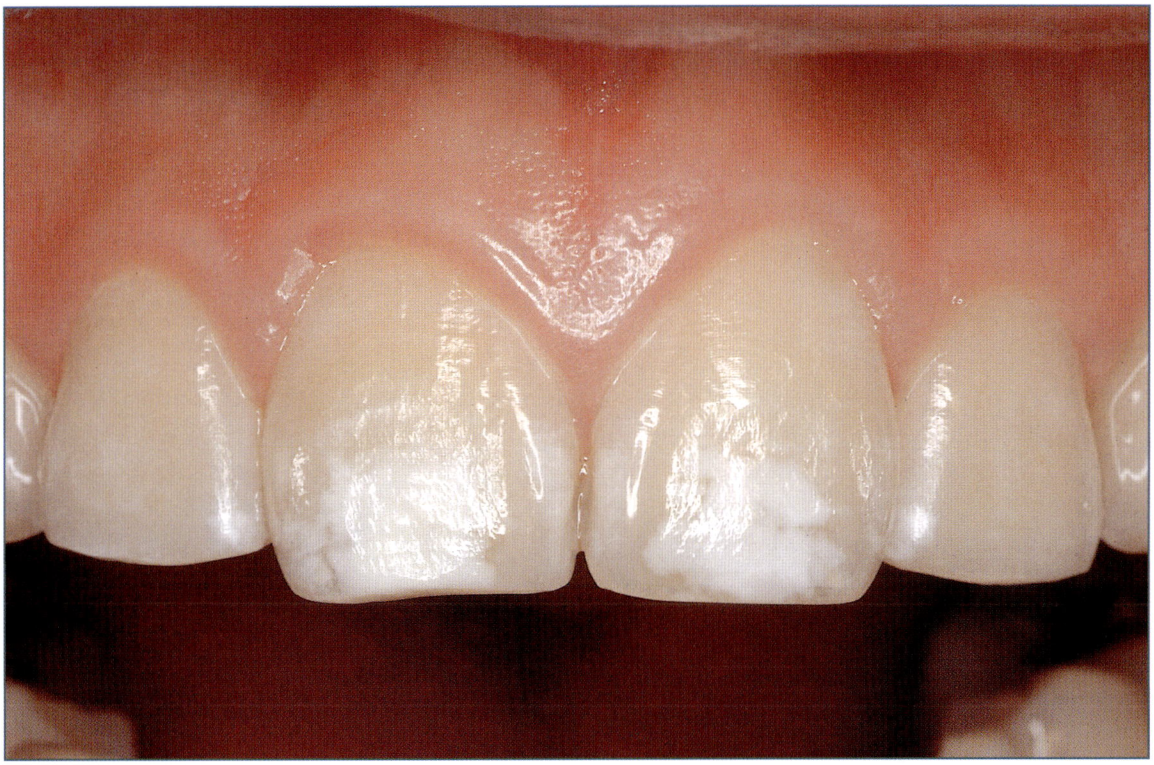

before treatment

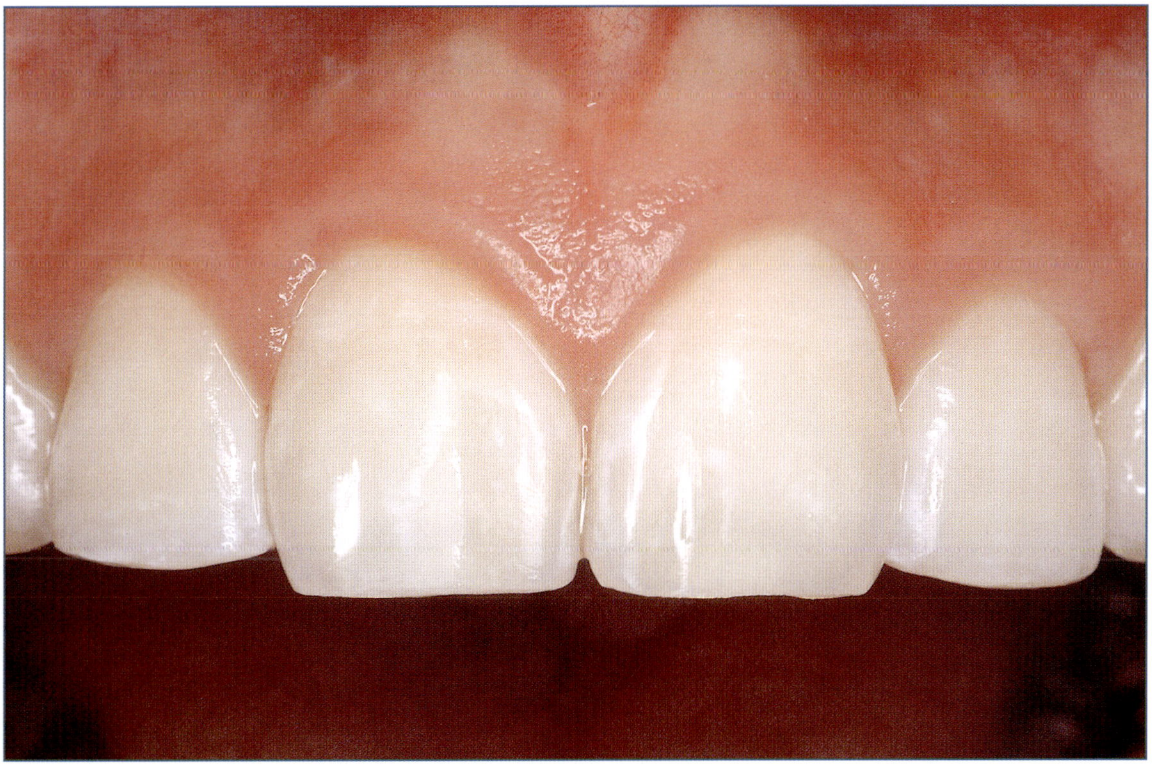

after treatment

14. Whitening in teeth with superficial decalcification

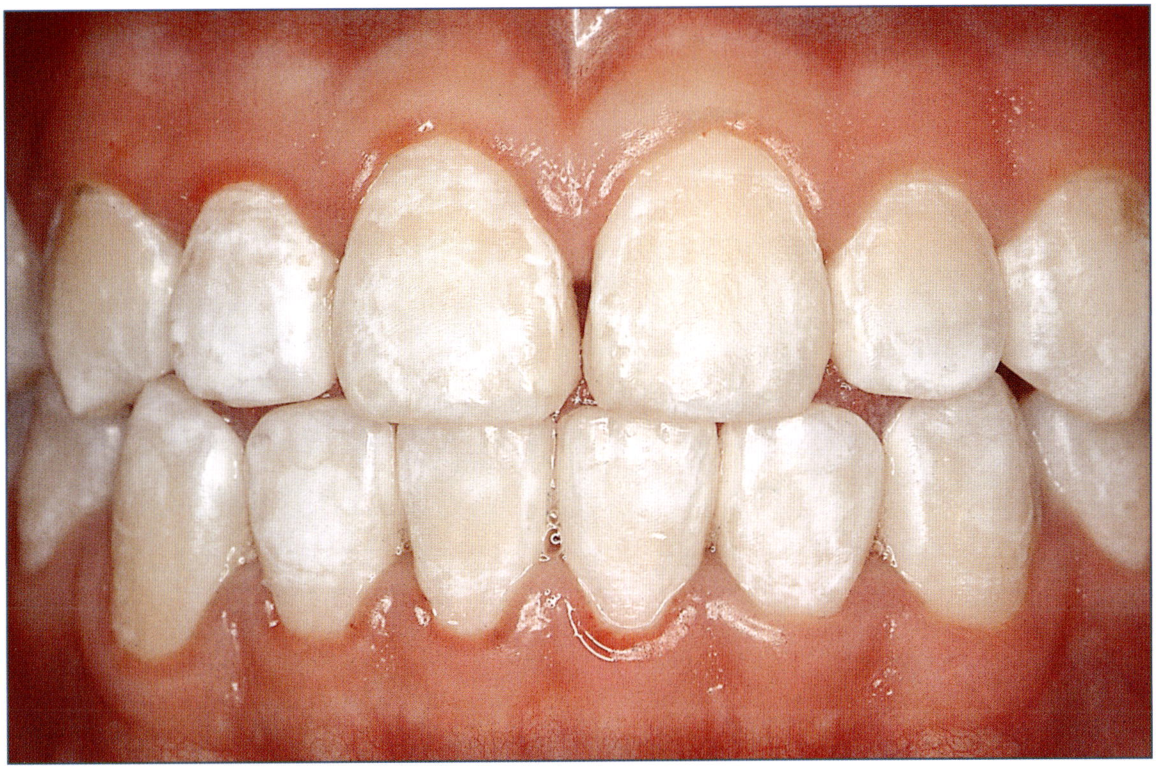

before whitening

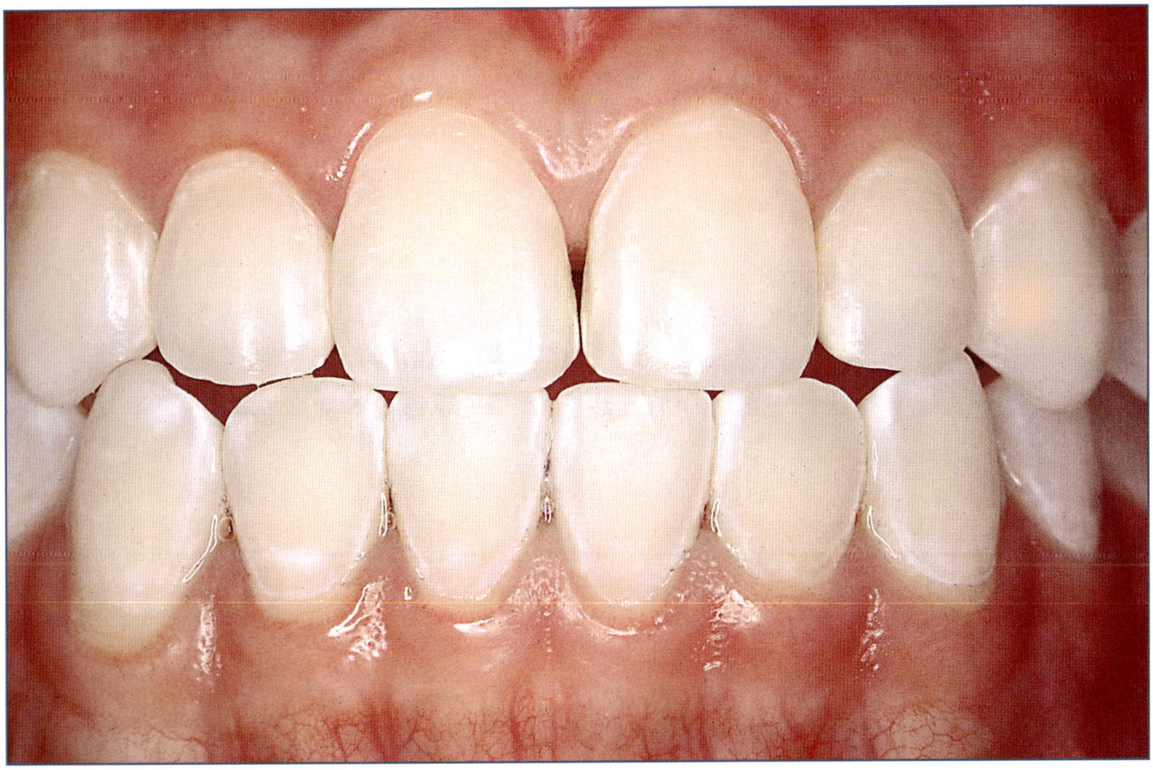

after microabrasion and whitening

15. Tetracycline discoloration

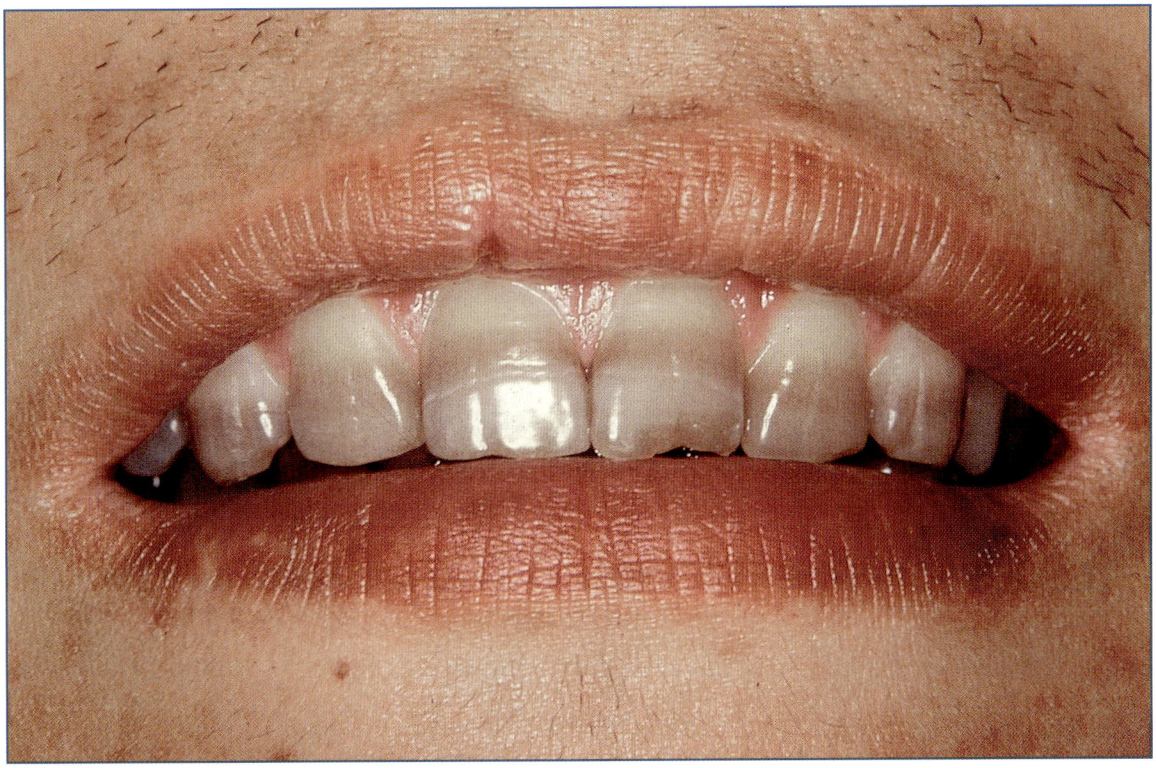

before whitening

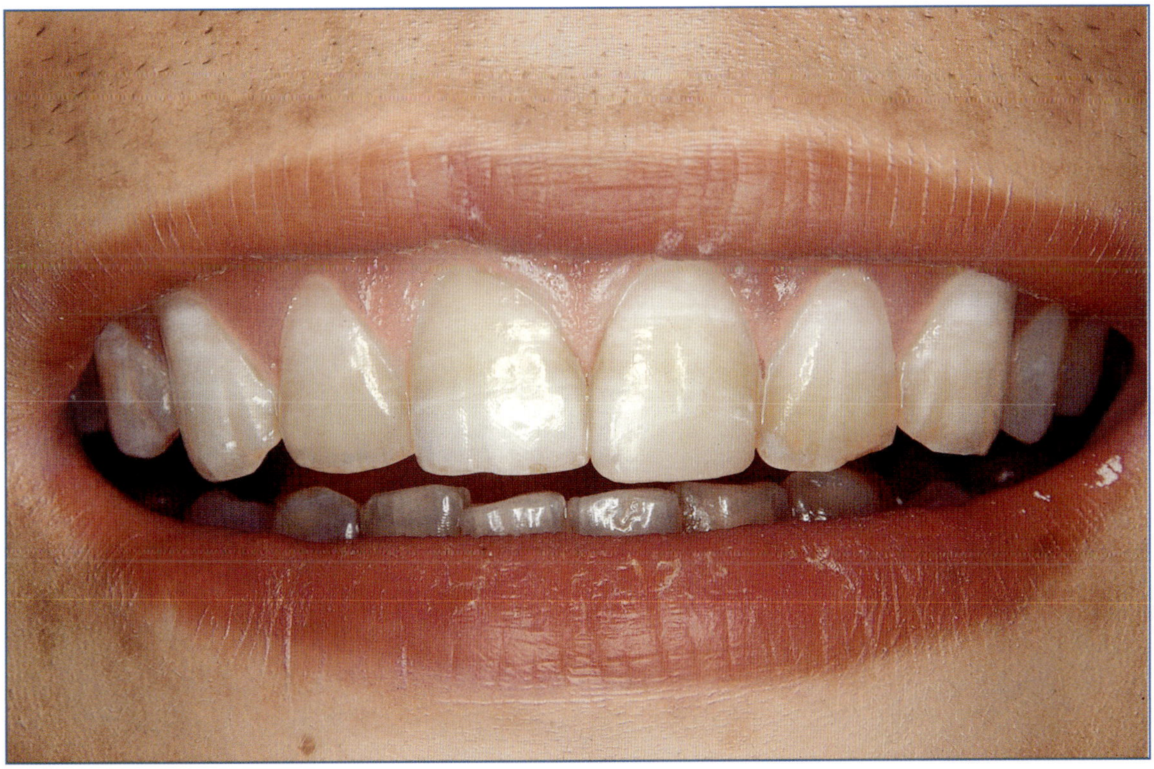

after whitening

16. Tetracycline discoloration with crack lines

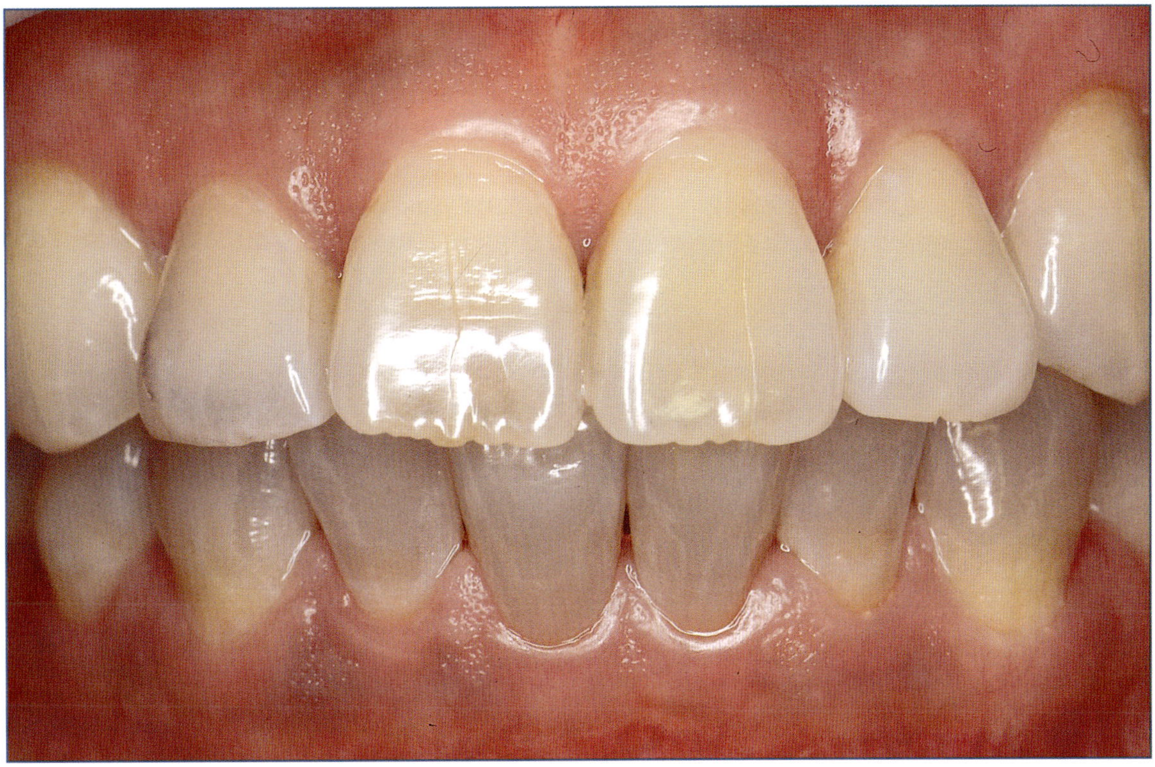

before whitening

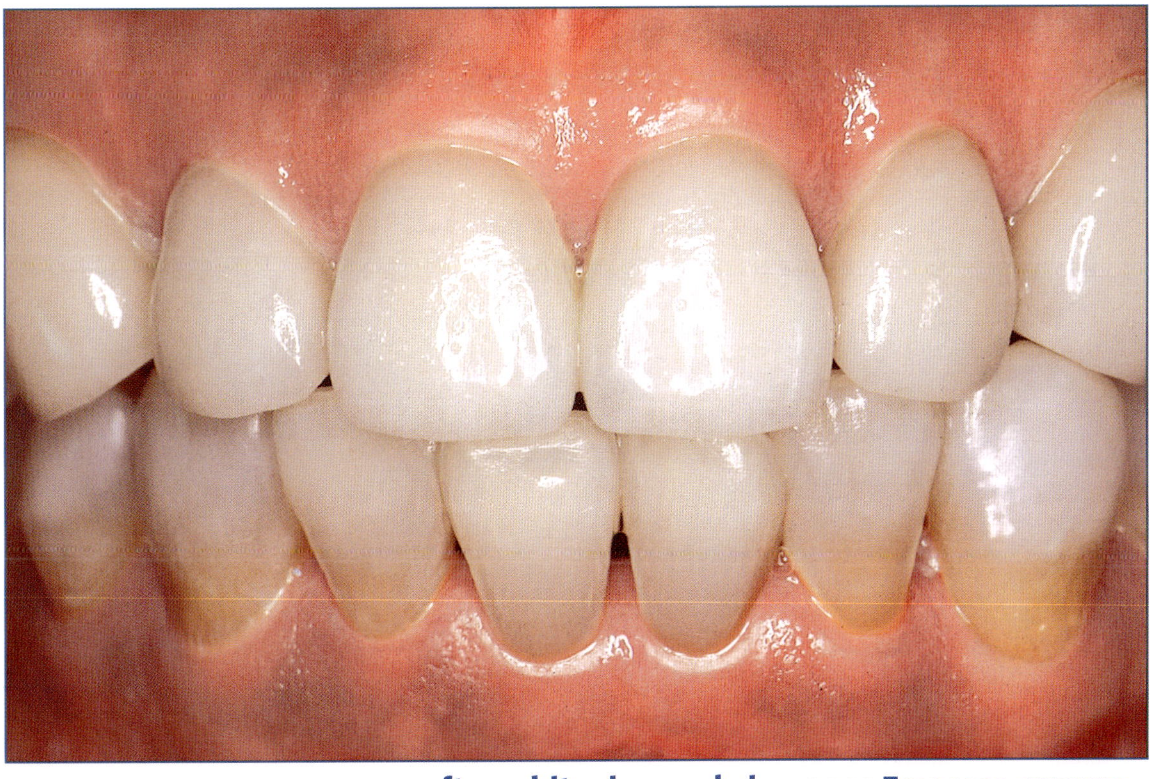

after whitening and six upper Empress crowns

17. Tooth jewelry

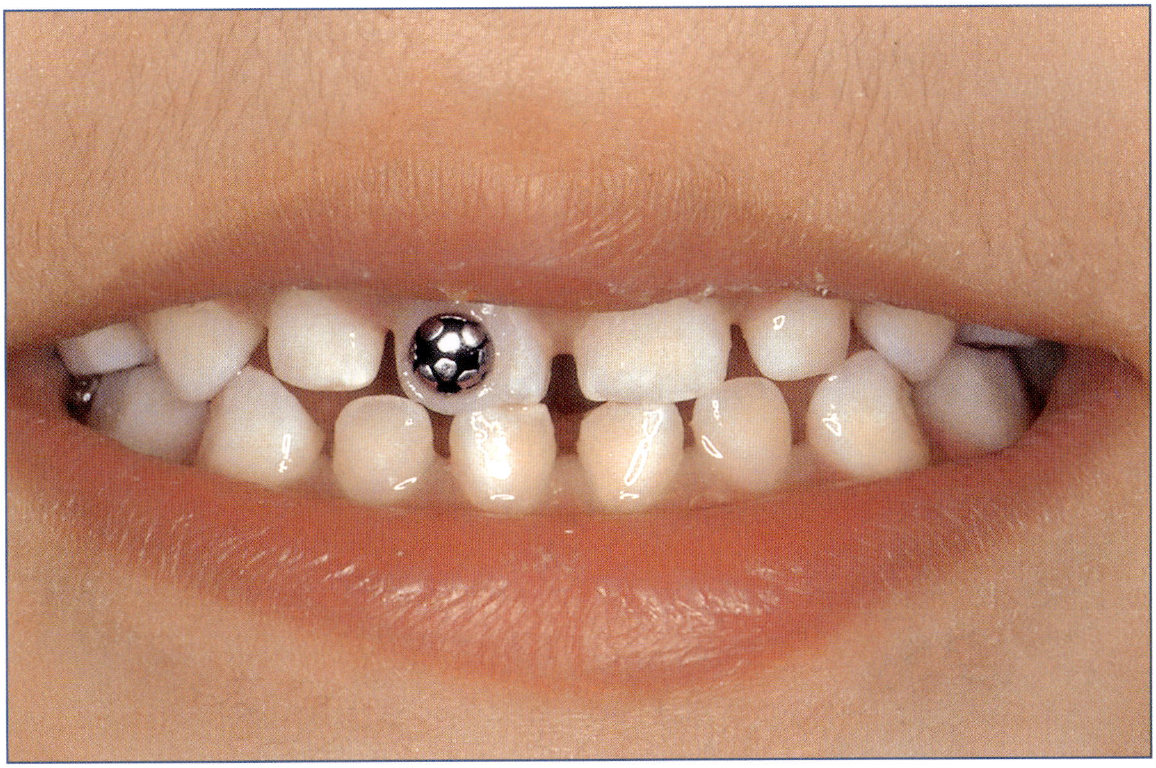

Soccer ball

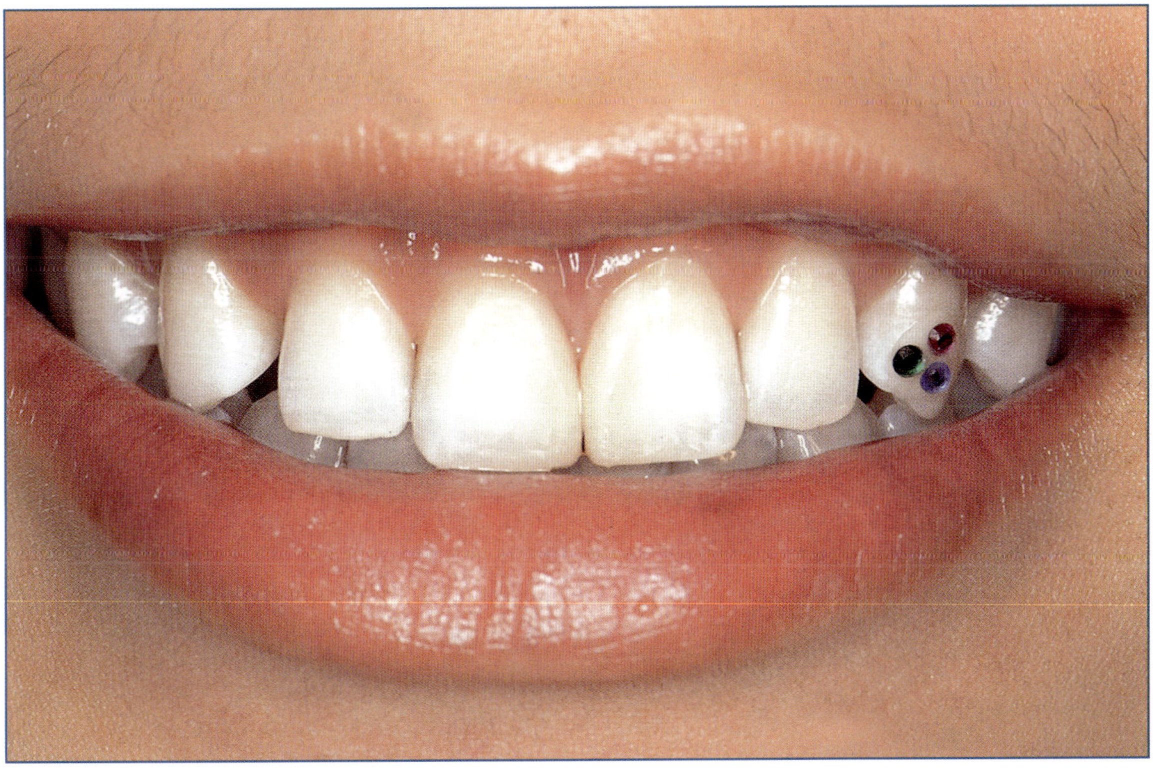

Ruby, sapphire, emerald

Tooth Whitening in Esthetic Dentistry

So-Ran Kwon
Seok-Hoon Ko
Linda H. Greenwall

Tooth Whitening in Esthetic Dentistry

Principles and Techniques

So-Ran Kwon
Seok-Hoon Ko
Linda H. Greenwall

With contributions from
Ronald E. Goldstein, DDS
Van B. Haywood, DMD
Hisashi Hisamitsu, DDS, PhD
Stephen J. Chu, DMD, MSD, CDT

quintessence books

Quintessence Publishing Co, Ltd
London, Berlin, Chicago, Tokyo, Barcelona, Beijing, Istanbul, Milan,
Moscow, Mumbai, Paris, Prague, São Paulo, and Warsaw

British Library Cataloguing in Publication Data
Kwon, So-Ran
Tooth Whitening in Esthetic Dentistry : principles and techniques
1. Teeth – Bleching 2. Dentistry – Aesthetic aspects
I. Title II. Ko, Seok-Hoon III. Greenwall, Linda
617.6
ISBN-13: 978-1-85097-177-1

quintessence books

Quintessence Publishing Co, Ltd
Grafton Road
New Malden
Surrey KT3 3AB
United Kingdom
www.quintpub.co.uk

Editor: Suzyon O'Neal Wandrey

ISBN-13: 978-1-85097-177-1
Printed in Singapore

Editors and Contributors

Editors

Dr. So-Ran Kwon, DDS, MS, PhD
Michigan Dental Clinic
Seoul, Korea

Dr. Seok-Hoon Ko, DDS, MS, MS
President
International Federation of Esthetic Dentistry
Seoul, Korea

Dr. Linda Greenwall
BDS, MGDS RCS, MRD RCS, MSc, FGDP
London, UK

Contributors

Ronald E. Goldstein, DDS
Clinical Professor of Oral Rehabilitation
School of Dentistry, Medical College of Georgia
Augusta, Georgia, USA

Van B. Haywood, DMD
Professor and Director of Dental Continuing Education
Department of Oral Rehabilitation
School of Dentistry, Medical College of Georgia
Augusta, Georgia, USA

Hisashi Hisamitsu, DDS, PhD
Professor and Chairman, Department of Clinical Cariology and Endodontology
Showa University School of Dentistry, Tokyo, Japan

Stephen J. Chu, DMD, MSD, CDT
Director, Advanced CDE Program in Aesthetic Dentistry
Clinical Associate Professor, Department of Periodontics and Implant Dentistry
New York University College of Dentistry, USA

Foreword

The publication of the English translation of Tooth Whitening in Esthetic Dentistry by the esteemed authors, Drs. Seok-Hoon Ko and So-Ran Kwon, is a major contribution to the dental literature. I have been so proud of the great progress that we have seen in esthetic dentistry in Korea, and so much of it is due to this dynamic husband and wife duo. Dr. So-Ran Kwon has become one of the most knowledgeable authorities on tooth whitening, as she has both researched and lectured considerably on the topic.

In most every study that we have seen regarding patient requests for dental services, tooth whitening is at the top of the list. And of tooth whitening options, certainly bleaching is the most conservative and economical treatment available. Of course, when bleaching isn't effective, composite resin bonding, porcelain laminates, or all-ceramic crowns are excellent alternatives. But the first and most conservative approach to any treatment plan should always be to consider whether bleaching can serve as the ideal treatment option - or at least aid in the whitening of adjacent or opposing teeth when laminates, bonding or crowns are selected.

This book dissects the subject quite well and gives both young and seasoned dentists alike an excellent approach to the topic. It deals not only with various whitening techniques, but also with the occurrence of sensitivity in certain situations and the maintenance required to keep the teeth as light as possible. Overall, this is a particularly well thought-out and beautifully illustrated text.

Another valuable inclusion in the book is the "Tooth Whitening Communication Tool," which consists of before and after bleaching results. It is a great demonstration tool, and patients will welcome the realistic pictures showing accurate bleaching shade changes in response to different types of tooth stains.

I compliment Drs. Seok-Hoon Ko and So-Ran Kwon on their ongoing research and clinical efforts, as well as on the tremendous amount of time they took to complete this textbook.

The international profession is indebted to you.

Ronald E. Goldstein, DDS

Preface

'Esthetic dentistry starts with tooth whitening'.

Fulfilling the desire and demand to have a bright and white smile is the ultimate goal. A bright smile not only presents a healthy and beautiful impression, but also increases one's interest in oral hygiene care and health, allowing a person to have more social self-confidence. Being able to make contributions to such a smile is one of the most precious privileges of the dentist.

This book is intended as a guideline for future and practicing dentists as well as dental hygienists. It demonstrates the wide scope of tooth whitening procedures and the challenges they pose with a multitude of clinical photographs and illustrations, emphasizing the efficacy and limitations of whitening treatments in various clinical situations.

The first chapter starts with a systematic approach to proper diagnosis and treatment planning, both of which are essential for successful whitening treatment. Chapters 2, 3 and 4 describe the basic principles and step-by-step procedures of non-vital tooth whitening, home whitening and power whitening and propose new and specific solutions for more efficient treatment. Chapters 5, 6 and 7 demonstrate how to combine tooth whitening with other treatment modalities, such as microabrasion, gingival bleaching and esthetic bonded restorations, to achieve ultimate esthetics in our daily practice. Specific safety and sensitivity issues have been addressed to help dentists prevent and overcome problems that can be encountered in certain situations. Recommendations on how to maintain the whitened tooth color after completion of treatment to ensure long-lasting patient satisfaction are also made. The last chapter, a valuable contribution from Dr. Linda H. Greenwall on the history of tooth whitening, provides a concise timetable of important events that have contributed to the advancement of tooth whitening. Finally, the supplementary volume provides before and after pictures, arranged according to different clinical situations, that show the dentist and the patient what can be expected after the treatment. It is one of the highlights of this book!

Tooth whitening is indeed a very conservative and economical treatment that can benefit both the patient and the dentist. It is our hope that this book will encourage the readers to incorporate tooth whitening more actively in daily practice, giving more patients a whiter and brighter smile.

Acknowledgements

It was a pleasure to write as a husband and wife team. However, our book would not exist without support and encouragement from many individuals, to whom we would like to express our highest appreciation:

Sincere thanks to our co-author, Dr. Linda H. Greenwall, for contributing a precious chapter on the History of Tooth Whitening and for reviewing the English translation. Her constant advice and support was invaluable.

Thanks, also to Dr. Ronald Goldstein for laying the foundation for Tooth Whitening and Esthetic Dentistry for all of us to grow roots on. He is a true pioneer and will be our precious mentor eternally. We are grateful to him, in particular, for the foreword and for other contributions.

We thank Dr. Van Haywood, Dr. Hisashi Hisamitsu and Dr. Stephen Chu for their friendship and significant contributions and for their continuous interest in furthering our activities.

Thanks for excellent guidance during the graduate program to Dr. Seung-Jong Lee and Dr. Chan Young Lee at Yonsei University from Dr. So-Ran Kwon, and to Dr. Brien Lang, Dr. William Kotowicz and Dr. Joseph Clayton at the University of Michigan from Dr. Seok-Hoon Ko.

We would also like to express our gratitude to:
– Our teachers, who exerted an extensive and positive influence not only on our thoughts on dentistry, but also on our personal lives: Prof. Masahiro Kuwata, Dr. Jae-Hyun Lee, and Dr. Heung-Ryul Yoon.

– Our colleagues, Dr. Dan Fischer, Mr. Dirk Jeffs, Dr. Ryuichi Kondo, Dr. Robert Dharma, Dr. Baldwin Marchack and Mr. Ken Beacham, who gave us their support and the chance to lecture in the field of Tooth Whitening and gave us insight into many other fields.

– The leaders of the International Federation of Esthetic Dentistry, whose friendship is of finest value to us: Drs. Takao Maruyama, Ronald Goldstein, Philippe Gallon, Peter Tay, Dan Nathanson, Jose Moura, Rafi Romano, Wynn Okuda and Akira Senda.

– Dr. Yoon Lee for performing the research on the sealed bleaching technique and for her support in initiating the book.

– Our dental staff, who quietly stood beside us all the way, giving us their unswerving assistance: Mr. Sang Woo Lee, Ms. Hae Sun Jung, Ms. Ji Young Oh.

– Our secretary, Ms.Yoo-Min Kim, without whom it would have been impossible to complete this book.

– Dr. Galip Gurel, our dearest friend, who gave us bounteous inspiration and was the vital force for publication of this book. He will be our special messenger forever to whom we are indebted.

Our abiding gratitude to Mr. Wolfgang-Horst Haase of Quintessence Publishing, who trusted in us and gave the final consent for publication of the book.

Sincere thanks to Mr. Bernd Burkart, Head of the Production Department, and the administrative and production staff of Quintessence Publishing Co. for their expertise in publication of the book.

We address our gratitude to Dr. Myung Oh, Immediate Past Deputy Prime Minister and Past Minister of Science and Technology of South Korea and current President of Konkuk University, for his long-term encouragement and for teaching us to become a personality, both socially and as a dentist.

Last but not least, our love to our parents, Yong Hyun Kwon & Che Sook Chang and Ahn-Soo Ko & Sun-Ok Na, who took us as we are and gave us their unconditional love and attention.

This book is dedicated to our precious children, Youngwon-Julia and Youngmin-Joseph. The best is for us to say that we thank God for them, the most beautiful gifts in our lives.

Finally, we sincerely thank God for His guidance and blessings in our life.

Dr. So-Ran Kwon (President, Korean Bleaching Society)
Dr. Seok-Hoon Ko (Past-President, International Federation of Esthetic Dentistry)

chapter

1

Diagnosis and treatment planning

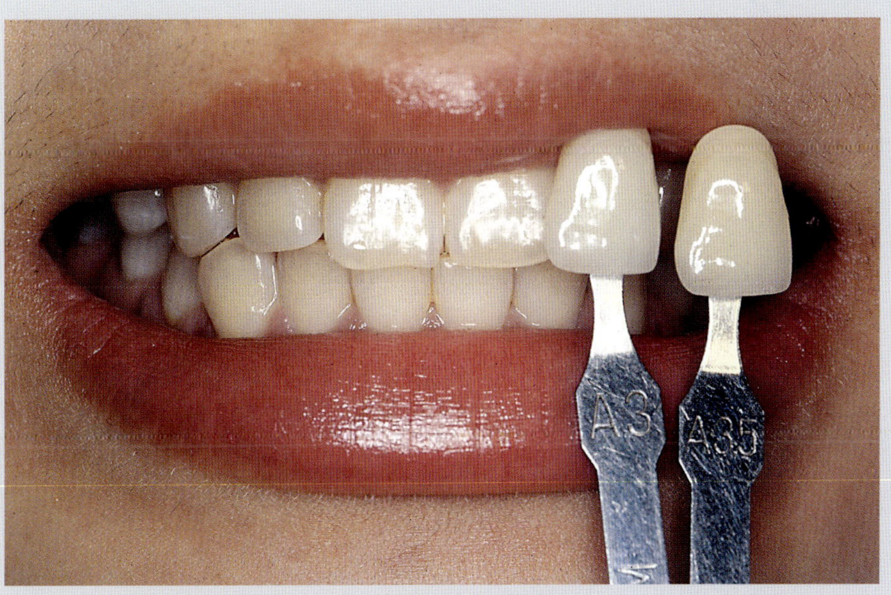

Tooth whitening flowchart

A systematic approach with special considerations for tooth whitening is most essential for successful diagnosis and treatment planning in tooth whitening. The tooth whitening flowchart (Fig. 1-1) systematically shows all the steps necessary, starting from a new patient's first visit to the final maintenance care. The first step of proper diagnosis and treatment planning is to carefully listen to the patient's chief complaint. The use of a specific tooth whitening questionnaire can help the dentist assess the patient's expectations and treatment outcome wishes and obtain valuable information on the cause of tooth discoloration. A comprehensive intraoral examination is followed by tooth shade evaluation and a smile analysis for a proper prognosis of the treatment outcome. A thorough consultation should include information on the patient's expectations, available treatment options, treatment fee and duration, treatment effectiveness and possible side effects, and the necessity of periodic touch-up whitening to maintain the color for a long time. A successful consultation can be completed by obtaining a signed informed consent form before initiating the tooth whitening treatment.

Diagnosis for tooth whitening

Chief complaint

More and more patients seek advice from their dentists about improving their smile rather than about relief of pain or recovery of function. Since 'beauty is in the eye of the beholder', it is important to listen carefully to the patient's chief complaint and expectations regarding the likely treatment outcome. For appropriate treatment planning, it is also helpful to check whether the patient has had any experience of tooth whitening (home whitening, power whitening or over-the-counter whitening) in the past. Record the factors that the patient is most concerned about (e.g., tooth shade, alignment, previous restorations, etc.) and how much time, expense and sacrifice the patient is willing to make in order to fully cooperate with the dental treatment.

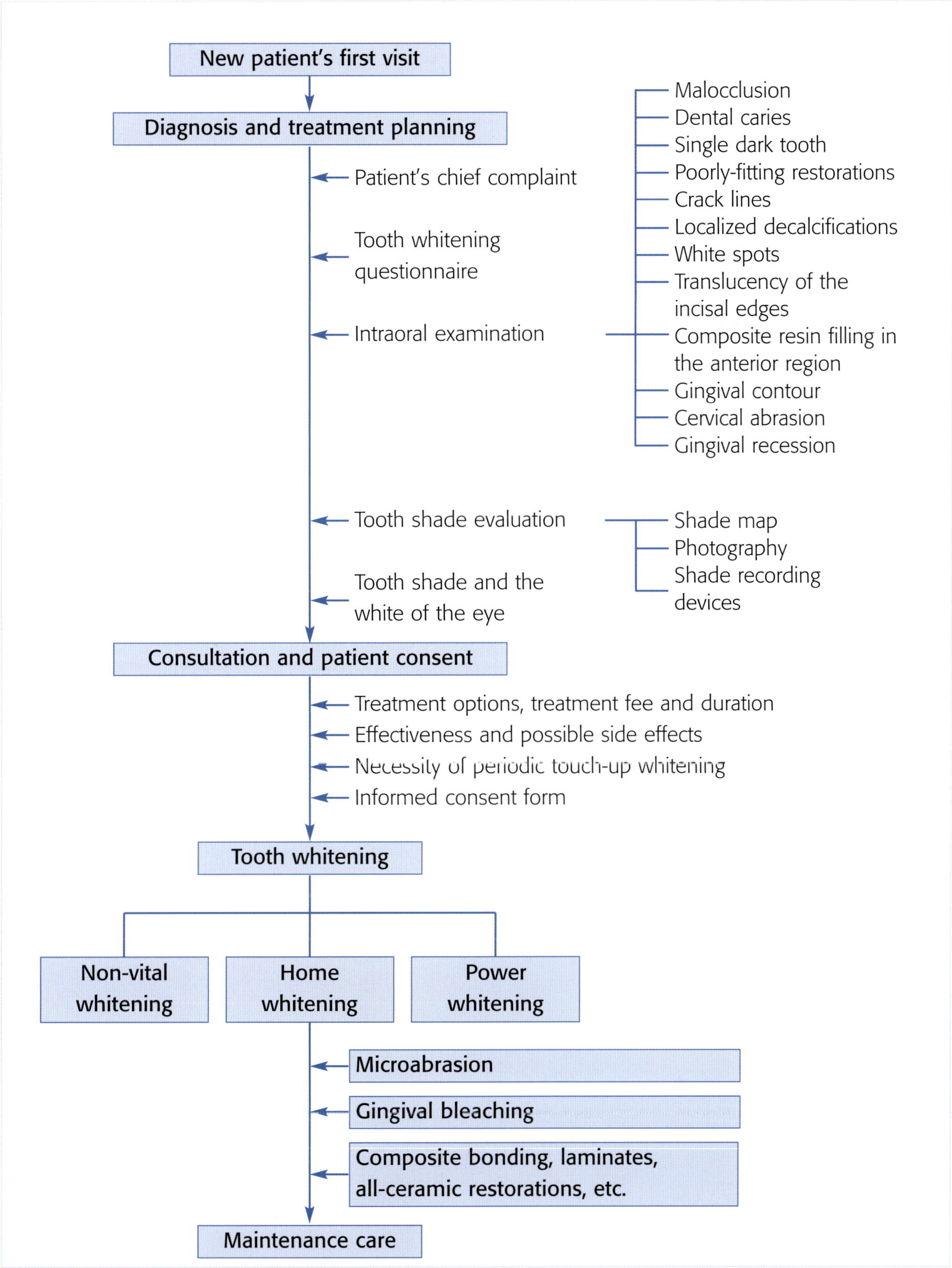

Fig. 1-1 Tooth whitening flowchart.

Tooth whitening questionnaire

A tooth whitening questionnaire (Fig. 1-2) is commonly used to record the medical, dental and behavioral history of the patient. The proper use of such a questionnaire provides the dentist with useful information on the etiology of the tooth discoloration and helps to propose the best treatment options available for the patient.

Tooth discoloration can be classified into three categories: extrinsic, intrinsic, and age-related.

1) Extrinsic discoloration (Fig. 1-3) due to excessive accumulation of stains is a very common problem seen in heavy smokers, wine lovers and tea drinkers, etc. It presents as a uniform yellow or brown discoloration covering the entire surface of the teeth. Teeth with this etiology generally respond very well to tooth whitening. It would, of course, be advisable to quit smoking or to reduce the intake of highly staining beverages and foods for proper maintenance of color, but this is not absolutely necessary.
2) Intrinsic discoloration (Fig. 1-4) is often caused by genetic conditions, presenting with various colors ranging from yellow, brown and grey to black. Since the stain is incorporated within the tooth matrix, the response to whitening varies greatly depending on the severity of the discoloration. A thorough analysis of the medical history in the questionnaire often reveals the etiology associated with intrinsic discoloration.
3) Discoloration due to aging (Fig. 1-5) is the result of long-term exposure to extrinsic stains and internal deposition of secondary and tertiary dentin. Teeth typically darken and become more yellow and brown with increasing age. This type of discoloration responds well to tooth whitening. As people live longer and want to look younger, there is an increased demand for tooth whitening in the aged population.

Intraoral examination

A thorough clinical examination of the soft and hard tissue is performed, even if a patient presents just for tooth whitening. Periapical and panoramic radiographs should be taken in order to identify apical lesions, which can be missed during visual inspection (Fig. 1-6). All teeth are checked for malocclusion, dental caries, single dark tooth, poorly-fitting restorations, crack lines, localized decalcification, white spots, translucency of incisal edges, composite resin fillings in the anterior region, gingival contour, cervical abrasion, gingival recession, etc. (Fig. 1-7).

- **Malocclusion:** If the teeth are in malocclusion, tooth whitening alone will not be sufficient to achieve a bright and white beautiful smile. Patients should be advised to start with orthodontic treatment first, followed by tooth whitening. If tooth discoloration is the only immediate concern for the patient, tooth whitening as an initial treatment may motivate the patient to continue with further esthetic treatment.

Tooth Whitening Questionnaire

Please, fill out the tooth whitening questionnaire regarding your medical, dental and behavioral history. If you have any questions regarding the form, please ask your dentist or the dental staff.

Name: ______________________ Birth date: ______________________

- **Are you happy with your tooth color?** ❑ Yes ❑ No ❑ Could be better

- **What kind of tooth color would you expect after tooth whitening?**
  ❑ Extreme white ❑ Natural white
  ❑ As recommended by dentist

Medical history

- Are you presently under the care of a physician? ❑ Yes ❑ No
  If yes, for what reason? ______________________
- Have you been under the care of a physician in the past for a prolonged time? ❑ Yes ❑ No
  If yes, for what reason? ______________________
- Are you presently taking pills or medicine? ❑ Yes ❑ No
  If yes, what kind? ______________________
- Have you taken medicine in the past for a prolonged time? ❑ Yes ❑ No
  If yes, what kind? ______________________
- Are you pregnant or nursing? ❑ Yes ❑ No
- Have you ever been told that you had any of the following medical conditions?
  ❑ Any genetic diseases ❑ Cerebral palsy
  ❑ Renal damage ❑ Severe allergies
- Have you ever lived in a highly fluoridated area? ❑ Yes ❑ No

Dental history

- Have you ever experienced a traumatic injury to your face or teeth? ❑ Yes ❑ No
- Do your gums bleed when you brush or floss your teeth? ❑ Yes ❑ No
- Have you ever experienced sensitivity to hot or cold foods or sweets? ❑ Yes ❑ No
- Have you ever whitened your teeth in the past? ❑ Yes ❑ No
- Do you have clicking or discomfort on your temporomandibular joints? ❑ Yes ❑ No

Fig. 1-2 Tooth whitening questionnaire (*continued next page*).

Behavioral history

- Do you smoke or use tobacco? ❑ Yes ❑ No
  If yes, how much? ______________________________
- Do you drink coffee, tea, wine or cola daily? ❑ Yes ❑ No
  If yes, how much? ______________________________
- Do you enjoy highly colored foods? ❑ Yes ❑ No
  If yes, what kind? ______________________________
- Do you prefer a whitening program at home? ❑ Yes ❑ No
- Would you like to have all the whitening procedure performed in the office?
  ❑ Yes ❑ No

Thank you very much for filling out the questionnaire.
We will provide you with the best customized whitening program based on the information above.

Fig. 1-2 Tooth whitening questionnaire (continued).

- **Dental caries:** Sensitivity or advanced carious lesions should be managed before starting tooth whitening. Carious lesions in the anterior region should initially be treated with a temporary filling material (e.g., light-cured glass ionomer) to ensure that there is no excessive leakage. After tooth whitening, the final composite or ceramic restoration can be placed to match the lighter color.
- **Single dark tooth:** Many times, patients are not aware of the presence of a single dark tooth. Pulp vitality of the single dark tooth should be tested.
- **Poorly-fitting restorations:** Poorly fitting restorations should be re-treated after tooth whitening.
- **Crack lines:** Crack lines are not an absolute contraindication to tooth whitening, but they should always be pointed out to the patient. Sensitivity to ice, air and hot stimuli should be performed to assess whether there is deeper cracking towards the pulp.
- **Localized decalcifications:** Localized decalcifications should always be identified during careful intraoral examination. Tooth whitening can lighten the background of these lesions so that they become invisible and blend in into the tooth.
- **White spots:** It is important to point out any white spots to the patient, regardless of whether shallow or slightly deeper. In some cases, the white spots become even more noticeable after whitening, upsetting both the patient and dentist. Therefore, possibility of further treatment to remove these lesions should always be considered before starting whitening.
- **Translucency of the incisal edges:** Some teeth look very grey, especially in the incisal area; this could be the result of translucency of the tooth. Diagnosis can easily be made by placing a white-gloved finger behind the incisal edge. If the tooth turns white, then it is translucent. This kind of translucency will remain even after whitening and can be masked by placing a composite restoration on the lingual surface, if needed.
- **Composite resin filling in the anterior region:** Composite resin fillings do not whiten after tooth whitening. They will blend in naturally with the whitened teeth in some cases, but in most cases, re-treatment of the composite resin fillings in the anterior region is required.
- **Gingival contour:** If there is asymmetry in the gingival contour or if the clinical crown appears prominently short, probing with a periodontal probe provides information on whether correction is possible with crown lengthening procedures.
- **Cervical abrasion:** Cervical abrasion lesions may become more sensitive after tooth whitening. Ideally, these lesions should be temporarily filled with a glass ionomer filling and finally treated with a composite resin filling.
- **Gingival recession:** Areas of gingival recession with dentin exposure are darker in color than the clinical crown. These areas will remain darker, even after whitening.

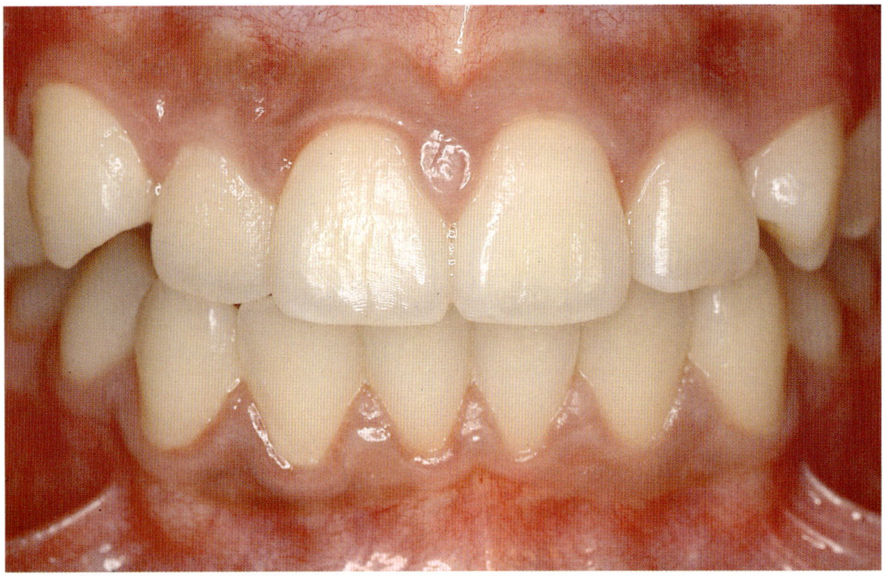

Fig. 1-3 Extrinsic discoloration due to excessive accumulation of stains, e.g., in heavy smokers or wine and tea lovers.

a. Generalized yellow discoloration prior to tooth whitening.

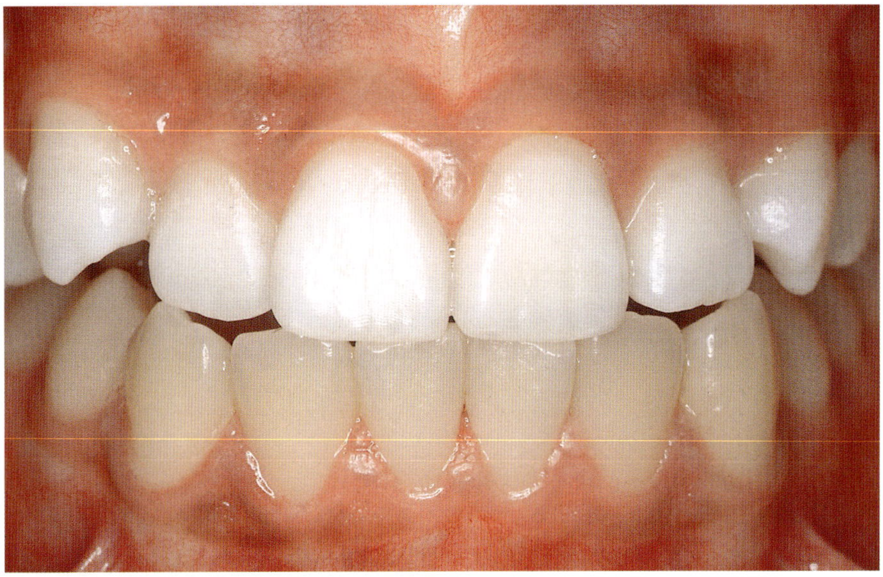

b. During tooth whitening.

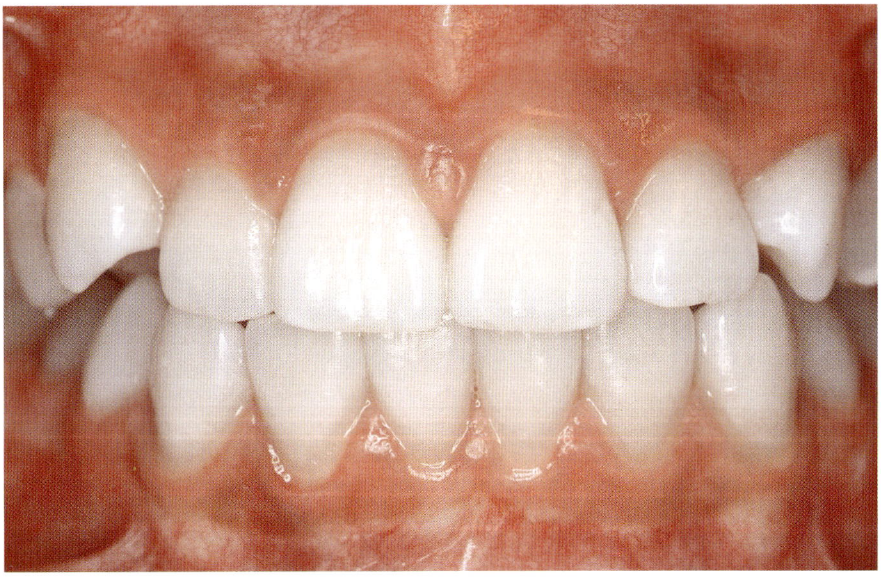

c. After tooth whitening.

Fig. 1-4 Intrinsic discoloration due to medication, especially tetracycline, taken during the tooth developmental stage.

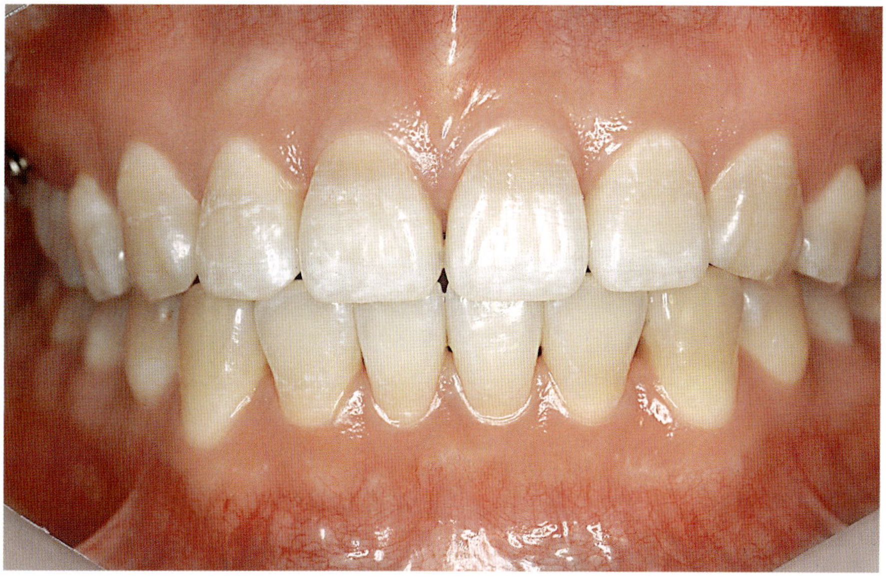

a. Tetracycline discoloration prior to tooth whitening.

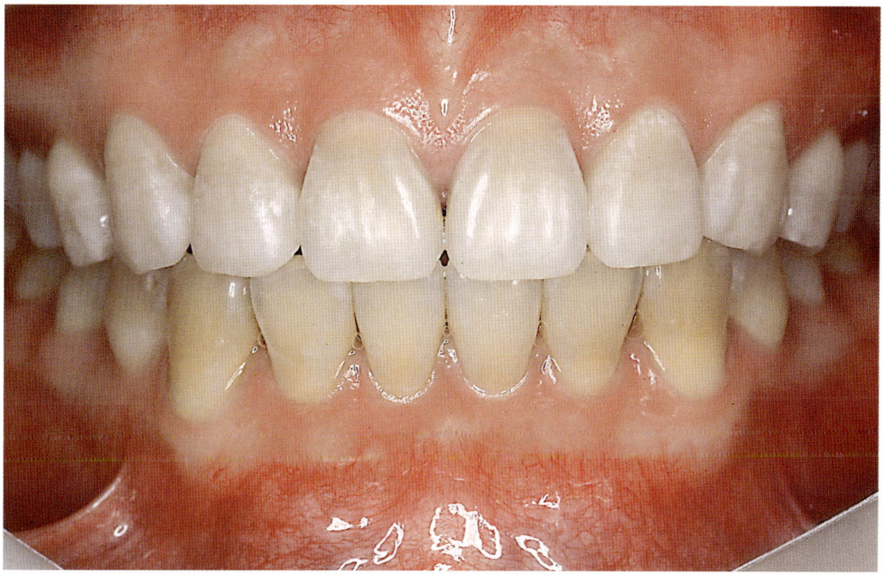

b. During tooth whitening.

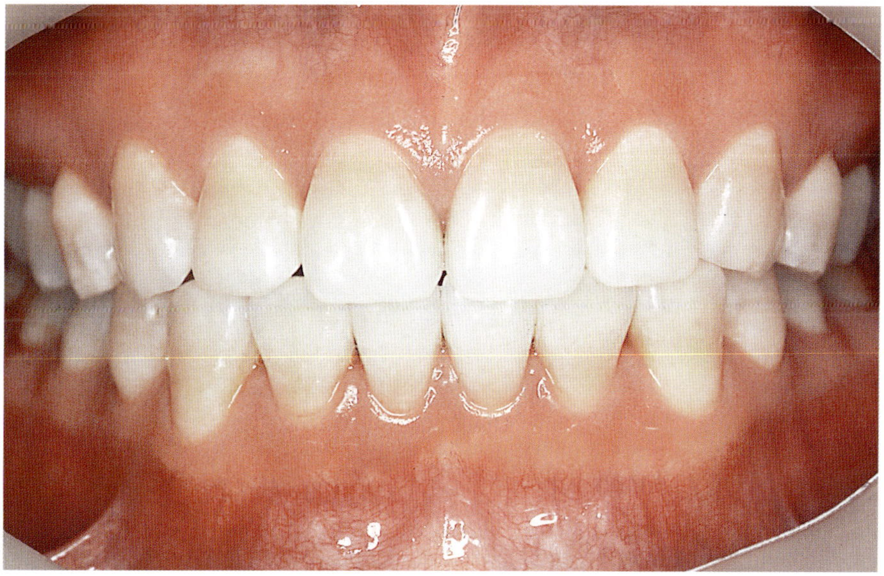

c. After tooth whitening.

Fig. 1-5 Discoloration due to aging is the result of long-term exposure to extrinsic stains and internal deposition of secondary and tertiary dentin.

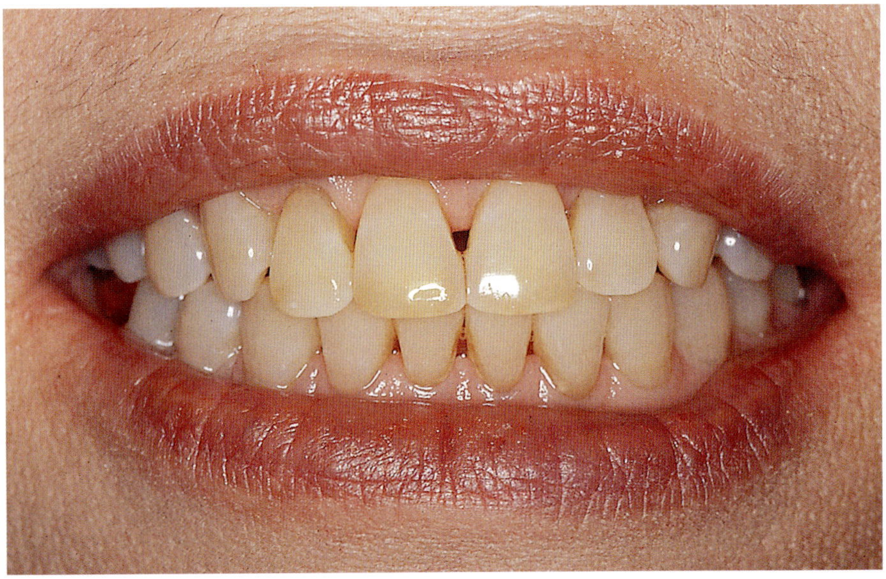

a. Generalized yellow to brown discoloration prior to tooth whitening.

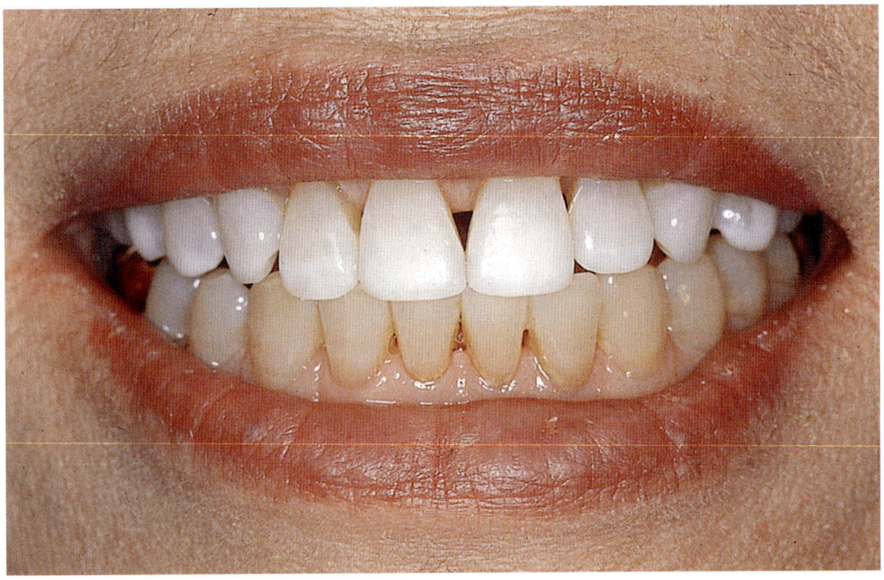

b. During tooth whitening.

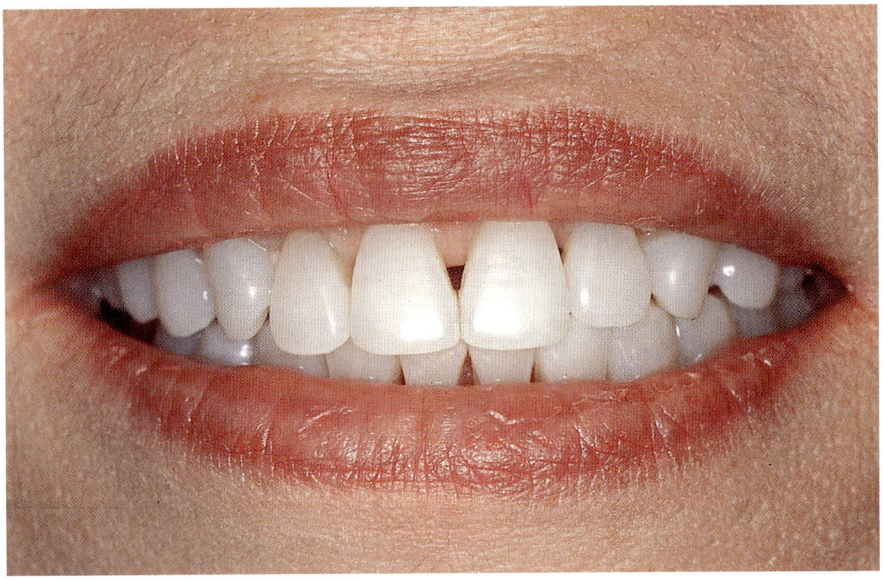

c. After tooth whitening.

Fig. 1-6 In order to identify apical lesions, which can be missed during visual inspection, a panoramic radiograph or periapical radiographs of the suspected lesion should be taken.

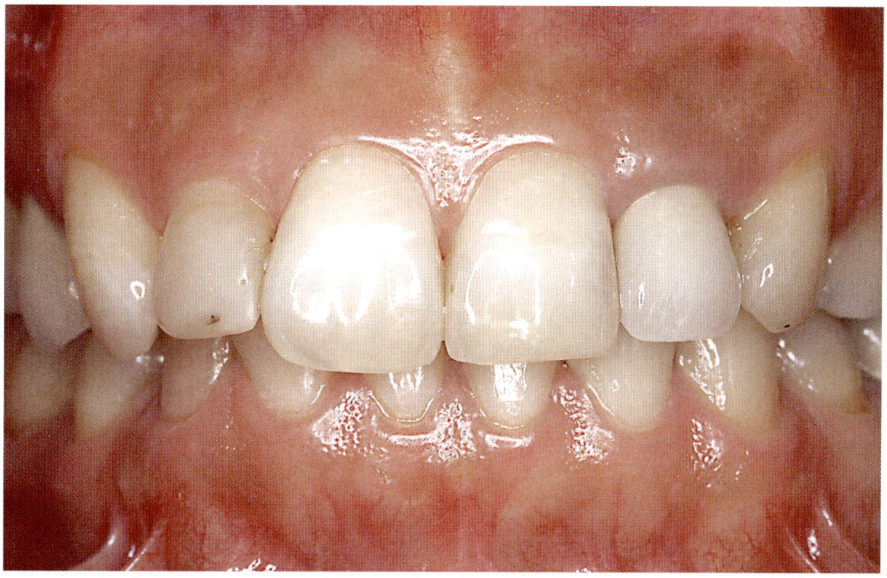

a. Intraoral view of a patient inquiring about tooth whitening.

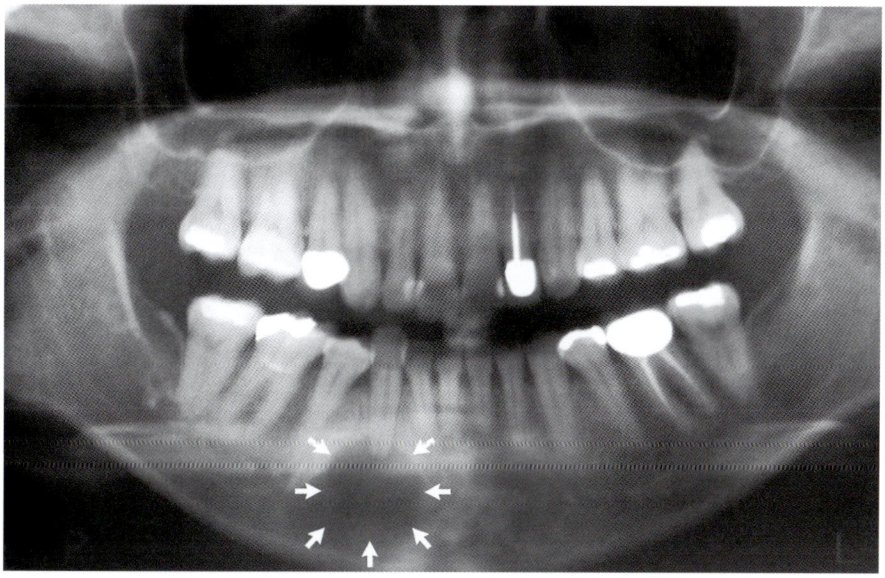

b. A routine panoramic radiograph revealed a large periapical lesion around the lower right canine.

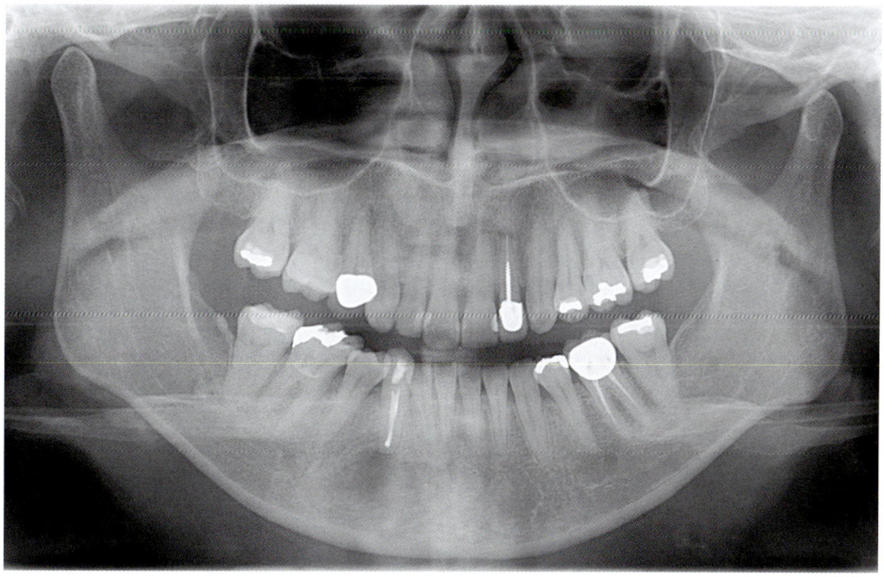

c. Treatment of the periapical lesion should precede tooth whitening.

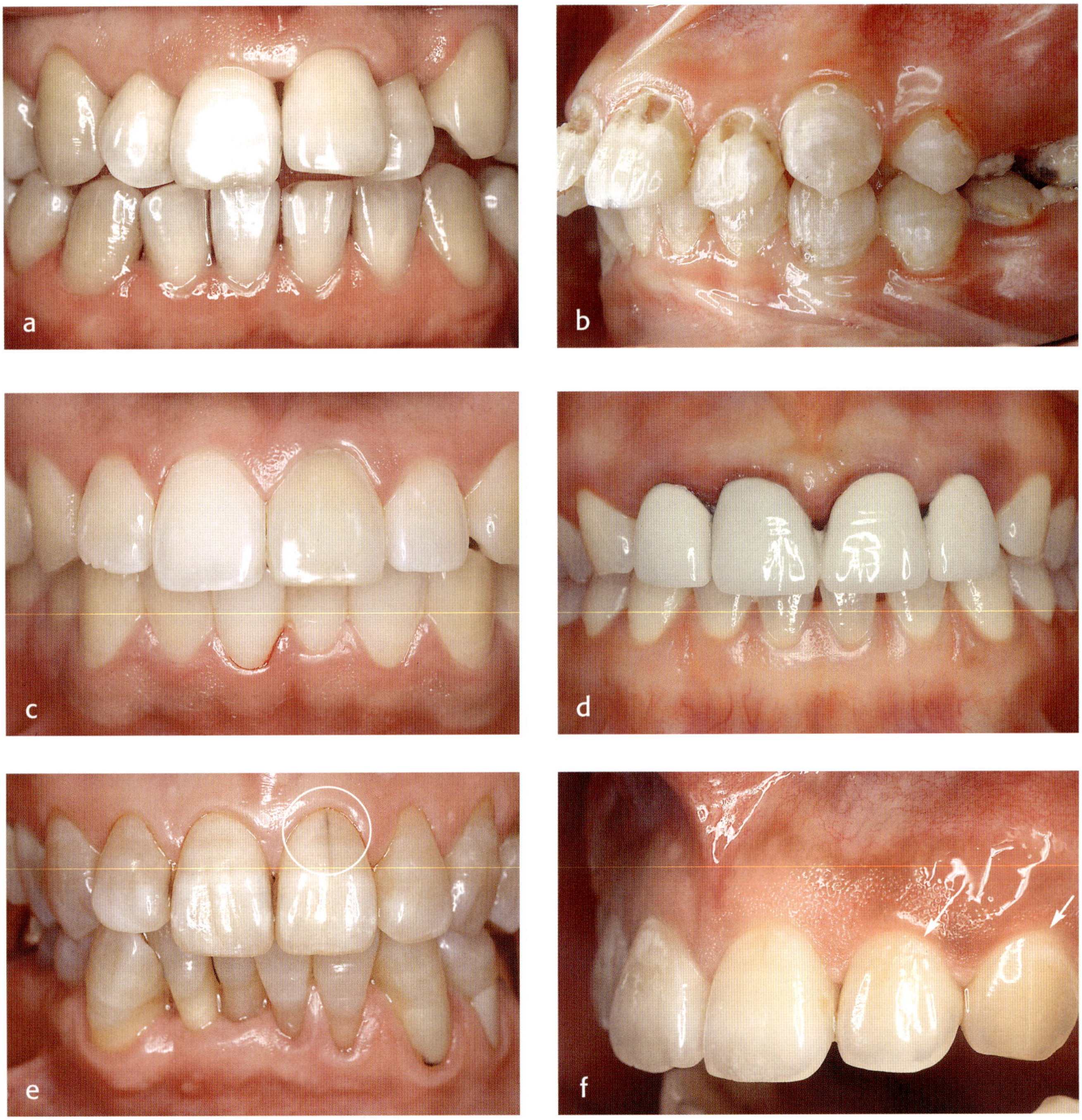

Fig. 1-7 A thorough oral examination is required before starting tooth whitening.

a. If the teeth are in malocclusion, tooth whitening alone will not be sufficient to achieve a bright and white beautiful smile.

b. Sensitivity or advanced carious lesions should be managed before starting tooth whitening.

c. Many times, patients are not aware of the presence of a single dark tooth.

d. Poorly-fitting restorations should be re-treated after tooth whitening.

e. Crack lines are not an absolute contraindication to tooth whitening.

f. Localized decalcifications should always be identified during careful intraoral examination.

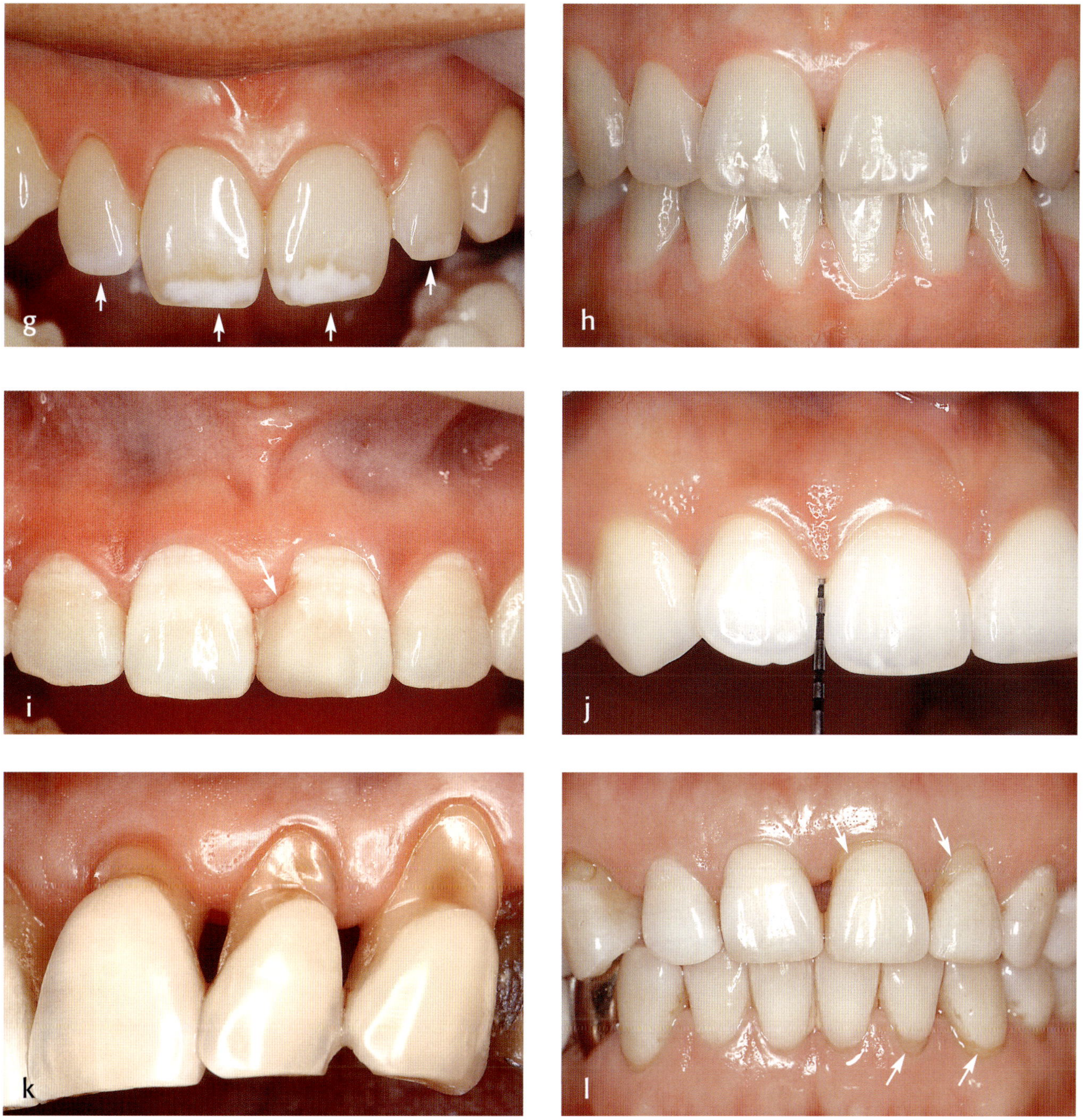

Fig. 1-7 A thorough oral examination is required before starting tooth whitening.

g. It is important to point out any white spots or markings to the patient, whether they are shallow or slightly deeper.

h. Some teeth look very grey, especially in the incisal area, which could be the result of translucency of the tooth.

i. Although composite resin fillings do not whiten after tooth whitening, in some cases they will blend in naturally with the whitened teeth.

j. If there is asymmetry in the gingival contour or the clinical crown appears prominently short, probing should be performed.

k. Cervical abrasion lesions may become more sensitive after tooth whitening.

l. Areas of gingival recession with dentin exposure are darker in color than the clinical crown.

Tooth shade evaluation

Recording the baseline shade before treatment is indispensable. This can be accomplished using a shade guide such as Classic Vita Shade Guide (Fig. 1-8) or Vitapan 3D Master Shade Guide (Fig. 1-9). Teeth usually become whiter than B1 on the Classic Vita Shade Guide and 1M1 on the Vitapan 3D Master Shade Guide, so additional bleaching guides are required. In these cases, the Bleach Guide (Ivoclar/Vivadent) (Fig. 1-10) or the Bleached Shade Guide (Vitapan 3D Master) (Fig.1-11) can be used. In terms of tooth color, yellow and orange (Vita Shade A&B) are good indications for whitening, whereas grey and dark brown (Vita shade C&D) have a guarded prognosis. The shade and characteristics of the gingival, body and incisal portions of the upper and lower teeth can be directly recorded as a shade map in the patient's chart (Fig. 1-12a). The easiest and simplest way of recording and evaluating the baseline shade is to take a photograph of the teeth along with the shade tabs and use this as a reference (Fig. 1-12b). Shade assessment using shade guides is very easy and simple but too much subjective; furthermore, slight nuances or subtle changes can be difficult to detect.

Vita Classical

Hue represented by letters.

- A: Orange
- B: Yellow
- C: Yellow / Grey
- D: Orange / Grey (Brown)

Chroma and value represented by numbers.

- 1: Least chromatic, highest value
- 4: Most chromatic, lowest value

Vitapan 3D Master Shade Guide

This improvement on the conventional Vita Classic Shade Guide allows the clinician to more objectively evaluate the shade in 3 steps.

- Value: Determine the lightness level (1: lightest to 5: darkest)
- Chroma: On the basis of the value determined, take the middle hue group (M) to determine the chroma (1: least chromatic to 3: most chromatic)
- Hue: Check whether the natural tooth is more reddish or yellowish.

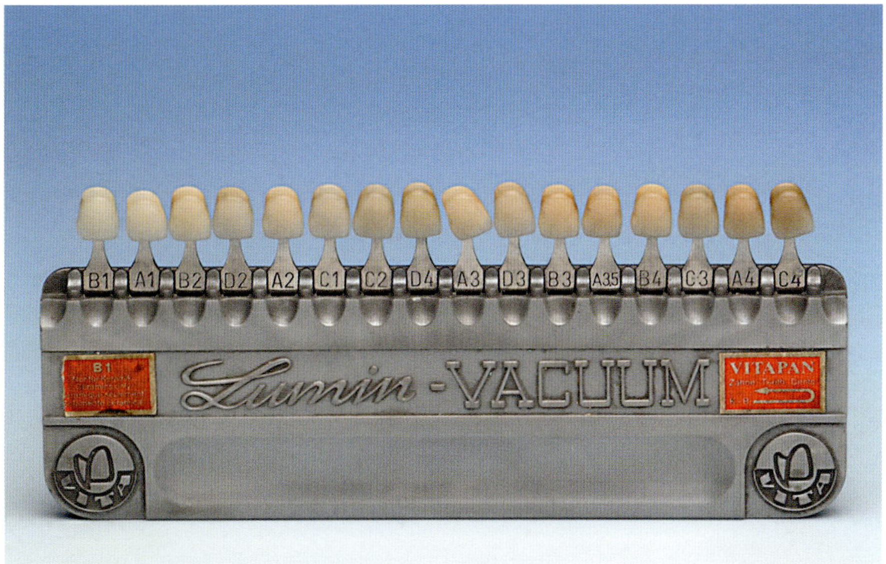

Fig. 1-8 Classic Vita shade guide.

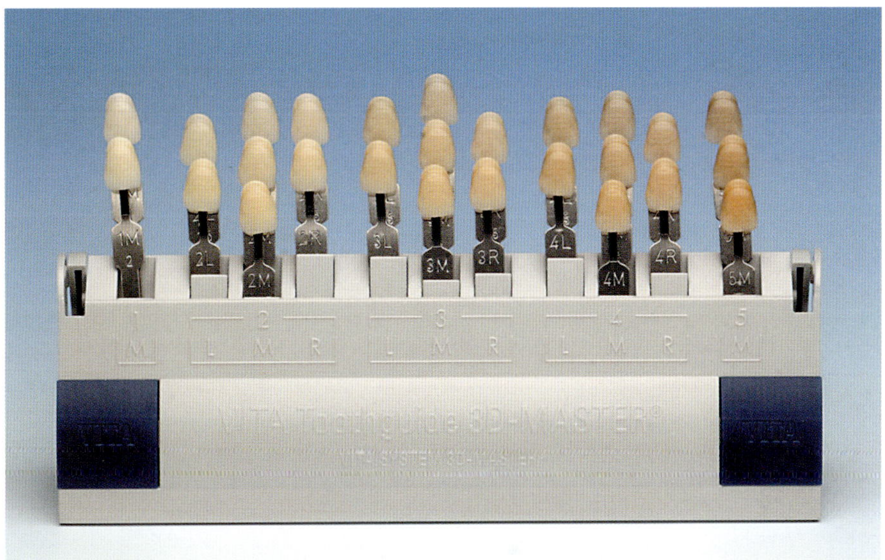

Fig. 1-9 Vita Tooth Guide 3D-Master shade guide.

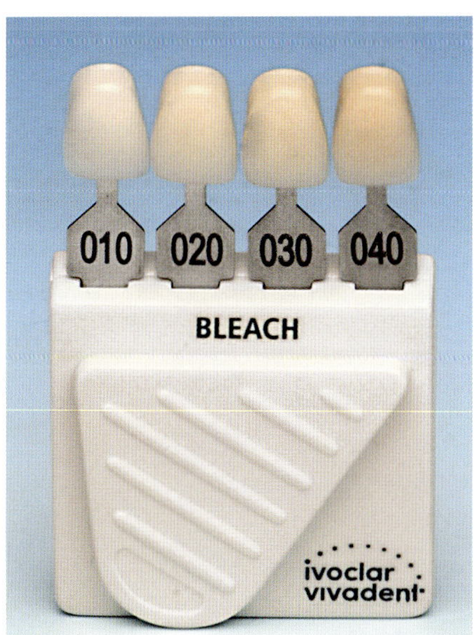

Fig. 1-10 Bleach Guide (Ivoclar / Vivadent).

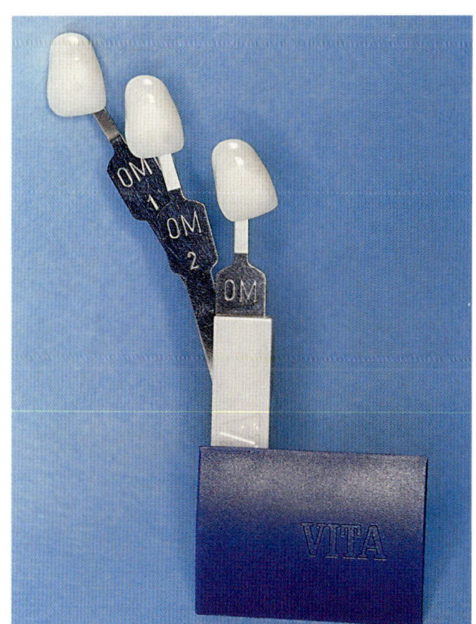

Fig. 1-11 Bleached Shade Guide (Vitapan 3D Master).

Fig. 1-12 Tooth shade evaluation.

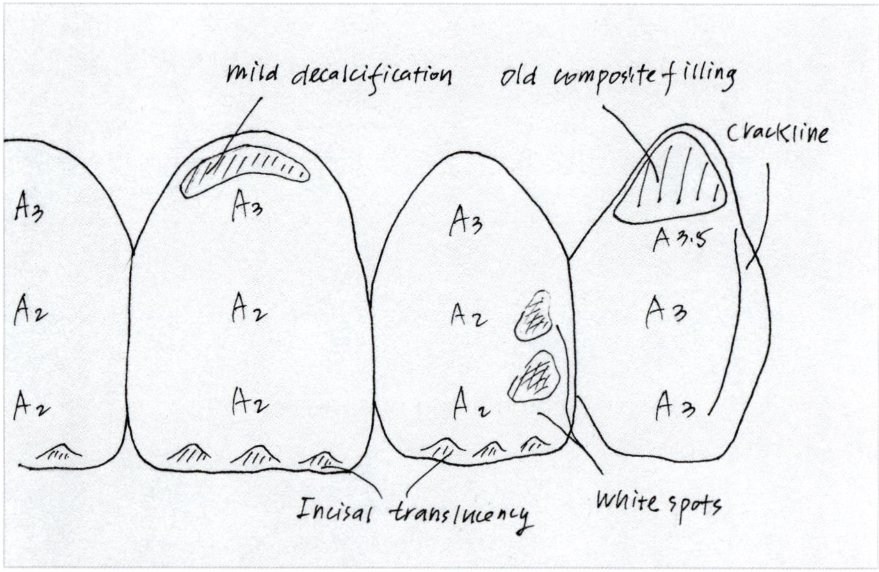

a. The shade and characteristics of the teeth are recorded as a shade map.

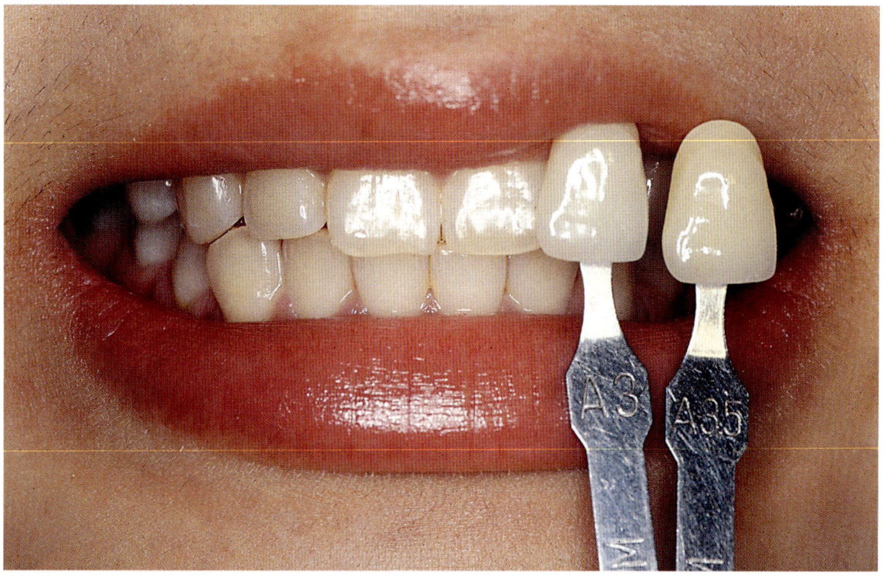

b. The easiest and simplest way of recording the baseline shade is to photograph the teeth along with the shade tabs as a reference.

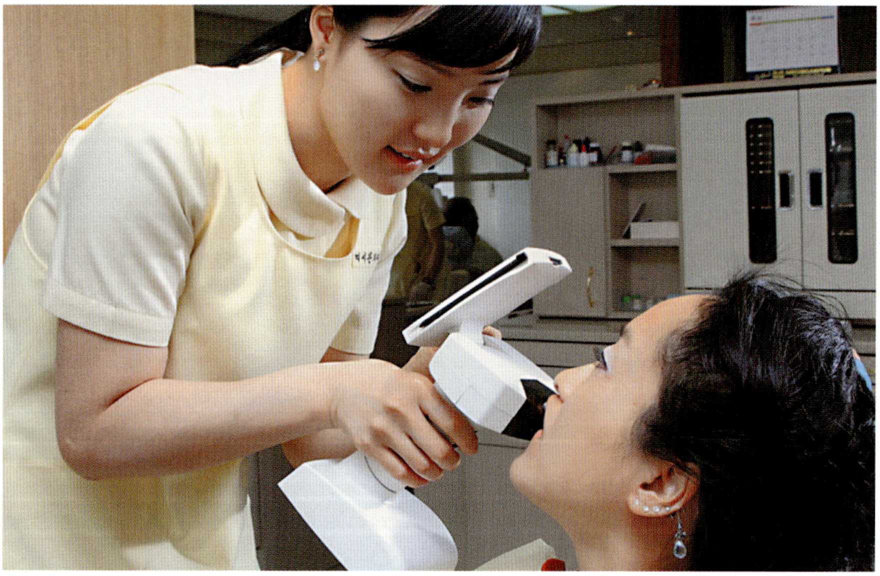

c. Use of specialized device for shade determination (Spectroshade, MHT Optic Research).

Advancements in technology have enabled the use of specialized devices for shade determination (Fig. 1-12c). The main advantages of technology-based shade determination are that measurements are not influenced by the human eye, environment or light source and that the results are reproducible. Clinical studies have shown that technology-based shade determination is more accurate and more consistent than human shade assessment. Shade systems can be broadly classified into three systems according to the underlying mechanism:

- RGB devices: acquire red, green and blue information to create a color image, like most video or digital cameras.
- Spectrophotometers: measure and record the amount of visible radiant energy reflected or transmitted by an object one wavelength at a time for each value, chroma and hue present in the entire visible spectrum, producing accurate and extensive color data.
- Colorimeters: measure color stimuli more directly and operate using three broad-band filters.

All of these devices can be further classified according to the area of measurement. Spot measurement (SM) devices measure a small area on the tooth surface, while complete-tooth measurement (CTM) devices cover the entire tooth. In terms of tooth whitening, spectrophotometers and complete-tooth measurement devices provide reliable data about the color map of the entire tooth. Spectrophotometer-based smile analysis permits visualization of a patient's entire set of teeth in order to obtain an overall view (Fig. 1-13). This is useful in recording an objective and accurate baseline shade and is useful for motivating the patient to initiate tooth whitening. However, the use of technology based instruments (Table 1-1) is more time-consuming and expensive, so that the overall cost-benefit ratio should be carefully considered.

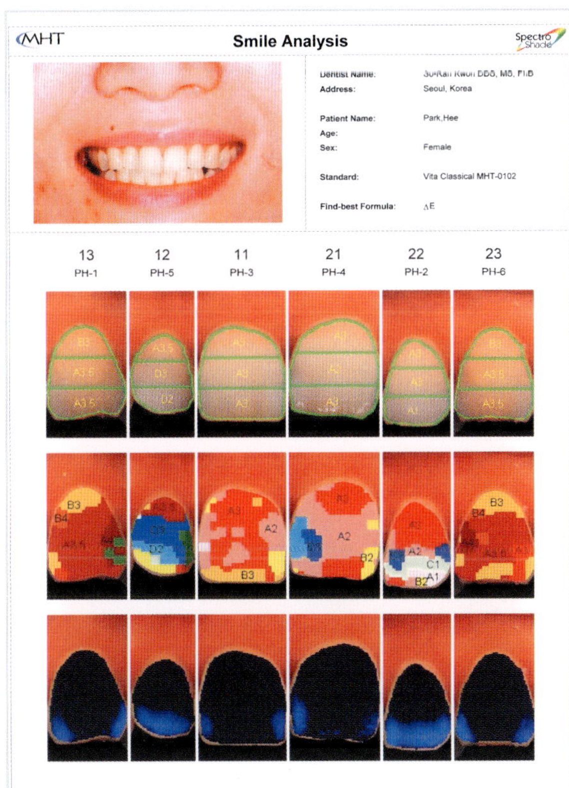

Fig. 1-13 Smile analysis with the aid of a spectrophotometer.

Table 1-1 Specifications for currently available technological shade systems.

Product	Company	Area of measurement	Underlying mechanism	Portable	PC image
Spectro Shade Micro	MHT Optic Research (Niederhasli, Switzerland)	Complete tooth	Spectro-photometer	Yes	Yes
Shade Scan	Cynovad (Montreal, Canada)	Complete tooth	RGB Digital Camera	No	Yes
Shade Vision	X-Rite (Grandville, MI)	Complete tooth	Colorimeter	Yes	Yes
Ikam	DCM (Leeds, UK)	Complete tooth	RGB Digital Camera	No	Yes
Shade Eye-NCC	Shofu (San Marcos, CA)	Spot	Colorimeter	Yes	No
Digital Shade Guide	Rieth (Schorndorf, Germany)	Spot	Colorimeter	No	No
Easyshade	Vita (Bad Sackingen, Germany)	Spot	Spectro-photometer	No	No

Table 1-1 continued (contribution from Stephen J. Chu, with permission from Quintessence Pub.)

Product	Advantages	Disadvantages
Spectro Shade Micro	• High-accuracy reference system • Measures difference between closest shade tab and actual shade (ΔE) • Nearly unlimited number of image captures • Can assess bleaching changes very accurately (vertical split-image software) • Restoration shade verification	• Large optical head can cause patient discomfort • Mildly susceptible to fogging • Difficult to image capture severely misaligned teeth
Shade Scan	• Good software • Enhanced image option • Organized printed report • Restoration shade verification	• Plastic lens protector is easily scratched, can distort images, fogs up, and must be sterilized (not disposable) • Difficult to get technical support • Difficult to capture images of severely misaligned teeth
Shade Vision	• Cordless • Good technical phone support • Good image quality • Automatically defaults to lighter shade to facilitate shade-matching correction • Good hue, chroma and value contrast maps • Images can be added from other files • Access to the anterior teeth is not limited • Disposable image capture tips • Restoration shade verification • Virtual try-in software program	• Only 8 images can be captured before downloading is required • LCD screen of optical device is black-and-white and sometimes hard to read • Image capture (especially of mandibular teeth can be difficult) • Difficult to capture images of severely misaligned teeth
Ikam	• Works with digital camera • Good image quality	• Difficult to position patient • Bulky device
Shade Eye-NCC	• No PC required • Direct printout • Easy handling • Three modes: tooth, porcelain, whitening • Comfortable for patient	• No overall information • Incisal measurement poor • System works best with Shofu ceramics
Digital Shade Guide	• Small device • Good price	• Design is not ergonomic • PC-dependent • No sterilization
Easyshade	• Easy handling • Comfortable for patient • Access to molar region • Tooth and ceramic mode	• Works only with Vita shade

Comparison of tooth shade with white of the eye

Haywood recommended using the white of the eye as a reliable reference point for evaluating patients for tooth whitening. If teeth are darker than the whites of the eyes, the patient's appearance is likely to be improved by tooth whitening (Fig. 1-14). It is very common that patients inquire about the possible final shade after tooth whitening. Rather than promising a particular shade to the patient, it would be more appropriate to suggest that the tooth shade after whitening may become whiter than the patient's white of the eye.

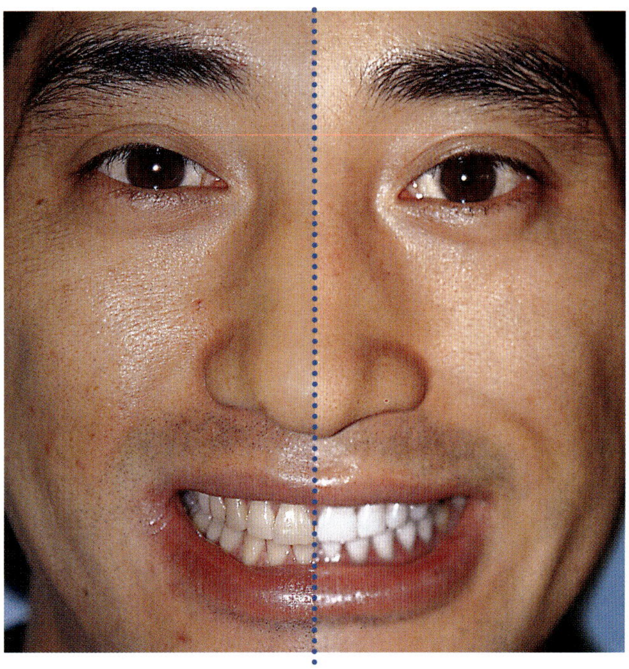

Fig. 1-14 Comparison of tooth shade with the white of the eye. Note that after tooth whitening (right side), the tooth color is whiter than the white of the eye.

Consultation and patient's consent

Once all preliminary examinations have been performed, the consultation with the tooth whitening questionnaire and the smile analysis sheet can be carried out. Consultation should be done in a consultation room rather than in a dental chair to provide a more comfortable atmosphere (Fig. 1-15). The expectations and requests of the patient should be addressed again so that the patient can be assured that his or her concerns are fully understood. A detailed explanation of the customized treatment plan with several options should be given. Accurate information regarding treatment duration and frequency, treatment fee, possible side effects and necessity of periodic touch-up whitening for maintenance should be provided before the patient signs the informed consent form (Fig. 1-16).

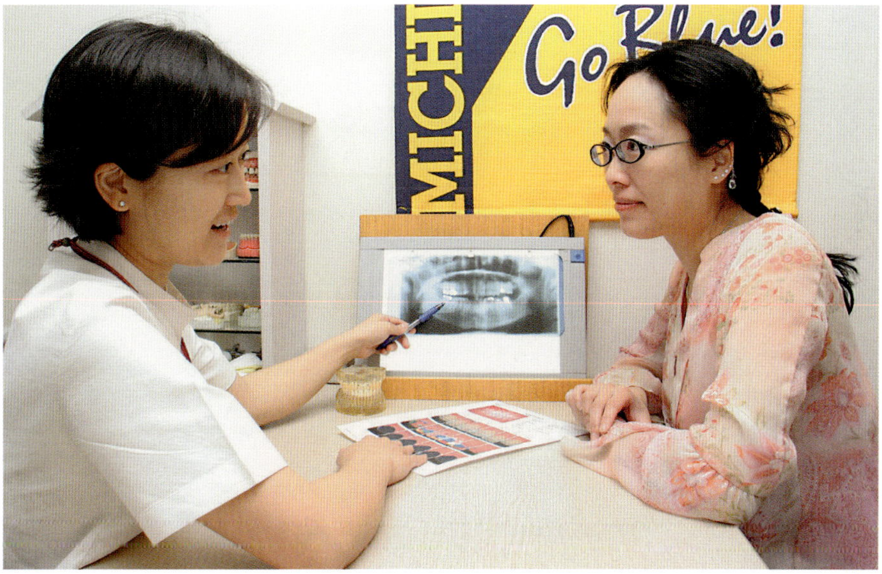

Fig. 1-15 Consultation and patient's consent.

••• Various factors must be considered during diagnosis and treatment planning in order to achieve successful tooth whitening. The use of a systematic approach gives confidence and satisfaction to the patient and successful results and rewards to the dentist.

Fig. 1-16 Tooth whitening informed consent form.

Tooth Whitening Informed Consent Form

Please carefully read the tooth whitening consent form, which provides important information on the procedure. If you have any questions regarding the form, please ask your dentist or the dental staff.

■ **How does whitening work?**

The tooth is a semi-permeable membrane, and the tooth whitening materials – carbamide peroxide and hydrogen peroxide – penetrate into the tooth, thus removing extrinsic and intrinsic stains.

■ **How white will my teeth look after whitening?**

There are individual variations since the color improvement depends on the cause of discoloration, tooth characteristics and your cooperation. In very rare cases, there may be no visible color change after whitening but, if you follow the instructions of your dentist, your teeth will definitely become whiter and brighter so that you should be happy with your smile.

■ **How long will it take?**

The duration of treatment depends on the degree of discoloration and your cooperation. Generally, tooth whitening takes 2 to 6 weeks. For severe discoloration, extended treatment times ranging from 3 to 6 months may be required.

■ **What kind of discomfort may I experience during whitening?**

Sensitivity to cold is a common discomfort during tooth whitening. It usually disappears in a few hours, but if it continues, please consult your dentist or dental staff for immediate relief. A burning sensation of the gums and, occasionally, a transient change of taste may occur.

■ **How do I maintain the shade after completion of tooth whitening?**

To maintain your white and bright smile for a long time, avoid food containing strong colorants that cause re-discoloration of your teeth. Proper prophylaxis every 6 months is recommended, and a simple touch-up whitening procedure may be repeated every 1 to 2 years.

I have read and understood the above information on tooth whitening and I consent to treatment.

Name: ______________________

Date: ______________________

Q&A

Question 1. Is it possible to whiten teeth with cracks and minor fractures?

Answer: The presence of cracks is not an absolute contraindication to tooth whitening. However, show the crack to the patient before the initiation of whitening and test for sensitivity to ice, air, and hot stimulus. Teeth with minor fractures may become sensitive during tooth whitening. Seal the fractured surface with a temporary filling material, and restore the fracture site after tooth whitening.

Question 2. How do you consult with patients who have blue to grey discolorations?

Answer: In patients with blue to grey discolorations, it is best to lower their expectations before initiating treatment. Rather than promising a particular shade, a lighter color than the baseline shade should be suggested. Treatment time for a favorable result maybe as long as 3 to 6 months.

Question 3. How do you take photographs before tooth whitening?

Answer: Recording the baseline shade before treatment is invaluable and can be accomplished with an analog or a digital camera. All photographs in this book were taken with a Nikon F-801s camera, 105mm macro lens, ring flash, and Kodak Professional Ektachrome transparency film E100.

Question 4. Do previous restorations get lighter during whitening?

Answer: Tooth whitening only affects the natural teeth. It does not change the shade of restorations. However, when there is discoloration around anterior composite resin fillings, as whitening removes the discoloration, the composite resin fillings may seem lighter. In addition, teeth with laminate veneers may become lighter by whitening from the lingual side.

Question 5. Is it absolutely necessary to use a shade measuring device prior to tooth whitening?

Answer: Shade measuring devices are useful in recording an objective and accurate baseline shade. However, overall cost-benefit ratio should be carefully considered.

References

Chu SJ et al. Fundamentals of color, Quintessence Publishing Co, Inc, 2004.

Douglas RD. Intraoral determination of the tolerance of dentists for perceptibility and acceptability of shade mismatch. J Prosthet Dent 2007; 97:200-8.

Guan YH. The measurement of tooth whiteness by image analysis and spectrophotometry: A comparison. J Oral Rehalbilitation 2005; 32:7-15.

Goldstein RE, Garber DA. Complete Dental Bleaching, Quintessence Publishing Co, Inc, 1995.

Goldstein RE. Esthetics in dentistry, 2nd Ed Vol 1: Principles, communications, treatment methods. BC Decker: Hamilton, Ontario, 1998.

Hattab FN, Qudeimat MA, Al-Rimawi HS: Dental discoloration: an overview, J Esthet Dent 1999;11:291.

Haywood VB. An examination for Night Guard Vital Bleaching. Esthet Dent Update 1995; 6(5): 51-2.

Jordan RE, Boksman L. Conservative vital bleaching of discoloured dentition. Compen Contin Educ Dent 1984; V(10):803-7.

Kwon S. Tooth Whitening State of the Art, Dental Publishing Co, Inc, 2004.

Nathoo SA. The chemistry and mechanisms of extrinsic and intrinsic discoloration. J Am Dent Assoc Suppl 1997; 128(4):6S-10S.

Paravina RD, Powers JM. Esthetic color training in dentistry, Elsevier Mosby, 2004.

Paravina RD. New Shade Guide for Evaluation of Tooth Whitening-Colorimetric Study. J Esthet Restor Dent 2007; 19:276-283.

chapter

2

Non-vital tooth whitening

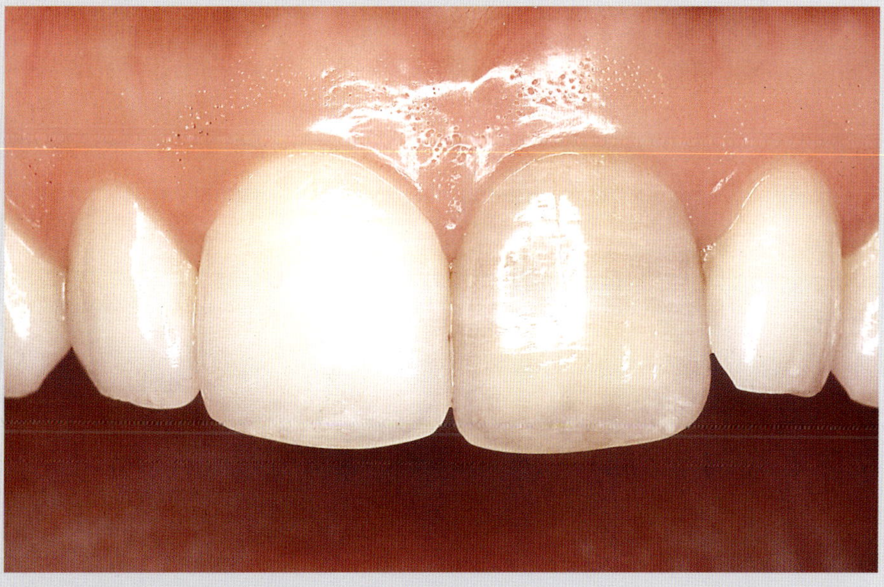

A single dark tooth can be very irritating to patients and present an esthetic challenge to dentists. The cause of single-tooth discoloration may be clinically classified into two categories: incomplete root canal treatment and pulp degeneration. Discoloration due to incomplete root canal treatment is caused by pulpal remnants remaining in the pulpal horn or by excessive root canal filling materials left in the pulp chamber. According to Grossman, pulp degeneration from trauma may cause hemolysis of red blood cells, resulting in the release of hemoglobin. Iron in the hemoglobin further reacts with hydrogen sulfide, a bacterial byproduct, to form iron sulfide, a strong pigment that affects the color of the offending tooth (Fig. 2-1). In some cases of minor trauma, the tooth may still be vital but mildly discolored due to the deposition of secondary and tertiary dentin in the pulp chamber; this is called calcific metamorphosis. If the discoloration occurs gradually over a long time period, the discoloration may go unnoticed until long after the actual trauma (Fig. 2-2). Very often, there are no clinical signs and symptoms, and the discoloration is discovered during a regular dental check-up as a periapical lesion on a routine radiograph (Fig. 2-3). The development of tooth discoloration during or following orthodontic treatment sometimes necessitates proper root canal treatment followed by further treatment (Fig. 2-4).

In the past, a single dark tooth was routinely prepared and restored with a porcelain laminate veneer or a full-coverage restoration to cover and conceal the discoloration. However, problems such as structural compromise of tooth structure due to excessive removal of healthy tooth structure, possible fracture or dislodgement of the restoration, and esthetic problems such as gingival recession were inevitable. This chapter provides guidelines for successful and safe whitening for various non-vital whitening techniques that achieve esthetic results without tooth reduction.

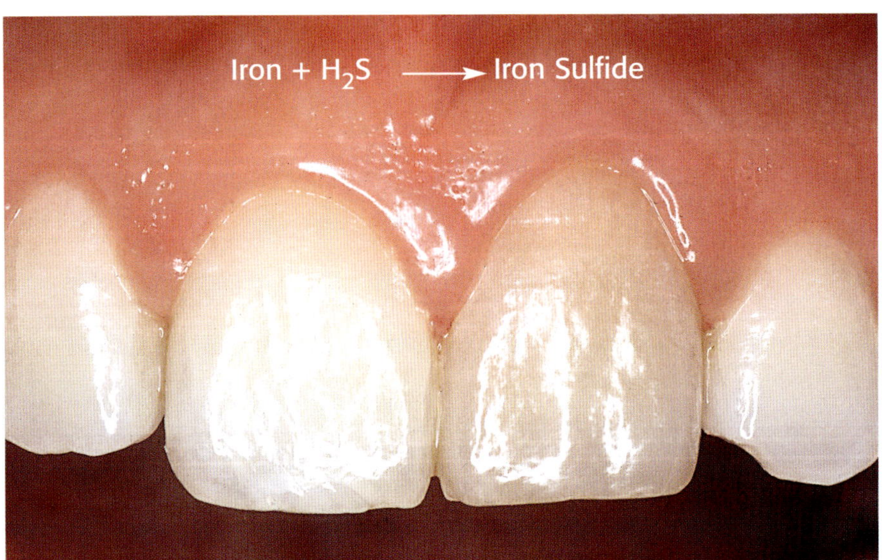

Fig. 2-1 Mechanism of a single-tooth discoloration.

Fig. 2-2 Single-tooth discoloration of the upper left central incisor.

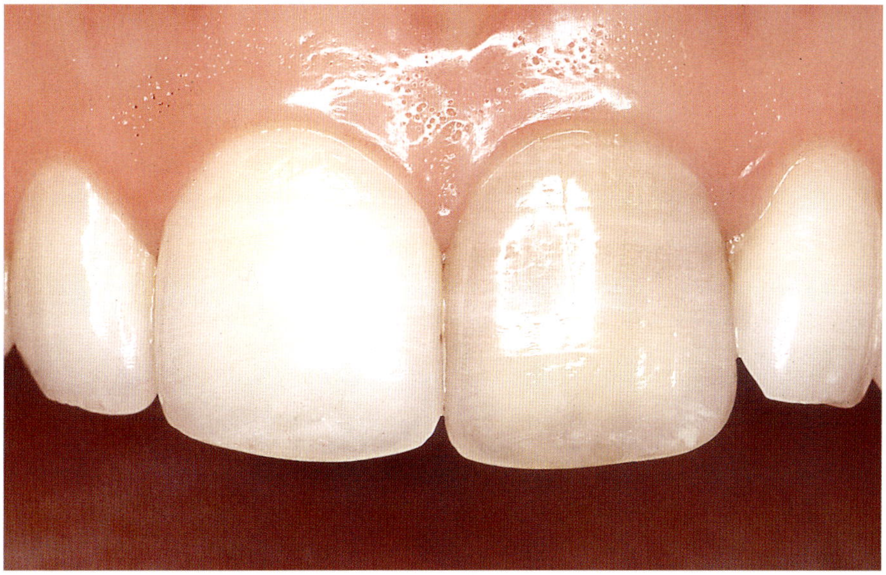

a. The discoloration was noticed long after the actual trauma.

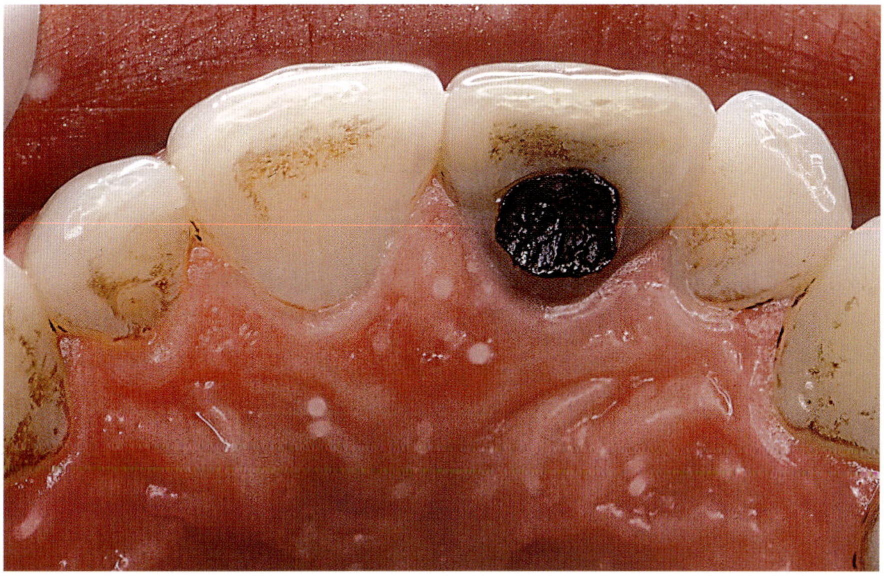

b. Lingual view showing the access cavity filled with amalgam.

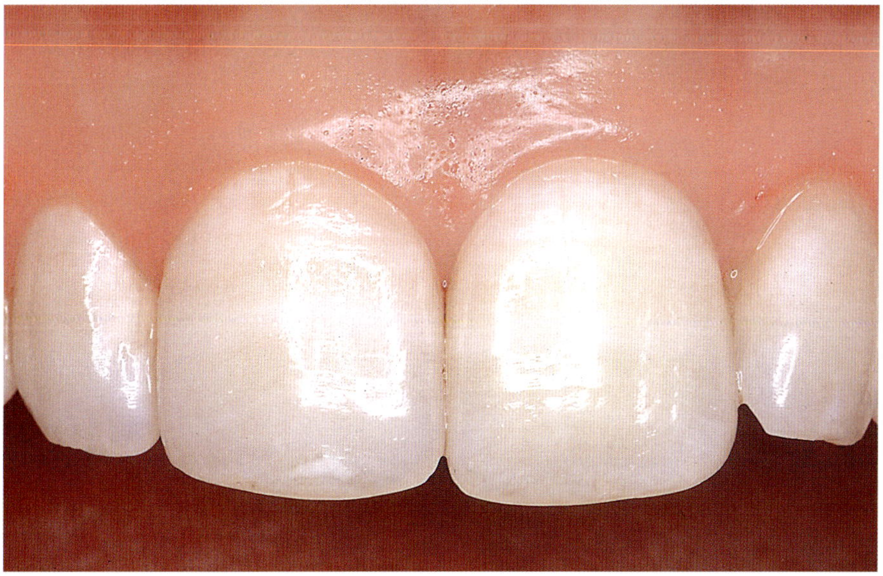

c. Result after walking bleach treatment.

Fig. 2-3 Single-tooth discoloration of the lower right canine.

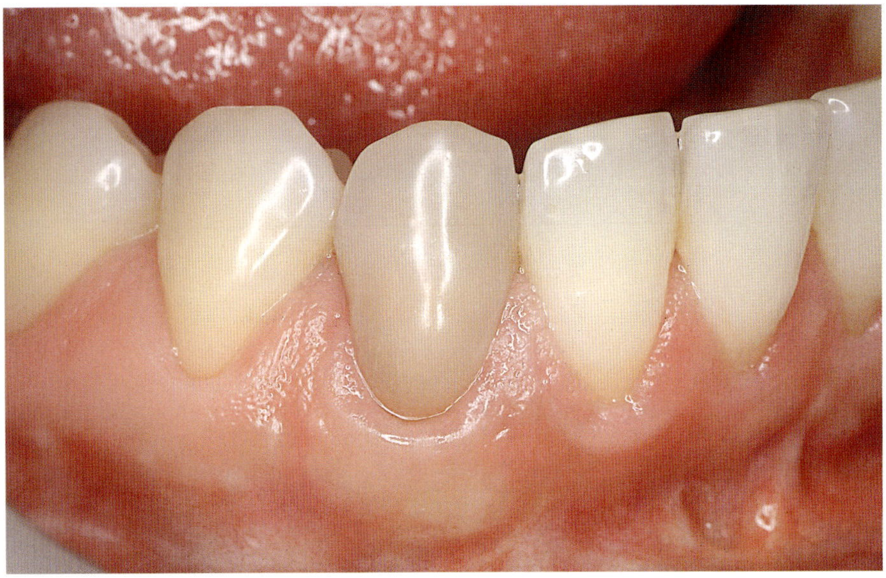

a. Very often, the patient is not aware of the discoloration.

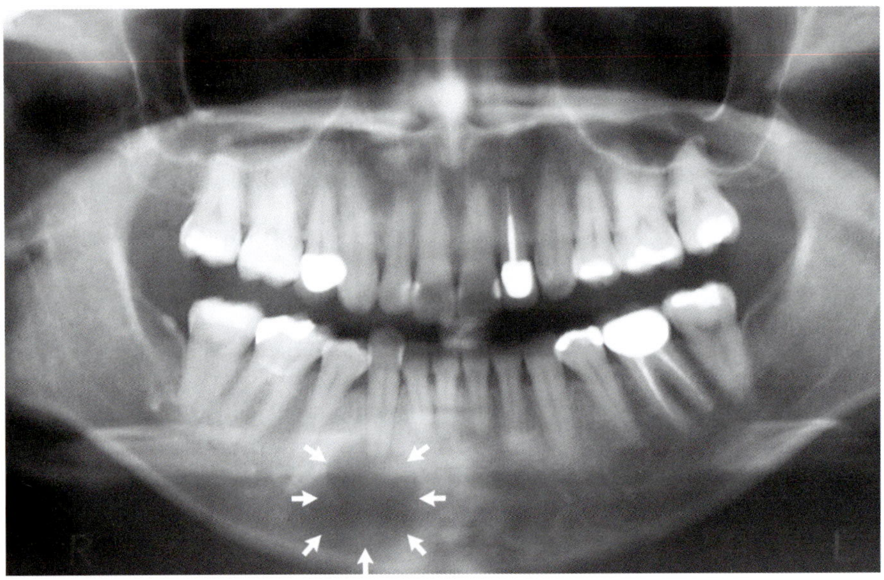

b. A periapical lesion was discovered during a routine dental check-up on a panoramic radiograph.

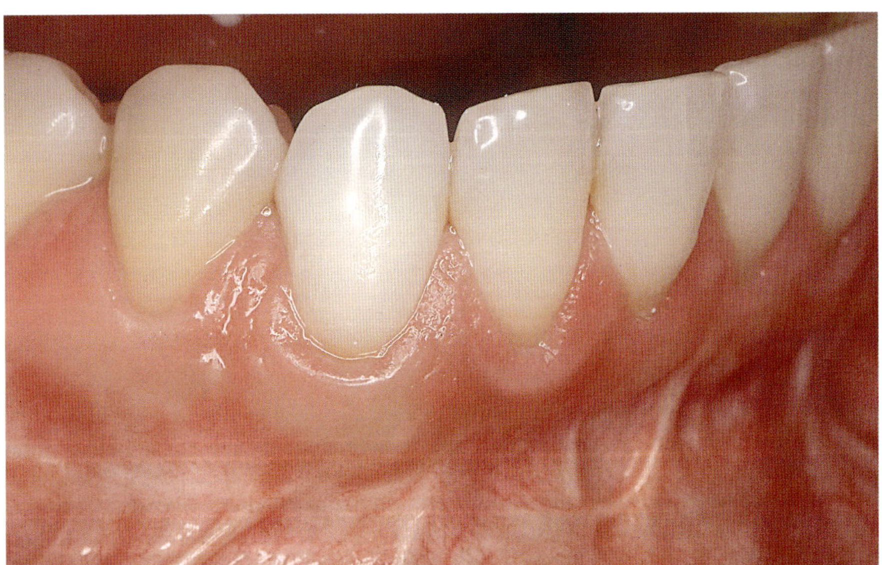

c. After root canal and walking bleach treatment.

Fig. 2-4 Single-tooth discoloration following orthodontic treatment.

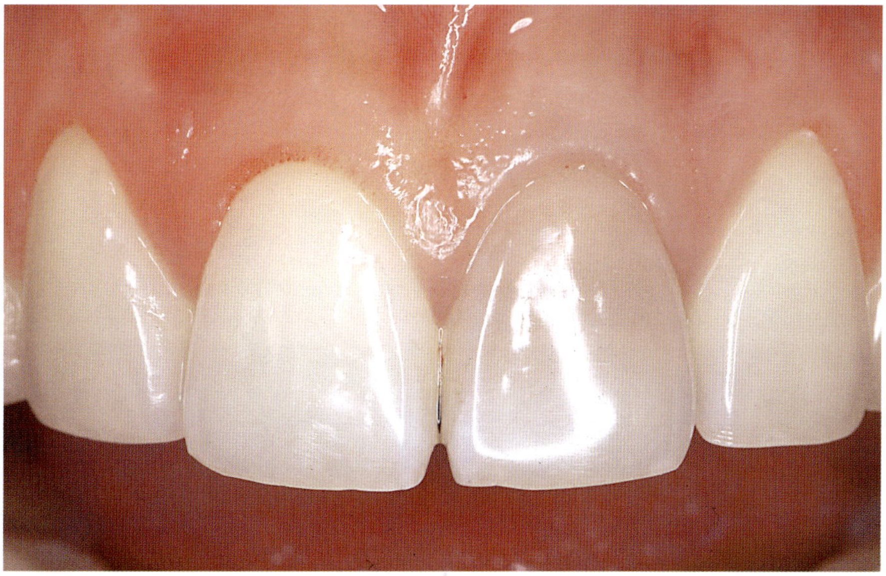

a. Discoloration of the upper left central incisor after orthodontic treatment.

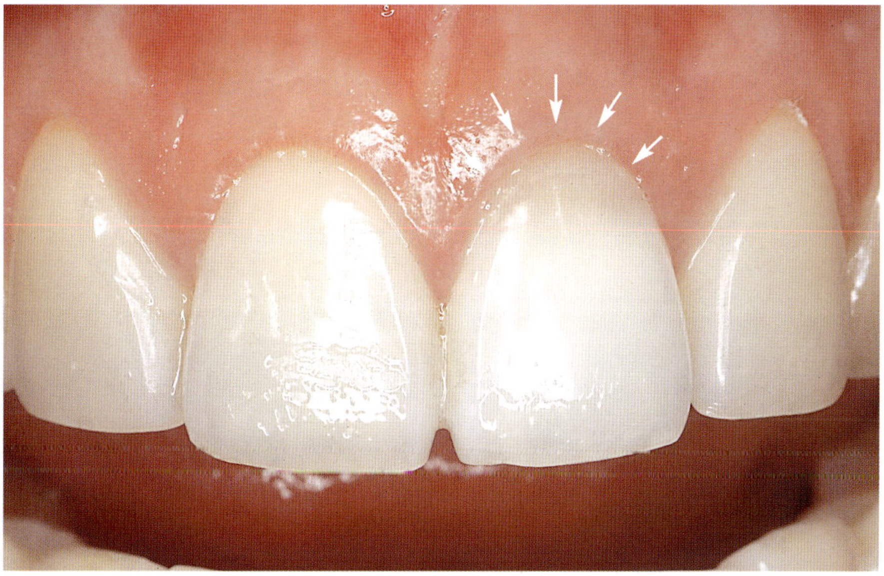

b. After two walking bleach sessions, the cervical discoloration remained due to a poorly-positioned barrier. The position of the barrier was therefore modified by removing part of the glass ionomer base with a slow-speed bur.

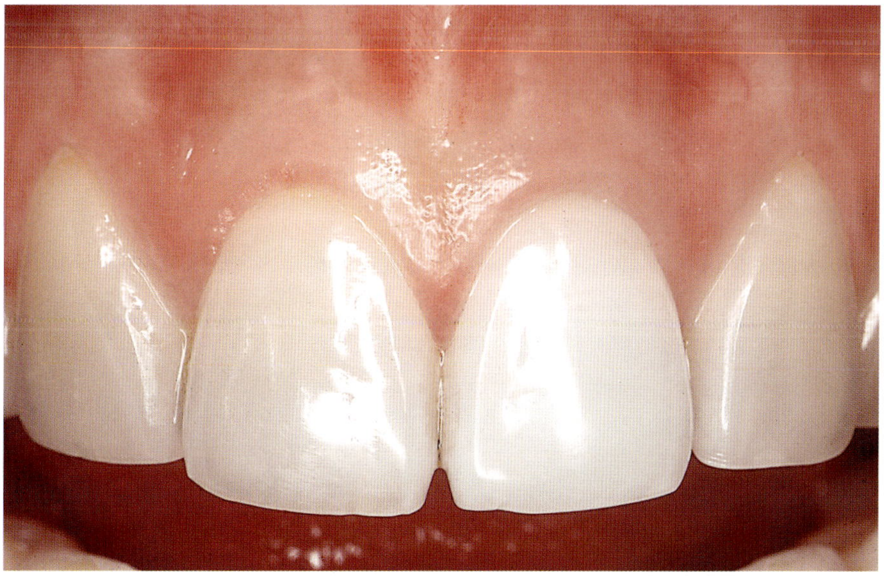

c. Walking bleaching was completed at an over-bleached state, after barrier modification.

Non-vital whitening techniques and materials

- Walking bleach technique
  - Sodium perborate + water
  - Sodium perborate + H_2O_2
  - 10–20% carbamide peroxide gel
  - 35% H_2O_2 gel (Opalescence Endo)
- Thermocatalytic bleaching
  - 30–35% H_2O_2 + heat
- Inside-outside bleaching
  - 10–15% carbamide peroxide gel + whitening tray
- Light- activated non-vital bleaching
  - 10% carbamide peroxide gel activated by light
  - Power whitening gel activated by light

Walking bleach technique

Since its introduction in 1961, the walking bleach technique has become one of the most commonly used methods for whitening endodontically treated teeth. A mixture of hydrogen peroxide and sodium perborate is placed in the pulp chamber and sealed with a temporary filling material. The whitening starts while the patient walks out of the office. Depending on the etiology and severity of the discoloration, the procedure is repeated 3 to 5 times until the color matches that of the adjacent teeth.

Walking bleach materials

The bleaching material most commonly used for the walking bleach technique is a paste consisting of 30 to 35% hydrogen peroxide (Superoxol) mixed with sodium perborate powder (Fig. 2-5a). Hydrogen peroxide is a very effective whitening material because of its strong oxidizing property. However, utmost care should always be taken to avoid soft tissue burns and contact with the patient's eyes or mucosa. Since hydrogen peroxide is a very reactive liquid, its oxidizing power decreases by 50% over a 6-month period, and regular replacement of the liquid may be necessary.

Sodium perborate is a white, odorless, water-soluble chemical compound that undergoes hydrolysis on contact with water, yielding hydrogen peroxide and borate. It produces less oxygen radicals but has a synergistic effect when combined with hydrogen peroxide. In very young patients, a mixture of sodium perborate with water can be used for a safer approach. A walking bleach method employing a lower hydrogen peroxide concentration (3%) was recently proposed and implemented.

For dentists who have difficulty in handling the mixture, 10% carbamide peroxide gel can be loaded into a syringe (Fig. 2-5b) and injected into the pulp chamber followed by the placement of a cotton pellet and temporary filling material. 35% H_2O_2 gel (Opalescence Endo, Ultradent Products Inc., Utah, USA) can also be sealed into the pulp chamber for the purpose of walking bleaching (Fig. 2-5c).

Fig. 2-5 Bleaching materials used for walking bleaching

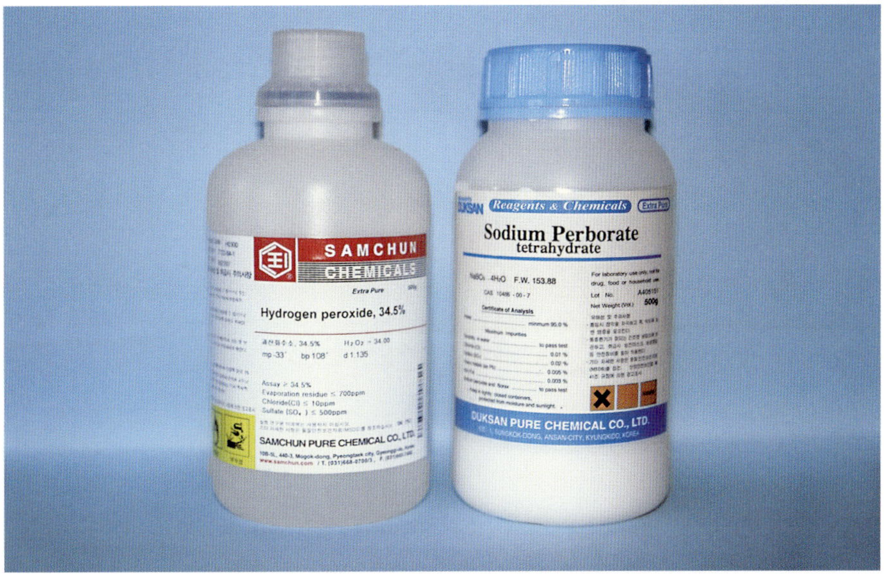

a. Sodium perborate powder and 35% hydrogen peroxide.

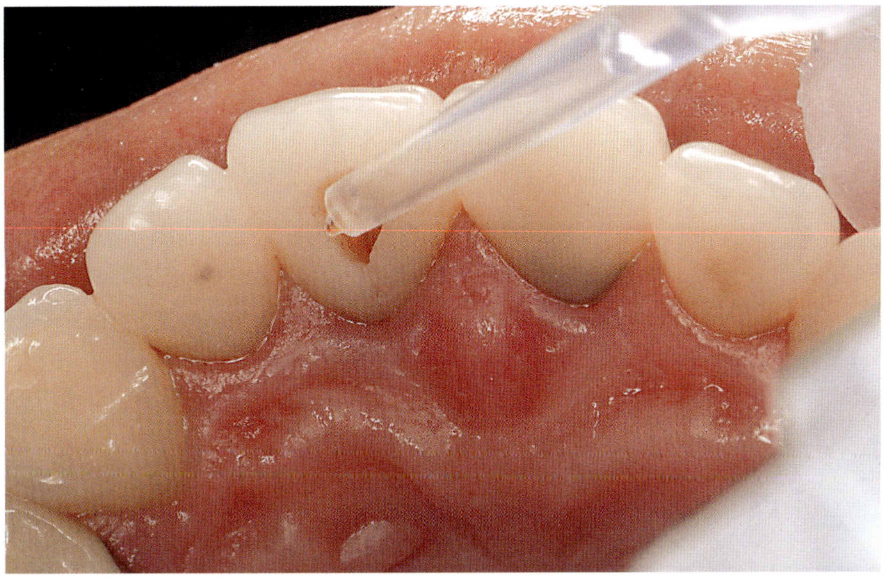

b. 10% carbamide peroxide gel is sealed into cavity.

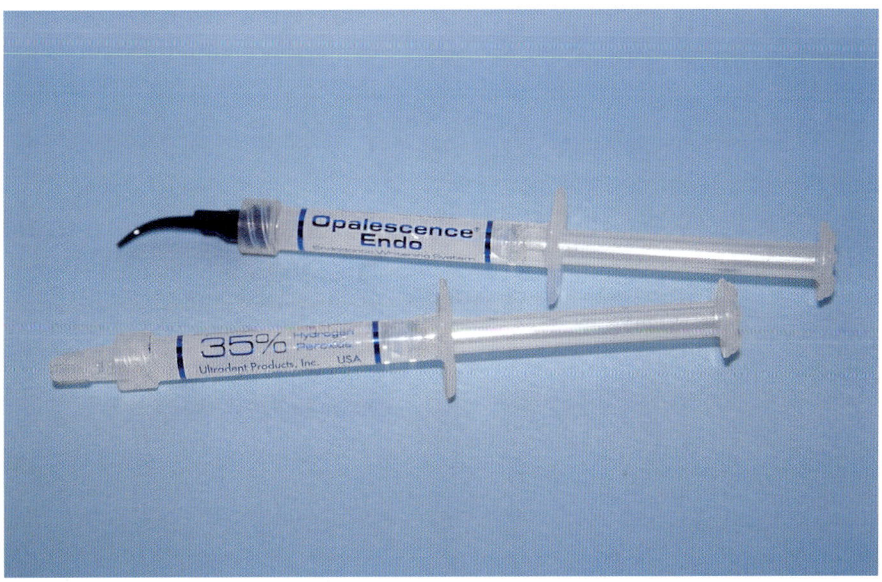

c. 35% H_2O_2 gel (Opalescence Endo, Ultradent Products Inc., Utah, USA)

Treatment technique (Fig. 2-6)

- **Diagnosis and root canal treatment:** Evaluate pulp vitality by means of thermal and electric pulp testing and confirm the periapical status by means of radiographs and adequacy of obturation in patients with previous endodontic treatment.
- **Shade assessment:** Take photographs and record the preoperative shade to obtain a reference for future comparison.
- **Placement of barrier:** On completion of root canal treatment, remove gutta percha and any root canal filling material to a depth of 2mm below the cemento-enamel junction (CEJ) using a slow-speed round bur, a Gates-Glidden drill or a heated instrument. Verify that the pulp horns as well as the access cavity are clean. Remove any remaining necrotic debris, root canal filling material or endodontic sealers. The barrier should be 2mm thick and should follow the outline of the CEJ. Consequently, the ideal morphology should be a 'bobsled tunnel outline' on the facial aspect and a 'ski slope' on the proximal aspect. Either glass ionomer, resin ionomer, intermediate restorative material (IRM), polycarboxylate cement or zinc phosphate cement can be used as the base material but, ideally, the material should bond to dentin. For ease of application, a light-cured glass ionomer can be dispensed with a syringe and metal tip to a thickness of 2mm (Fig. 2-7).
- **Application of bleaching material:** A thick paste of sodium perborate mixed with either hydrogen peroxide or water is used. The mixture is applied to the pulp chamber with an applicator or an amalgam carrier. By compressing the mixture with a dry cotton pellet, excessive moisture is removed and space is created for the temporary filling material.
- **Sealing with temporary filling material:** For adequate sealing, the minimum thickness of the temporary filling material should be 2mm. As the whitening material releases oxygen radicals, the resulting pressure may cause the temporary filling material to pop out. To prevent this, glass ionomer may be used as a temporary filling material.
- **Shade evaluation:** Recall the patient in 3 to 5 days and compare the shade with the adjacent teeth or instruct the patient to return earlier should whitening occur faster. Depending on the etiology and severity of the discoloration, the procedure generally has to be repeated 3 to 5 times (Fig. 2-8). Treatment should be completed when the tooth becomes a little lighter than the adjacent teeth. This 'overbleaching' provides some compensation for the rebound of color that occurs as the shade stabilizes.
- **Final composite resin filling:** It is best to wait an extra 2 weeks after the last walking bleaching to allow for color stabilization, oxygen dissipation and recovery of the bond strength. The cavity is filled with a cotton pellet and a temporary filling material, and the patient is recalled after 2 weeks. At that time, the cavity can be etched, primed and bonded for the final restoration. If time is a factor for the patient, rinsing the cavity with catalase or a calcium hydroxide dressing for 2 days has been proposed instead of waiting 2 weeks.

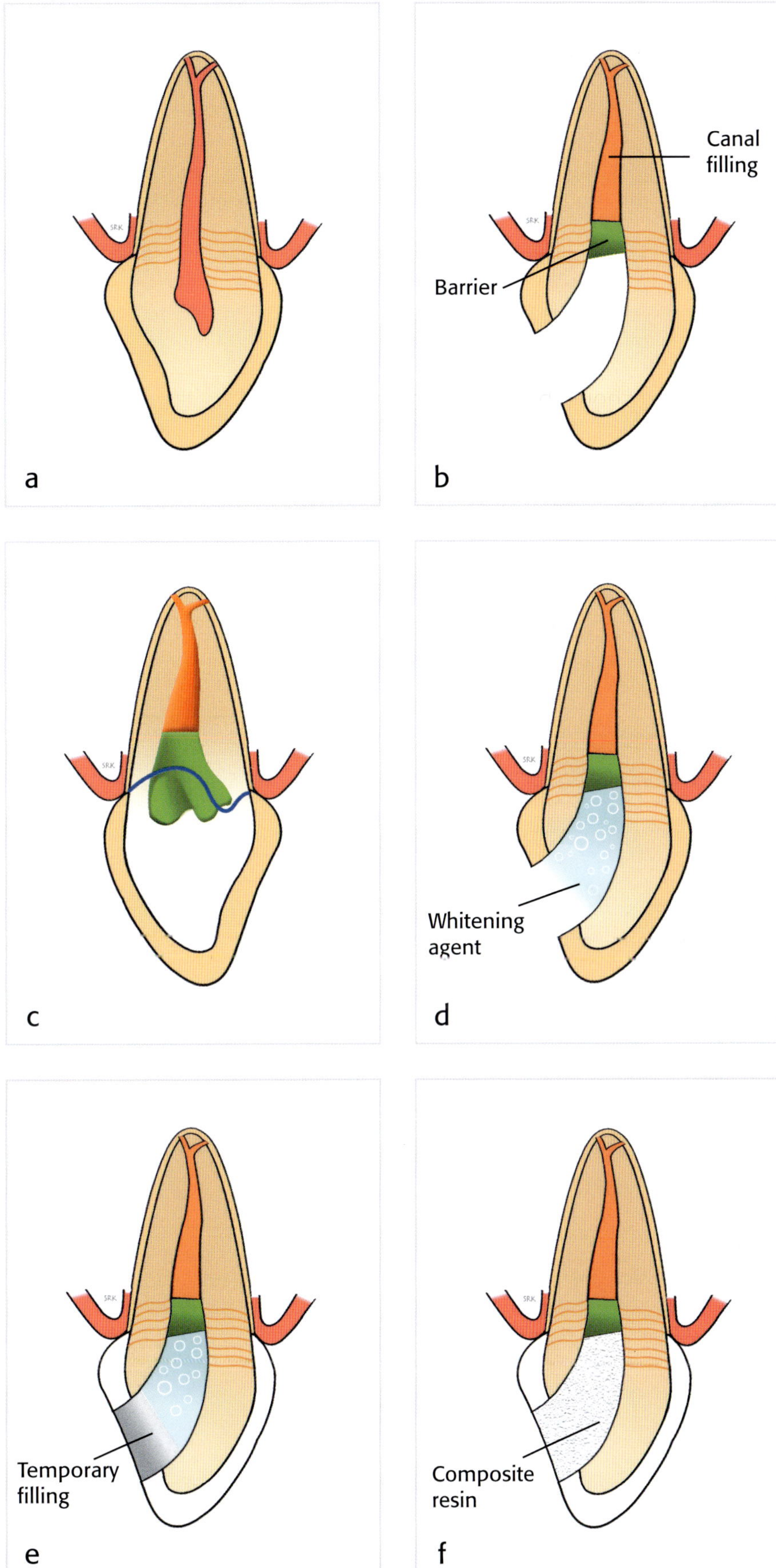

Fig. 2-6 Walking bleach diagram.

a. Discoloration due to pulp necrosis and bacterial by-products.

b. Root canal filling and barrier placement

c. Ideal morphology of the barrier should be a 'bobsled tunnel outline'.

d. Application of bleaching material.

e. Temporary filling.

f. Final restoration with composite resin.

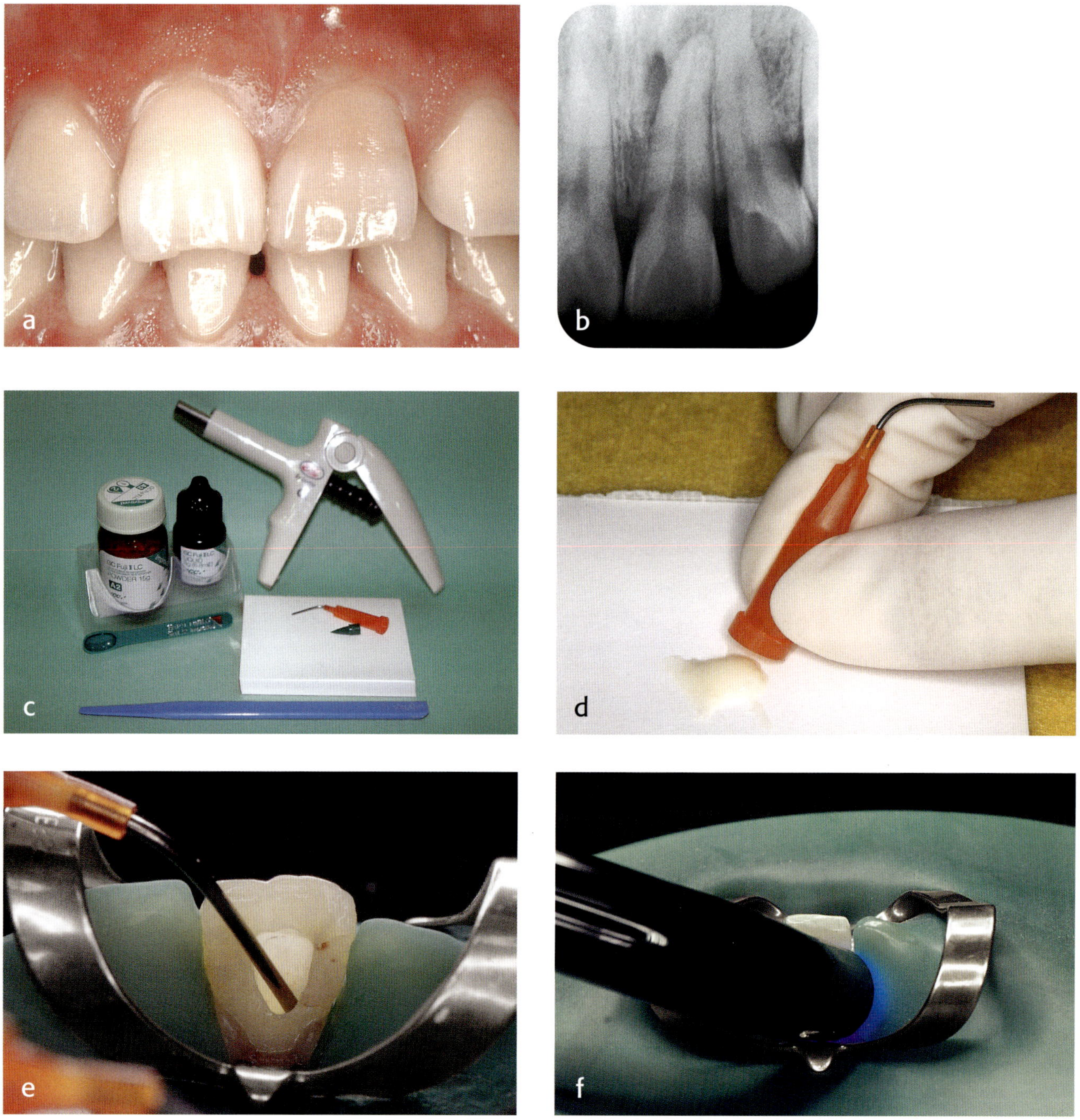

Fig. 2-7 Treatment of the upper left central incisor discolored due to trauma.
a. Single-tooth discoloration with sinus tract formation.
b. Periapical radiolucency is visible on the preoperative radiograph.
c. Light-cured glass ionomer (GCFuji II LC, GC, Japan) and Centrix syringe with a metal tip.
d. Glass ionomer mixture is inserted into the metal tip.
e. Barrier placement with the use of a metal tip.
f. Light curing of the barrier.

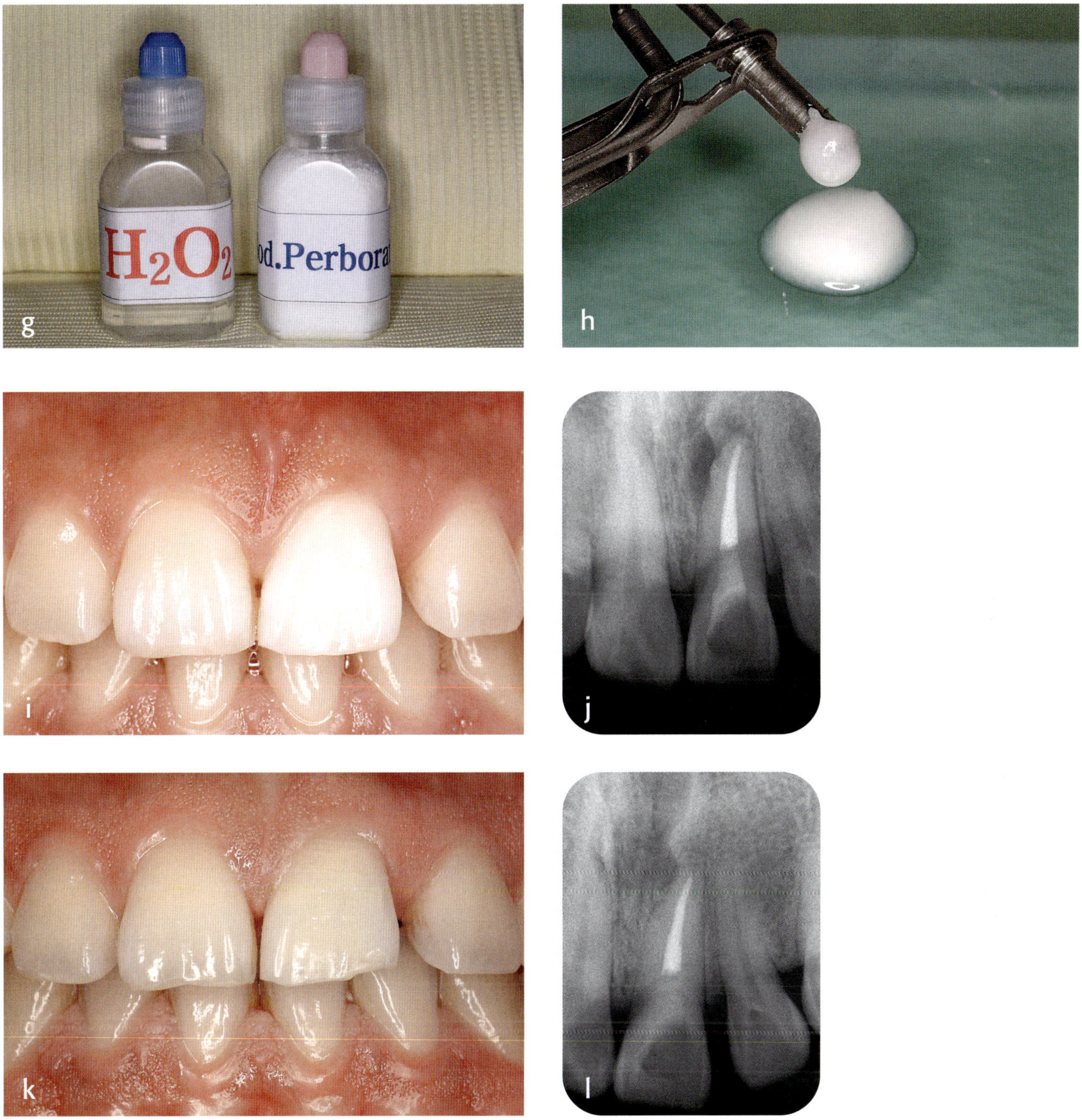

Fig. 2-7 Treatment of the upper left central incisor discolored due to trauma.

g. Hydrogen peroxide and sodium perborate.

h. The mixture of hydrogen peroxide and sodium perborate is placed into the pulp chamber with an amalgam carrier.

i. After 5 sessions of walking bleaching, the tooth is overbleached compared to the adjacent teeth.

j. Radiographic view after root canal treatment, barrier placement, and completion of walking bleaching.

k. At the 5 year follow-up, the treated tooth still matches the color of the adjacent teeth.

l. At the 5 year follow-up, the periapical radiograph shows that the apical lesion has healed.

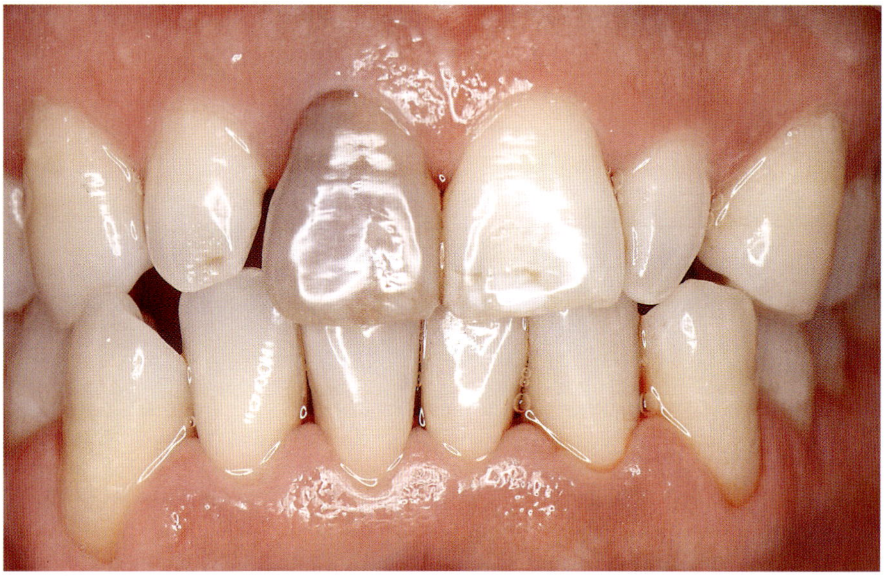

Fig. 2-8 Dark brown discoloration of the upper right central incisor.

a. Esthetic treatment was required for single-tooth discoloration and peg lateralis on the right and left side.

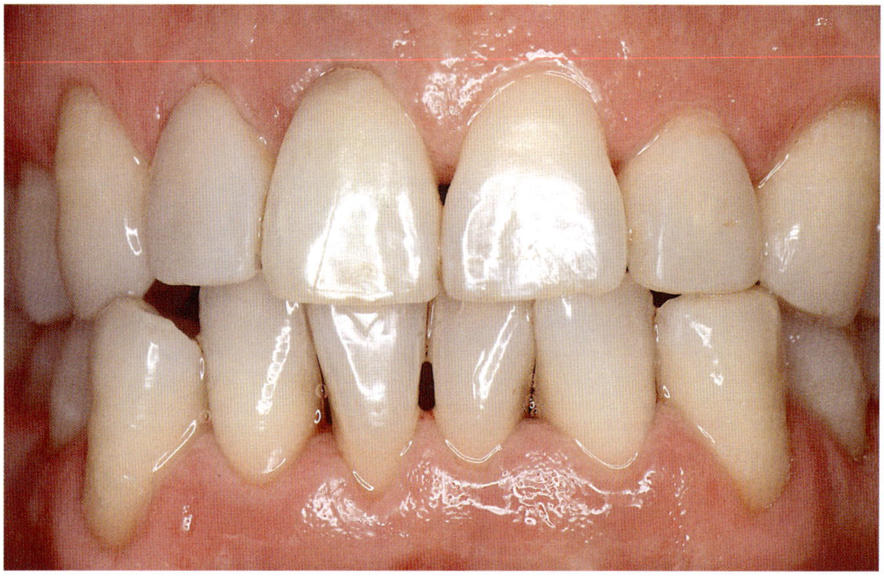

b. Walking bleach treatment of the upper right central incisor and composite restorations of both peg lateralis were performed. The 5 year follow-up photograph shows well-maintained color and esthetics.

Advantages

- Simple and effective.
- The bleaching material is sealed into the access cavity and continues to be effective until the next visit.
- Easier for the patient to comply.
- Short chair time.

Disadvantages

- The temporary filling material can easily pop out.
- Improper placement of the barrier can lead to remaining cervical discoloration.
- Use of acidic bleaching material can lead to cervical root resorption.

Side effects

- **Cervical root resorption:** Cervical root resorption related to walking bleaching has been reported in patients with pulp necrosis before the age of 25 and in cases in which heat was used with hydrogen peroxide. The etiology and mechanism of cervical root resorption has not been fully explained yet. It has been postulated that the whitening material may diffuse through patent dentinal tubules into the periodontal ligament and initiate an inflammatory reaction, foreign body reaction or a decrease in pH, thereby activating osteoclastic activity, leading to resorption. Consequently, there is a special risk factor in young patients with relatively wide open dentinal tubules and in patients with a defect between the cementum and enamel at the level of the CEJ. In order to prevent the leakage of whitening material into the perialveolar tissue, barrier formation is of utmost importance. In young patients, sodium perborate mixed with water is a safe alternative. Cervical root resorption can be managed with a calcium hydroxide dressing in the initial stage. If the resorption has progressed, exposure of the lesion with a crown lengthening procedure or forced eruption followed by an appropriate filling is required (Fig. 2-9)
- **Tooth fracture:** Tooth fractures generally occur due to previous trauma, but they may also be caused by excessive tooth reduction during access cavity opening. Therefore, caution should be taken to minimize the size of the opening, and proper postoperative instructions should be given to the patient (Fig. 2-10).
- **Color relapse:** Color relapse after walking bleaching usually occurs due to marginal leakage of the coronal restoration and should be prevented by minimizing the size of the access cavity. The cavity should be restored 2 weeks after the last walking bleach procedure to allow all the residual oxygen to dissipate. A full-coverage restoration should be recommended if the size of the access opening is too large (Fig. 2-11).

Mechanism of cervical root resorption

- Leakage of H_2O_2 through the dentinal tubule → Inflammatory reaction → **resorption**
- Protein denaturation → Foreign body reaction → **resorption**
- Decrease in pH by H_2O_2 → Activation of osteoclasts → **resorption**

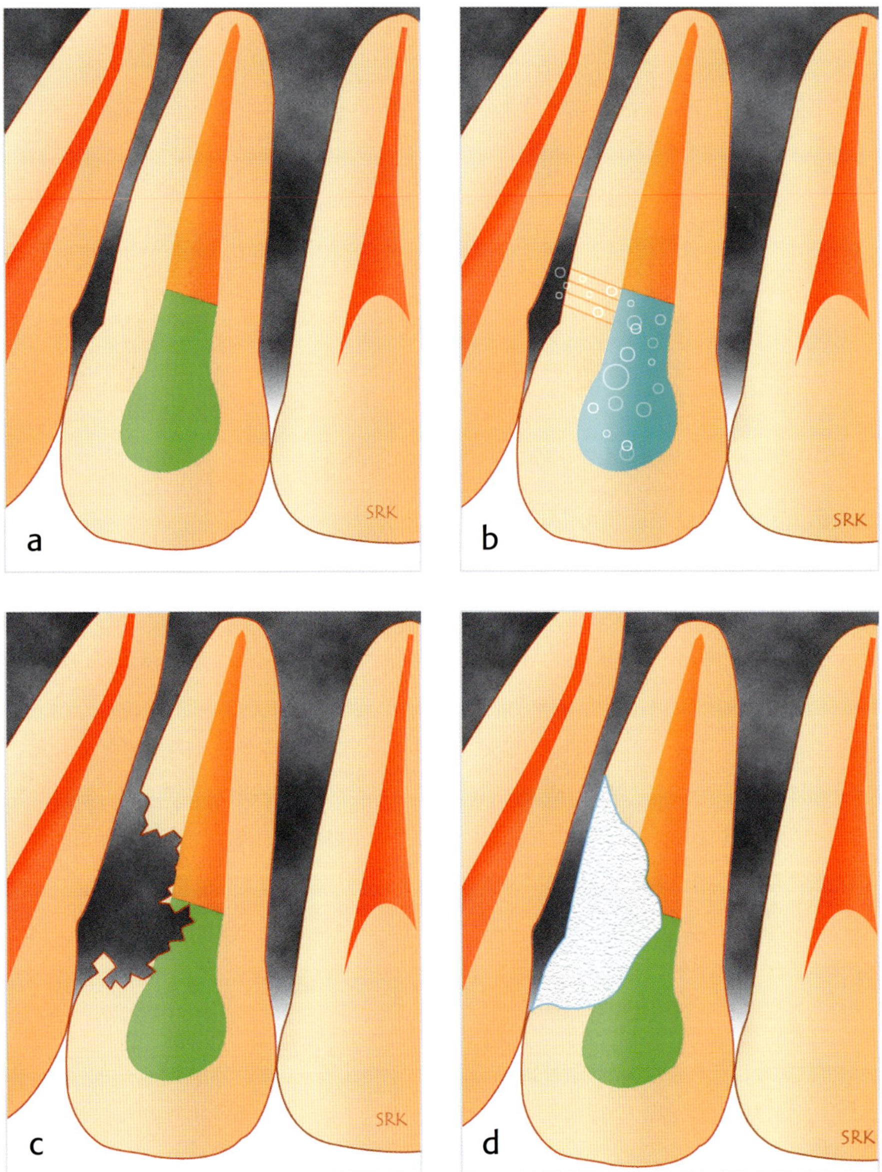

Fig. 2-9 Mechanism of cervical root resorption.

a. After root canal treatment.

b. Leakage of whitening material through the dentinal tubules can occur if it is inserted without proper barrier placement.

c. Cervical root resorption due to the leakage of whitening material.

d. The resorption area is sealed with a glass ionomer filling.

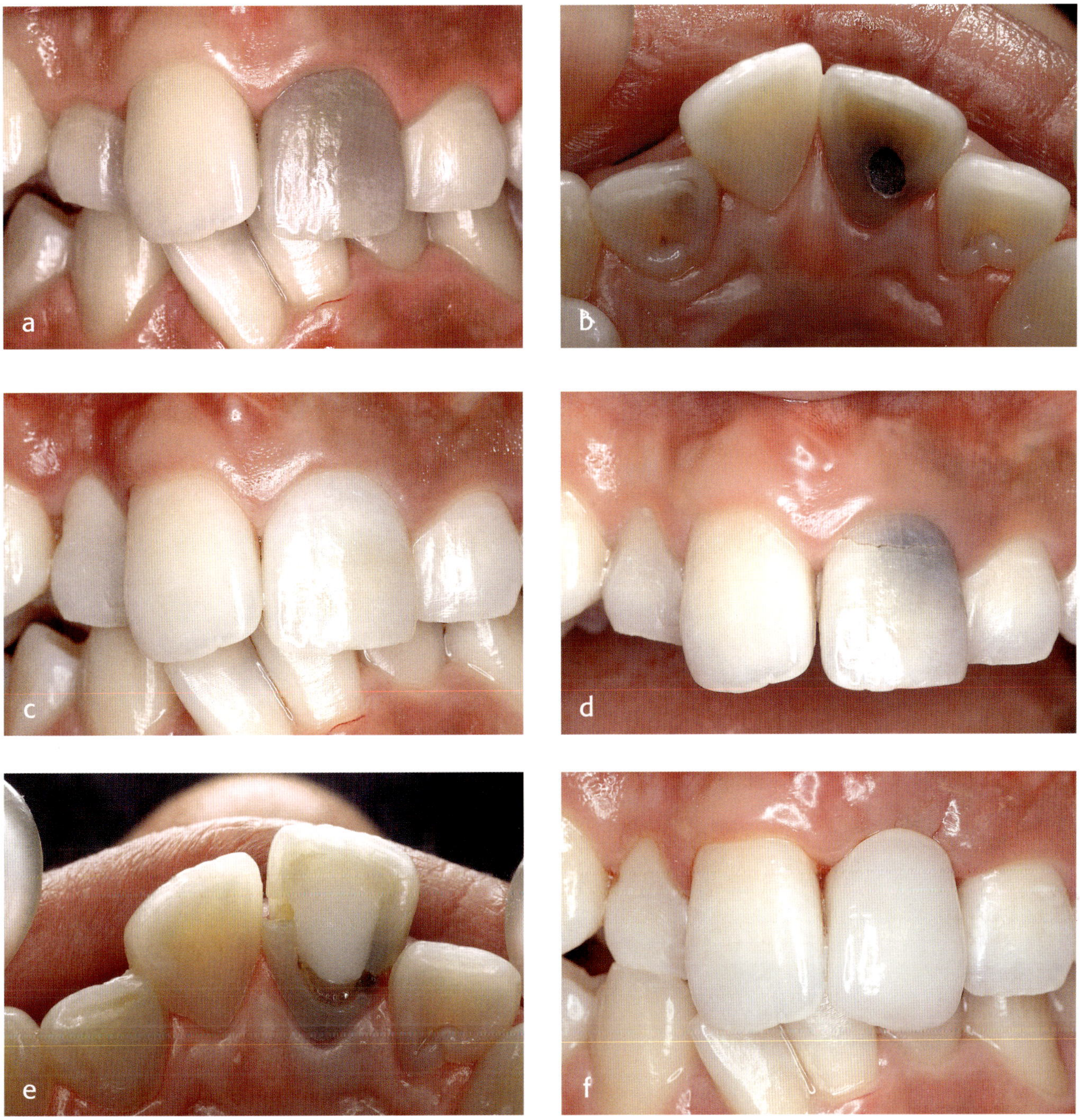

Fig. 2-10 Single-tooth discoloration of the upper left central incisor due to a traumatic injury to the face.

a. Dark brown discoloration of the upper left central incisor.

b. Palatal view showing previous root canal treatment and amalgam filling.

c. The amalgam filling was removed, and 5 sessions of walking bleaching were performed.

d. Another trauma 3 years after treatment resulted in fracture of the central incisor.

e. Palatal view of the fracture.

f. The tooth had to be restored prosthodontically.

Fig. 2-11 Color relapse.

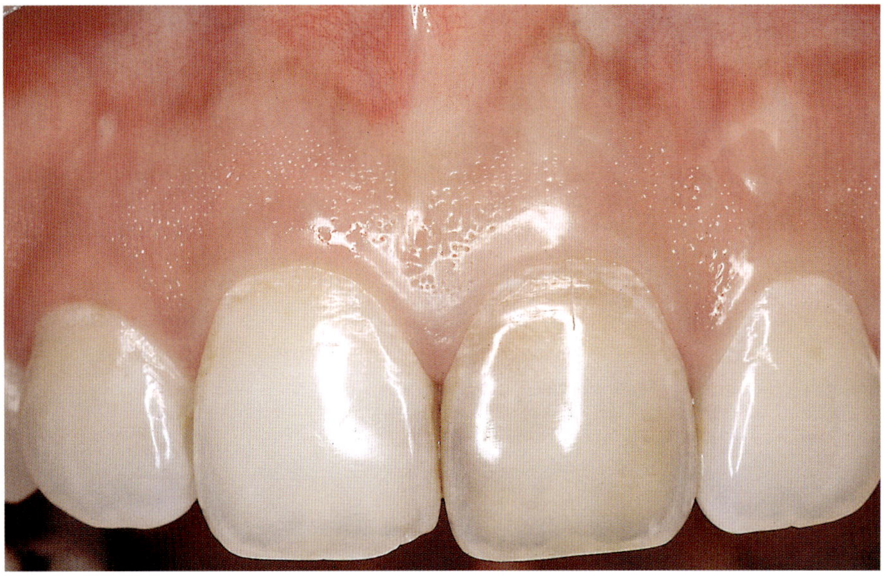

a. Color relapse after walking bleaching.

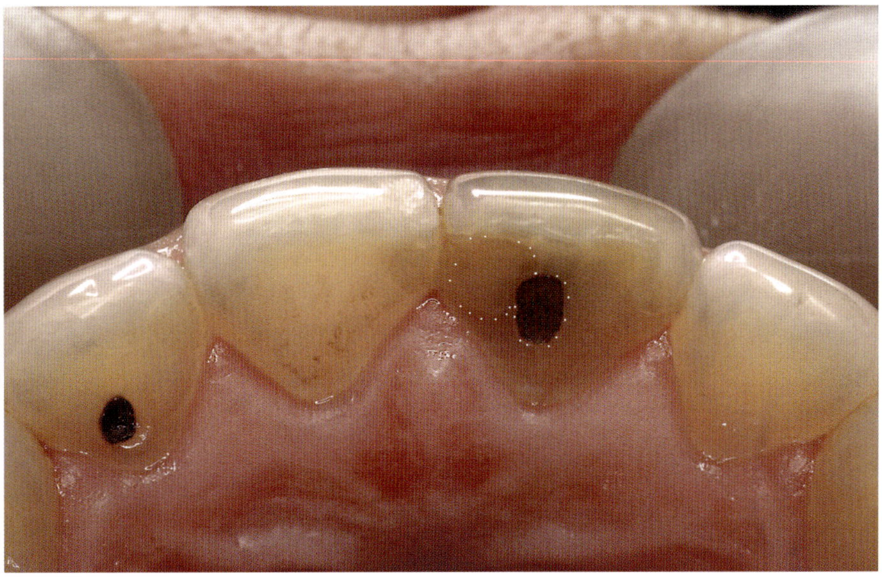

b. Palatal view showing the extensive outline of the margin.

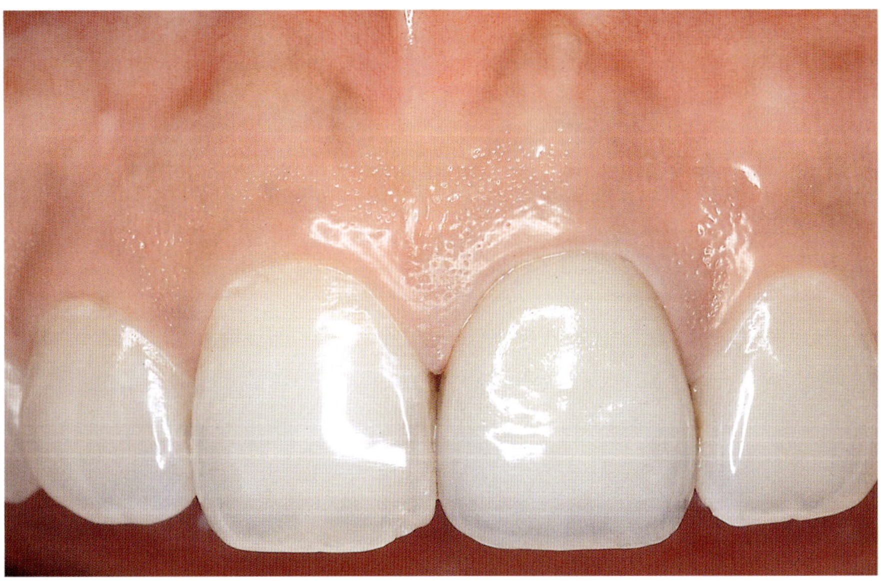

c. After placement of a full-coverage restoration.

Thermocatalytic bleaching

Thermocatalytic bleaching is similar to walking bleaching but has an additional step using a heated instrument. After proper barrier placement, 35% hydrogen peroxide is inserted into the access cavity and heated with a specialized heating device or light source (Fig. 2-12). The temperature (50–60 °C) should be comfortable to the patient without anesthesia. After heating, the procedure can be complemented with walking bleaching, if necessary. Although this procedure is very effective, the rate and efficacy of bleaching seems to be indirectly proportional to the safety of the procedure.

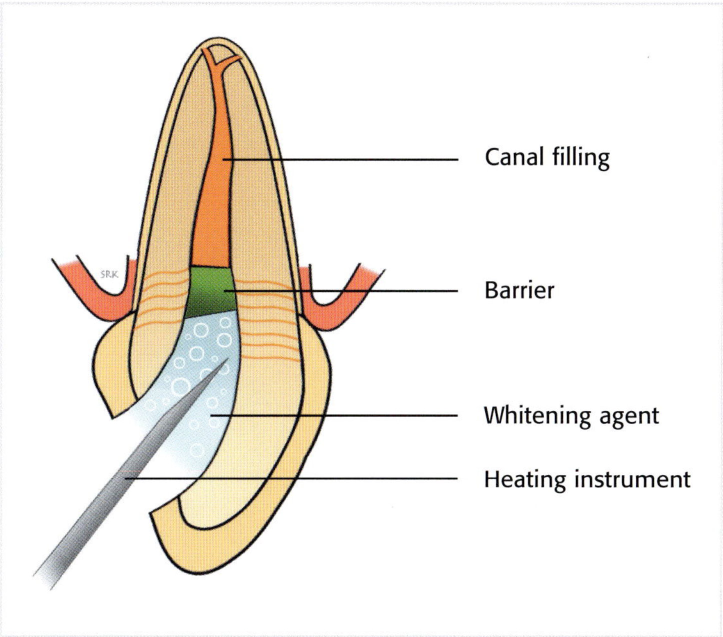

Fig. 2-12 Thermocatalytic bleaching.

Inside-outside bleaching

This technique was first described by Settembrini and Liebenberg in 1997. After proper root canal treatment and barrier placement, the access cavity is left open, and 10 to 20% carbamide peroxide gel is applied into the cavity directly and retained with a home whitening tray (Figs. 2-13 and 2-14). The advantage of this procedure is that the bleaching material acts both internally and externally at the same time. Since the carbamide peroxide gel used for the procedure has a neutral pH, the potential risk of root resorption seems to have been removed. However, there have not been any studies supporting this hypothesis.

Advantages

- The whitening material acts internally and externally.
- Use of whitening material of neutral pH.
- Once the optimal shade is achieved, the treatment can be stopped immediately.
- No need to use heat.

Disadvantages

- The method is technique-sensitive as it relies on patient compliance.
- The periodic insertion of whitening material and cleaning of access cavity can be burdensome for the patient.
- If the patient uses the whitening material overzealously, excessive bleaching may occur.
- The tongue can be irritated from the margins of the open access cavity.

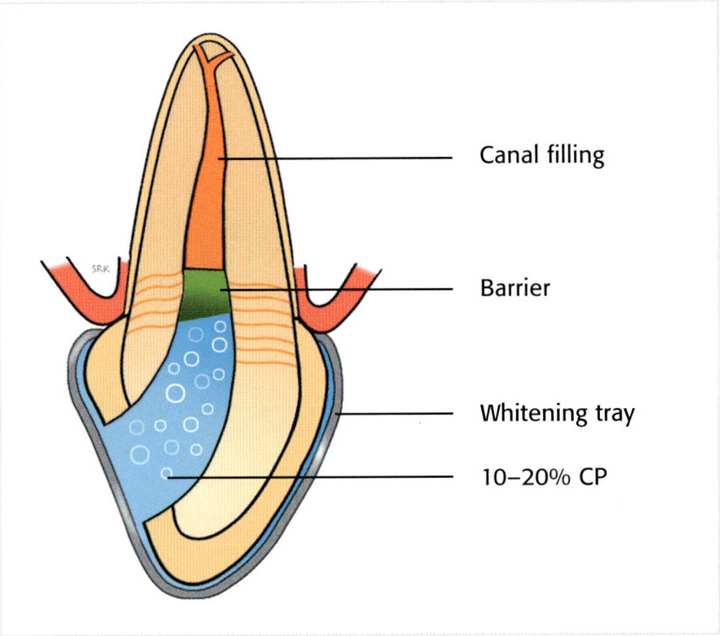

Fig. 2-13 Inside-outside bleaching.

Fig. 2-14 Inside-outside bleaching.

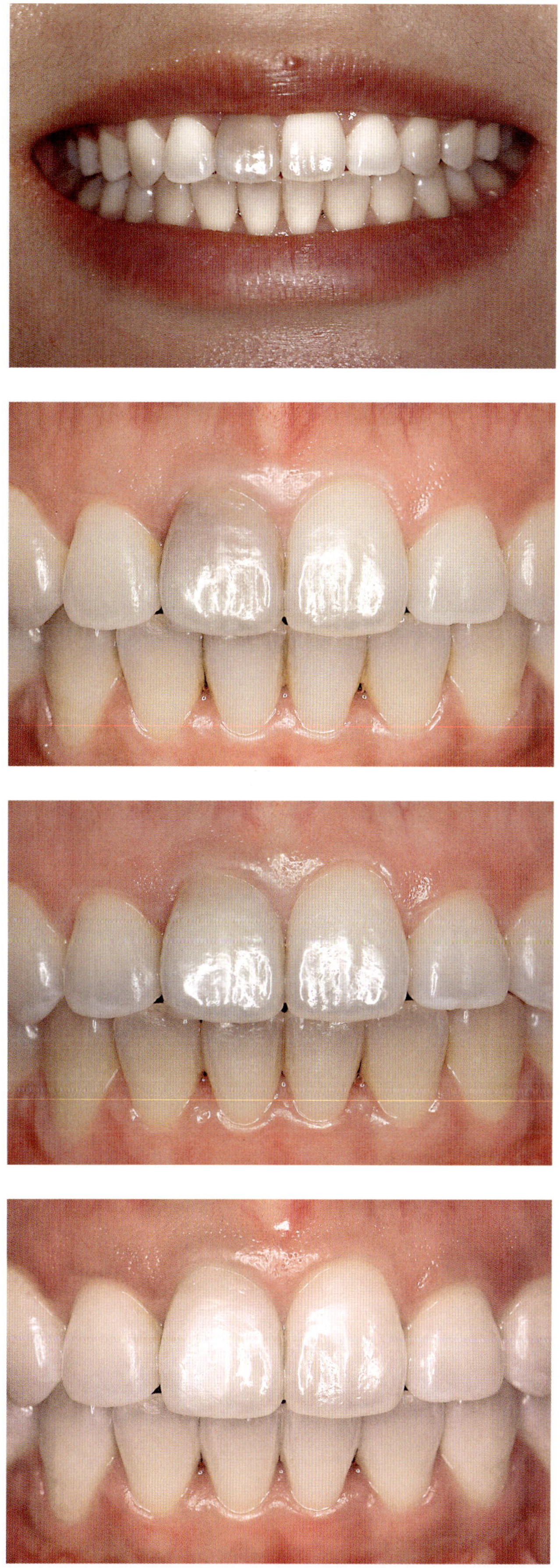

a. The patient was worried about the single dark tooth when smiling.

b. Dark brown discoloration of the upper right central incisor and generalized yellow discoloration.

c. Inside-outside bleaching was performed on the upper right central incisor in combination with home whitening of the upper arch.

d. After completion of whitening of both arches.

Light-activated bleaching of non-vital teeth

CP irradiation method (contribution from Hisashi Hisamitsu)

A 10% carbamide peroxide gel is placed on the labial surface and into the access cavity of the non-vital tooth and light activated from the buccal and lingual side (Fig. 2-15). This technique is termed the "CP irradiation method" or "Hisamitsu method" after its developer. The advantage of this technique is that the discoloration of the non-vital tooth improves on the day of treatment, dispensing with the need for multiple visits (Figs. 2-16a and b). The mechanism of shade improvement through light activation is unclear. It has been suggested that the increase in temperature due to irradiation catalyzes the breakdown into hydrogen peroxide and permeation into the dentin.

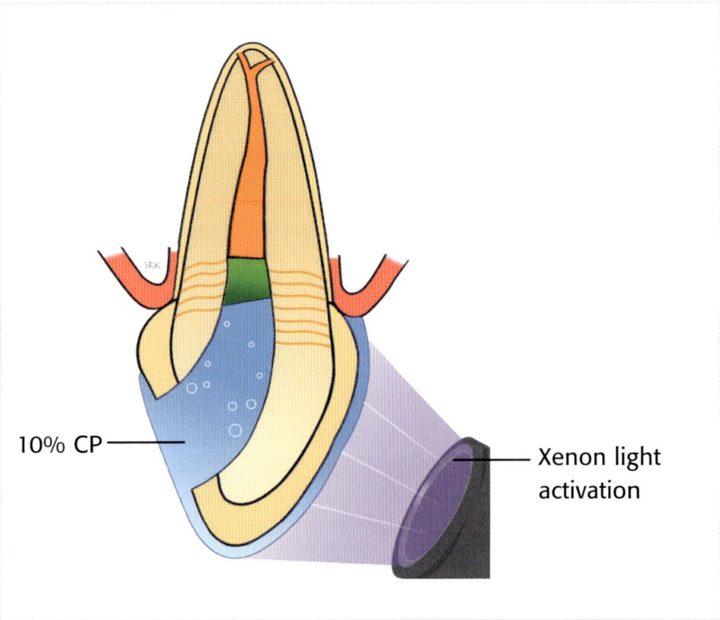

Fig. 2-15 CP irradiation method.

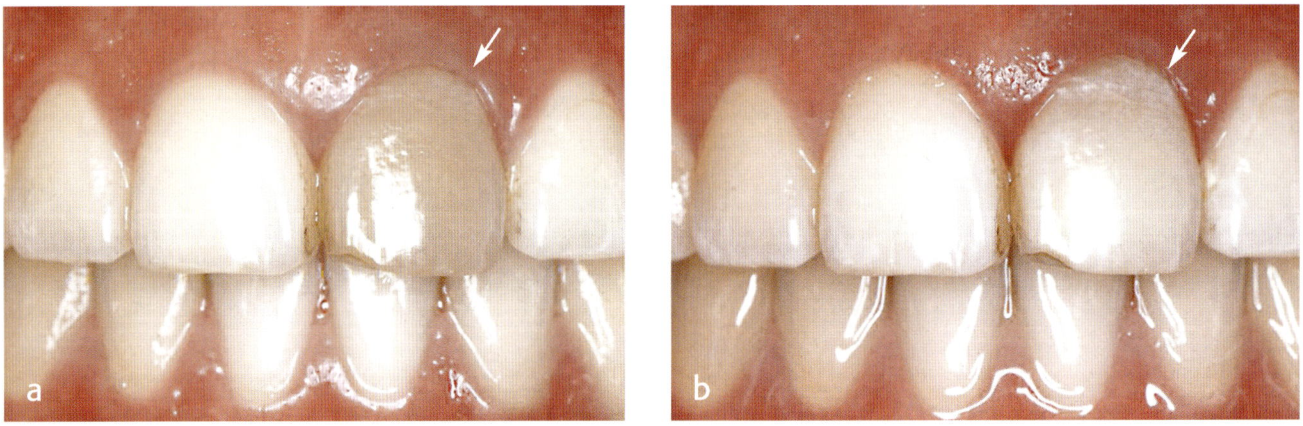

Fig. 2-16 Discoloration of the upper left central incisor.
a. Before CP irradiation.
b. After CP irradiation (same day).

Light activation with power whitening gels

Discolored abutment teeth or discolored roots can be a dilemma to the esthetic dentist. In these delicate situations, a resin barrier can be placed around the non-vital abutment tooth followed by application of a power whitening gel, which is then activated with a light source (Figs. 2-17 and 2-18).

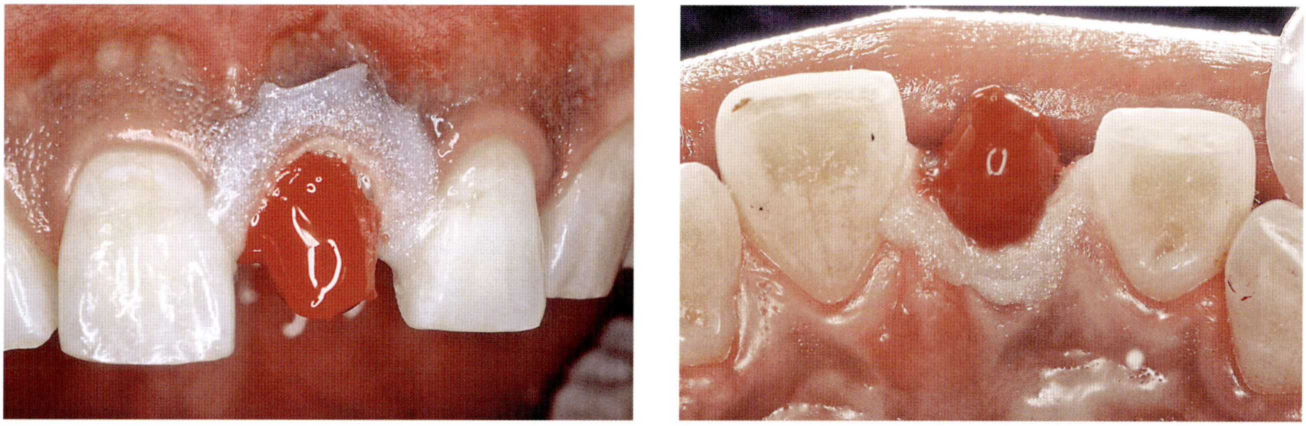

Fig. 2-17 Power whitening gel with light activation.
a. Power whitening gel is placed on the discolored abutment tooth after proper resin barrier placement.
b. Palatal view.

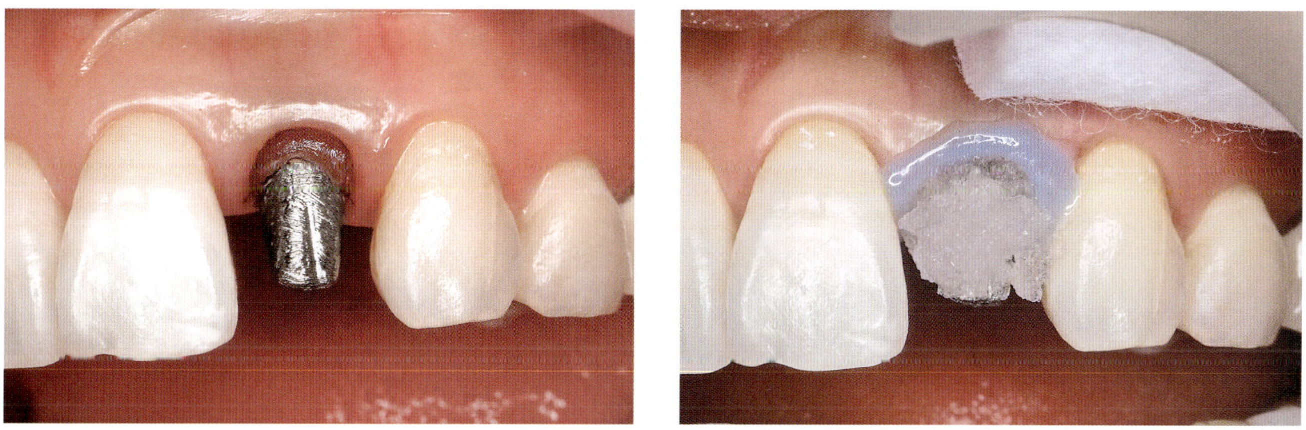

Fig. 2-18 Discoloration of abutment tooth.
a. Dark abutment tooth with a metal post and core.
b. After proper isolation of the gingiva, a highly concentrated bleaching gel is placed onto the tooth and activated with a light source.

••• Non-vital bleaching techniques include the walking bleach technique, thermocatalytic bleaching, inside-outside bleaching, and light-activated bleaching methods. If the protocols are followed properly, all of these techniques provide safe and effective bleaching results with minimal tooth reduction.

Q&A

Question 1. If a post is placed after walking bleaching, the barrier would need to be removed for conventional post placement. Would this affect the maintenance of the bleaching result?

Answer: The role of a barrier is to prevent the leakage of whitening material through the dentinal tubules. Therefore, removing the base after walking bleaching should not affect the maintenance of the bleaching result.

Question 2. How do you detect cervical root resorption after walking bleach treatment? What kind of signs or symptoms does the patient show?

Answer: Taking a periodic radiograph every six months is of great help in early detection of cervical root resorption. The patients usually complain of discomfort and gingival swelling, but there may be no symptoms.

Question 3. How should a discolored tooth be treated if the pulp chamber and root canal seems to have been obliterated?

Answer: In a discolored tooth with calcified pulp chamber and canals, pulp vitality should be evaluated. If the tooth is non-vital, root canal treatment should be performed followed by barrier placement and walking bleach treatment (Fig. 2-19). If the tooth is vital, whitening should be performed externally either by home or power whitening (Fig. 2-20).

Question 4. How do you charge for walking bleach treatment?

Answer: The walking bleach fee should include the fee for barrier placement, internal whitening sessions and placement of the final access cavity restoration. This should be approximately one-half to two-thirds the fee for a full-coverage restoration.

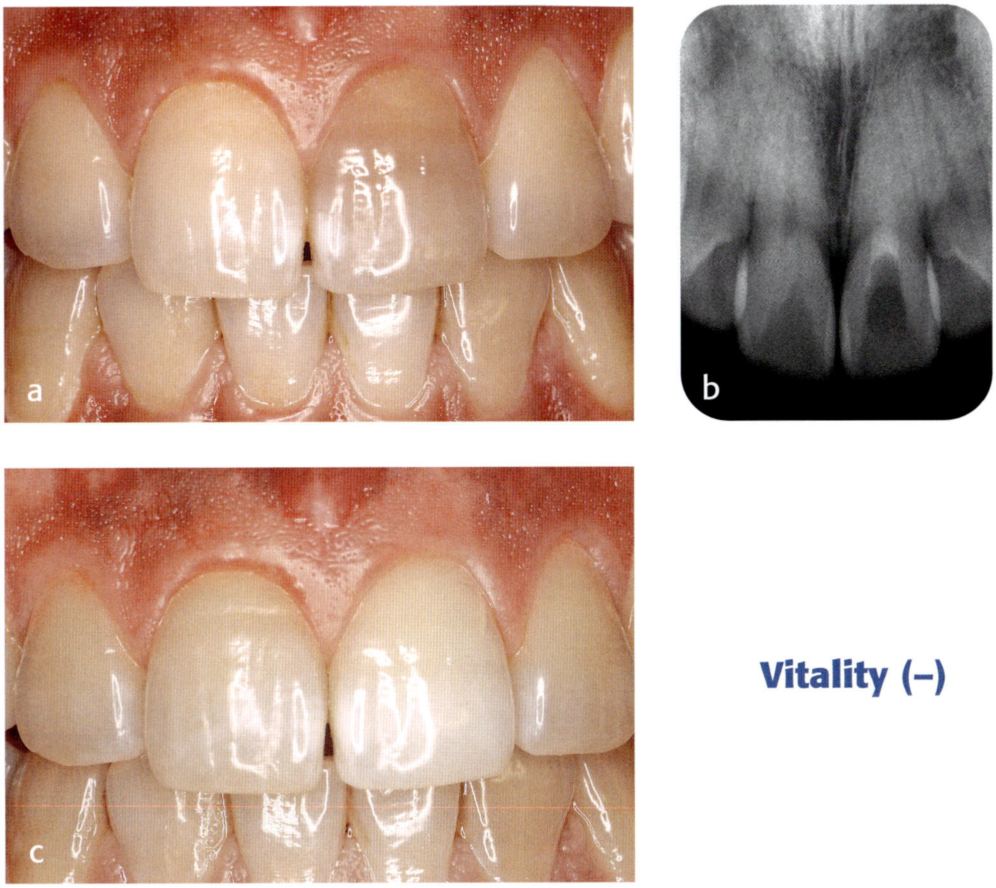

Fig. 2-19 Single-tooth discoloration with a calcified pulp chamber and canal.

a. A discolored upper left central incisor with negative pulp vitality.

b. Although the periapical radiograph showed an obliterated pulp chamber and canal, root canal treatment was performed and the canal negotiated to half of the root.

c. After barrier placement, walking bleaching was performed to an overbleached state.

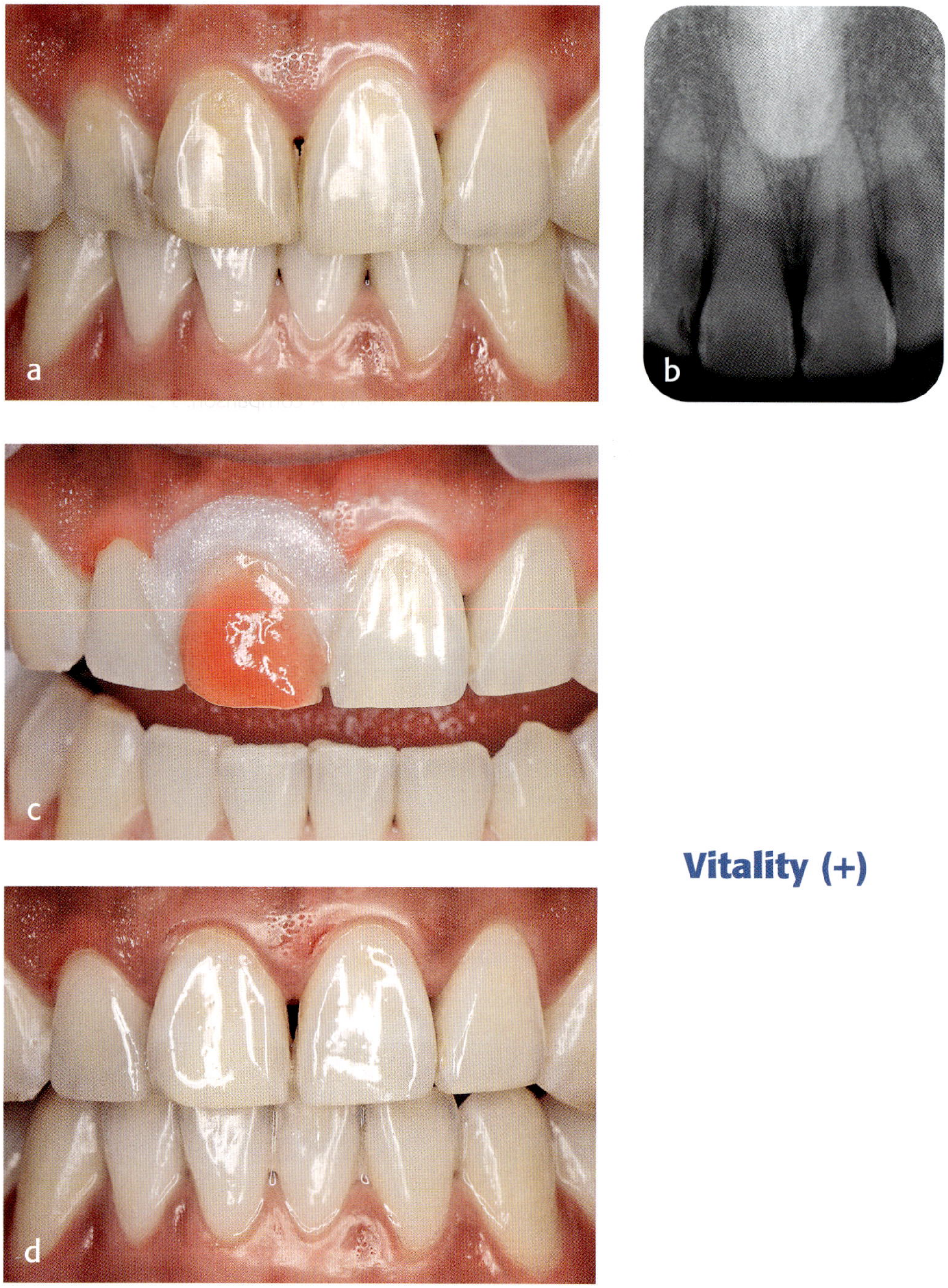

Fig. 2-20 Single-tooth discoloration with a calcified pulp chamber and canal.

a. A discolored upper right central incisor with positive pulp vitality.

b. The periapical radiograph showed an obliterated pulp chamber and canal. However, the tooth was still vital.

c. Power whitening of the discolored tooth with proper gingival isolation.

d. After power whitening.

References

Cvek M, Lindvall AM. External root resorption following bleaching of pulpless teeth with hydrogen peroxide. Endodont Dent Traumatol 1985; 1:56.

Deliperi S. Two-Year Clinical Evaluation of Nonvital Tooth Whitening and Resin Restorations. J Esthet Restor Dent 2005; 17(6); 369-379.

Douglas RD. Intraoral determination of the tolerance of dentists for perceptibility and acceptability of shade mismatch. J Prosthet Dent 2007; 97:200-8.

Friedman S, Rotstein I, Libfeld H, Stabholz A, Heling I. Incidence of external root resorption and esthetic results in 58 bleached pulpless teeth. Endodont Dent Traumatol 1988; 4:23.

Goldstein RE, Garber DA. Complete Dental Bleaching, Quintessence Publishing Co, Inc, 1995.

Greenwall LH. Bleaching techniques in restorative dentistry, Martin Dunitz, 2001.

Grossman LI. Endodontic Practice, 5th Ed. Philadelphia: Lea and Febiger, 1960.

Guan YH. The measurement of tooth whiteness by image analysis and spectrophotometry: A comparison. J Oral Rehalbilitation 2005; 32:7-15.

Gultz J. Inside/Outside Nonvital Tooth Bleaching. Con Esthet Resor Practice 1998.

Hara AK. Nonvital tooth bleaching: A 2-year case report. Quintessence Int 1999; 30(11):748-754.

Harrington GW, Natkin E. External resorption associated with bleaching of pulpless teeth. J Endodont 1979; 5:344.

Hisamitsu H, Toko T. Tooth Whitening basics and clinical techniques. Quintessence Japan, 2004.

Holmstrup G, Palm AM, Lambjerg-Hansen H. Bleaching of discoloured root-filled teeth. Endodont Dent Traumatol 1988; 4197.

Liebenberg WH. Intracoronal lightening of discolored pulpless teeth: a modified walking bleach technique. Quintessence Int 1997; 28:771-7.

Madison S, Walton RE. Cervical root resorption following bleaching of endodontically treated teeth. J Endodont 1990; 16:570.

Paravina RD. New Shade Guide for Evaluation of Tooth Whitening-Colorimetric Study. J Esthet Restor Dent 2007; 19:276-283.

Rotstein I, Mor C, Friedman S. Prognosis of intracoronal bleaching with sodium perborate preparations in vitro: 1 year study. J Endodont 1993; 19:10.

Rotstein I, Torek Y, Lewinstein I. Effect of bleaching time and temperature on the radicular penetration of hydrogen peroxide. Endodont Dent Traumatol 1991; 7:196.

Rotstein I, Torek Y, Misgav R. Effect of cementum defects on radicular penetration of 30% H_2O_2 during intracoronal bleaching, J Endodont 1991; 17:230.

Rotstein I. Role of catalase in the elimination of residual hydrogen peroxide following tooth bleaching. J Endodont 1993; 19:567.

Settembrini L, Gultz J, Kaim J, Scherer W. A technique for bleaching non-vital teeth: inside/outside bleaching. J Am Dent Assoc 1997; 128:1283-4.

Shinohara MS. Shear Bond Strength Evaluation of composite Resin on Enamel and Dentin after Nonvital Bleaching. J Esthet Restor Dent 2005; 17:22-29.

Steiner DR, West JD. A method to determine the location and shape of an intracoronal bleach barrier. J Endodont 1994; 20:304.

chapter 3

Home whitening

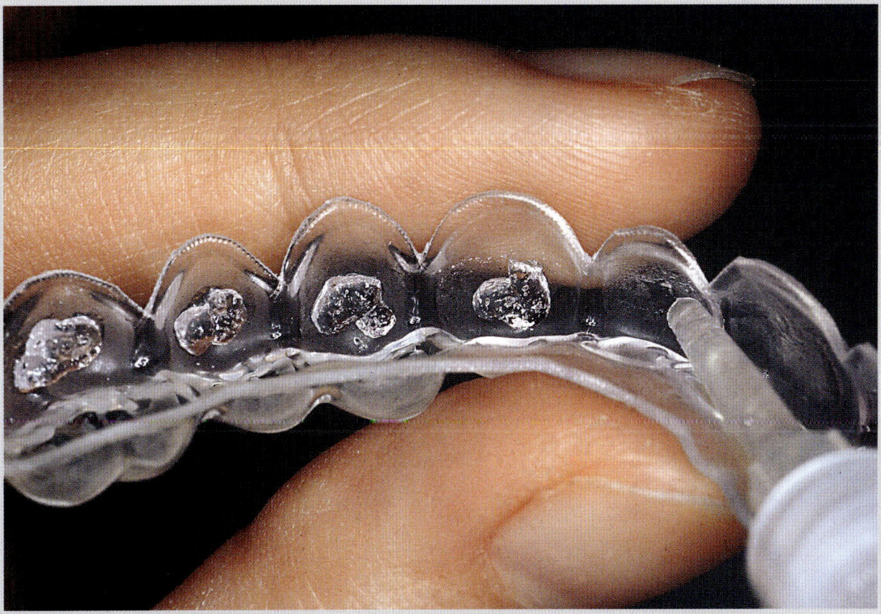

The technique of home whitening can be traced back to 1968, when Klusmier, an orthodontist in Arkansas, recommended placing an over-the-counter oral antiseptic containing 10% carbamide peroxide (Gly-oxide, Marion Merell Dow) into an orthodontic retainer at night to overcome gingival irritation. He noted an improvement in tissue healing and, more interestingly, a lightening of tooth color. Thereafter, he started using this technique for tooth whitening and presented his findings at several dental meetings. This technique spread to other study groups and was first reported in the dental literature by Haywood and Heymann, in 1989. A survey published by Clinical Research Associates showed that, by 1990, only 52% of dentists surveyed had incorporated this method of whitening into their practices. The reason for this hesitation at that time was fear of an unknown procedure and fear of change. Now, 18 years after its first publication, the technique has become one of the most widely accepted procedures amongst dental professionals. This acceptance is based on well-documented long-term studies that confirm its safety, efficacy and success under dental supervision.

Mechanism of tooth whitening

The exact mechanism of tooth whitening is not fully understood, but it has been mostly attributed to an 'oxidation' reaction. Hydrogen peroxide, the most commonly used whitening agent, is a strong oxidizing agent with the ability to produce highly reactive oxygen (O•) and perhydroxyl (HO_2•) radicals (Fig. 3-1). In an acidic environment, more oxygen radicals are formed, whereas in a basic environment, more perhydroxyl radicals with a higher oxidizing power are formed. During the process of whitening, these highly reactive radicals penetrate into the organic matrix of the enamel and dentin, reaching the pulp in 5 to 15 minutes. These radicals not only change the color of the enamel by removing extrinsic stains, but also change the color of dentin affected by intrinsic stains. According to Albers in 1991 (Fig. 3-2), during the initial whitening process, highly pigmented carbon-ring compounds are opened and converted into chains of lighter color. Existing carbon double-bond compounds, usually pigmented yellow, are converted into hydroxyl groups, which are usually colorless. As this process continues, the tooth continually lightens. However, the process eventually reaches a saturation point at which continued whitening does not affect the tooth color anymore. Care should be taken that treatment is stopped at that point. Excessive whitening beyond the saturation point could affect the tooth structure, inducing tooth brittleness and increased porosity. For safe tooth whitening, the entire procedure should therefore be performed under the supervision of a dentist.

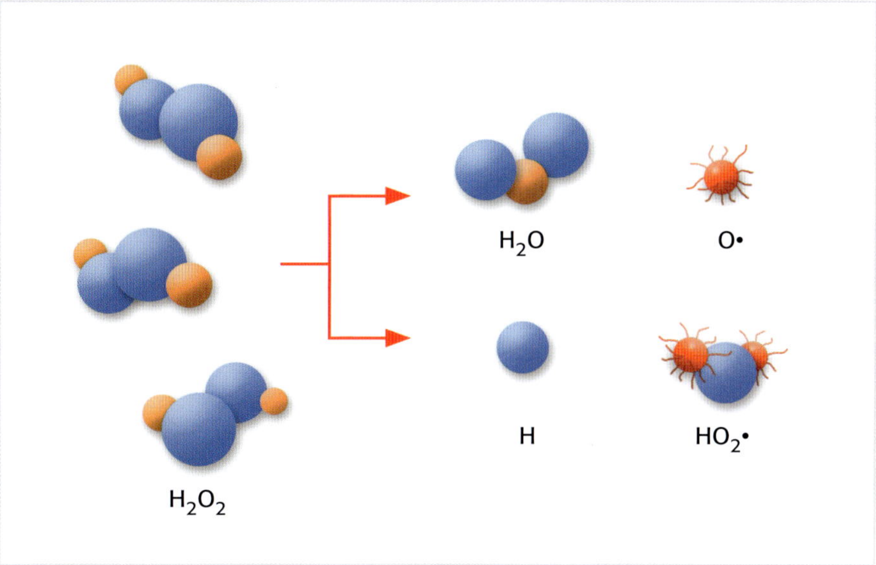

Fig. 3-1 Disassociation of hydrogen peroxide.

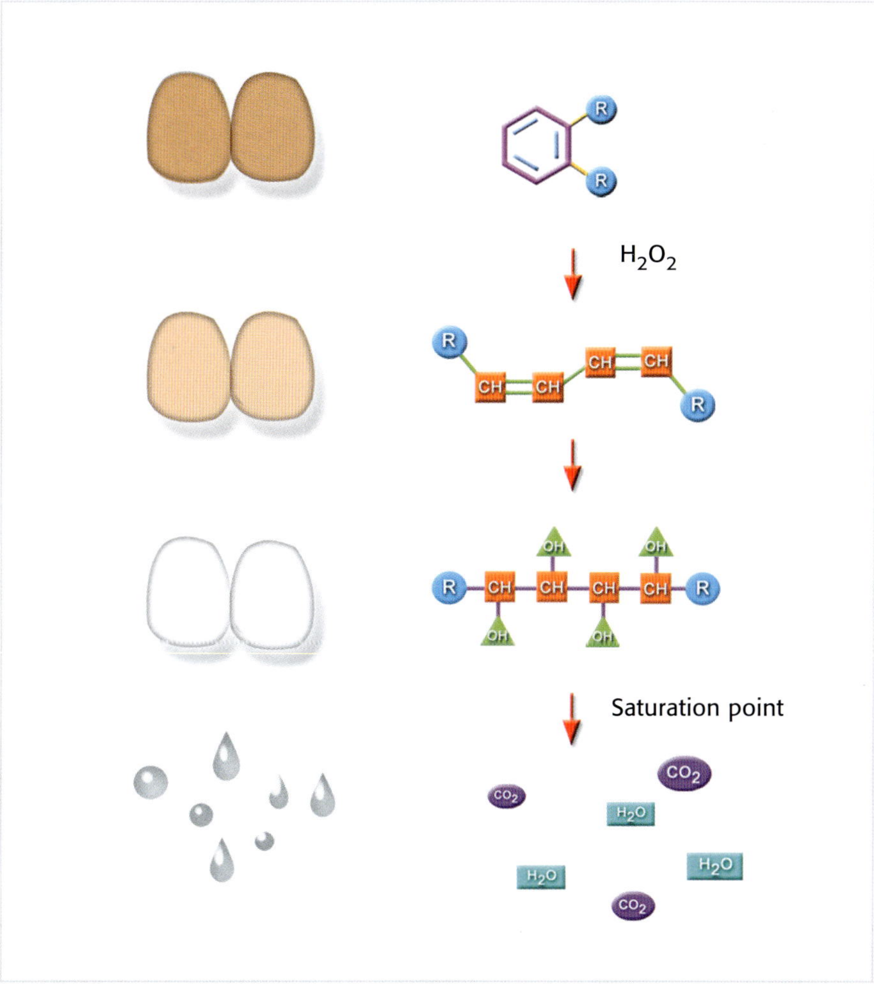

Fig. 3-2 Mechanism of tooth whitening (Albers 1991, ADEPT Report).

Home whitening materials

The most commonly used active ingredients in peroxide-containing tooth whitening materials are hydrogen peroxide and carbamide peroxide. 10% carbamide peroxide ($CH_6N_2O_3$) chemically decomposes into 3.35% hydrogen peroxide, 6.65% urea, carbon dioxide, and ammonia (Fig. 3-3). Both hydrogen peroxide and carbamide peroxide have been accepted by the US Food and Drug Administration (FDA) as an oral antiseptic. Products containing 10 to 15% carbamide peroxide along with 1.5 to 3% hydrogen peroxide are classified as category I, which are generally recognized as safe and effective in tooth whitening. There are a wide variety of home whitening products available on the market. Generally, the concentration of carbamide peroxide varies from 10 to 22%. The more highly concentrated, thicker, more viscous materials produce a lightening effect more quickly than the less concentrated, less viscous materials. However, in the end, there is no significant difference in their whitening efficacies. The choice of material depends on a number of factors, including efficacy, safety, cost, concentration, ease of application, pH (neutral), viscosity, flavor, treatment time and package design.

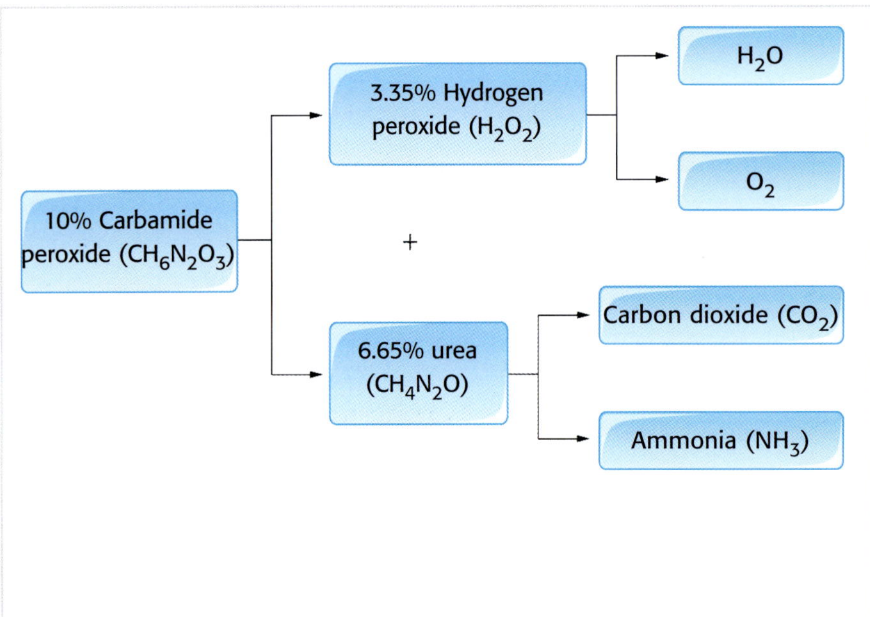

Fig. 3-3 Decomposition of carbamide peroxide.

Over-the-counter (OTC) products

Over-the-counter whitening kits (Fig. 3-4) can be easily purchased through stores and mail order without the prescription of a dentist. In the past, OTC products contained a 3-step system consisting of an accelerator, a gel and a whitening tooth paste. The accelerator and the gel usually contained different concentrations of acids that dissolve tooth minerals. The third step, the whitening toothpaste, contained titanium dioxide, which is an ingredient usually found in paint or correction fluid. With the recent introduction of hydrogen peroxide strips in 2000, OTC systems have improved in terms of material and delivery system, making them more effective and user-friendly. The strips contain various concentrations of hydrogen peroxide. They are preloaded flexible polyethylene strips designed to deliver hydrogen peroxide in gel form directly to the labial surface of the anterior teeth without the need for tray fabrication. Other delivery methods include paint-on-pens, capsules and mouthpieces with activating lights. The main problem with OTC products is that patients may misdiagnose their dental conditions, leading to abuse and overzealous use of the product.

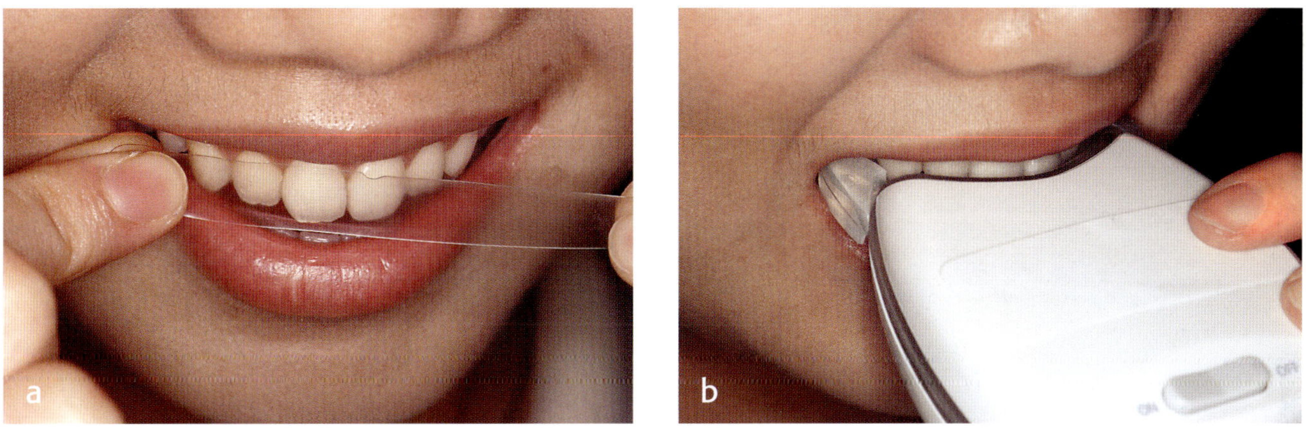

Fig. 3-4 Over-the-counter products.
a. Preloaded flexible polyethylene strips.
b. Mouthpiece with activating light.

Indications and contraindications of home whitening

Indications

- Generalized yellow, orange or light brown discoloration
- Age-related yellow discoloration
- Mild tetracycline staining
- Superficial brown fluorosis stains
- Discoloration due to smoking, coffee, tea and other chromogenic foods
- Patients with genetically yellow or grey teeth
- Patients wanting shade improvement with minimally invasive treatment
- Yellow discoloration of single vital anterior teeth

Contraindications

- Amelogenesis imperfecta and dentinogenesis imperfecta
- Severe tetracycline discoloration
- Discoloration due to restorative materials (e.g., amalgam)
- Pregnant or nursing women
- Severe surface damage due to attrition, abrasion or erosion
- Lack of compliance
- Inability to tolerate the tray or the taste of the product
- Unrealistic expectations
- Teeth with severe pre-existing sensitivity

Home whitening technique

Home whitening can be initiated following proper diagnosis and treatment planning and after the patient's informed consent has been obtained. There may be subtle changes according to the patient's character and the nature of the discoloration, but the main appointment set-up for home whitening can be divided into three phases: initiation, review and termination.

It is important to have a basic set-up, which ensures that every patient can be successfully treated according to a regular regime and that all staff members are aware of their role and balanced assignment in tooth whitening.

Initiation phase

The tooth surface is cleaned and accurate impressions reproducing the upper and lower teeth are taken so that whitening trays can be made. The whitening trays can be fabricated in the office or in the laboratory while the patient waits. Therefore, fabrication and delivery of the whitening kit and tray can be managed at the same visit. During the delivery procedure, proper loading of the whitening gel into the tray and placement and removal of the tray can be demonstrated to acquaint the patient with the home whitening procedure. In addition to the demonstration, the patient should be given written instructions (Fig. 3-5), which should be verbally explained step-by-step. Detailed explanations on possible discomforts and precautions are given at that time (Fig. 3-6).

- **Information on home whitening kit:** Home whitening kits differ according to the manufacturer. The dental staff should be familiar with the specific product used. The contents of the kit are shown and demonstrated to the patient (e.g., whitening syringes, tray, tray case, desensitizing agent, shade guide, instruction sheet).
- **Try-in of the tray:** The retention, comfort and fit of the tray is evaluated in the patient's mouth. The tray is modified and corrected if the borders are overextended or impinging on the gingiva.
- **Tray-loading:** Demonstrate gel loading into the tray. Usually, 2 to 3 drops of gel is placed into the labial surface of each tooth in the tray. The amount may vary according to tooth size and presence or absence of reservoirs. It is best to demonstrate loading half of the tray and to leave the other half for the patient to perform.
- **Removal of excess whitening material:** Emphasize the importance of tooth cleaning to the patient, since the whitening material acts on the tooth surface. After placement of the loaded tray, excess whitening material is wiped off with cotton swabs.
- **Home whitening in the office:** The first home whitening procedure should be performed in the office, so that the patient can be acquainted with the full procedure from the beginning to the end. While the patient is wearing the tray, the instruction sheet can be reviewed again, and further information on the wearing time and treatment interval can be given. For maximum effects, home whitening should be performed overnight on each day of the recommended treatment period. If sensitivity is encountered, the tray may be worn every other day for 2 hours during the daytime.
- **Removal of tray and rinsing:** After removal of the tray, the teeth should be rinsed with cold water and gently brushed with a toothbrush. The tray should be rinsed under running water using a bactericidal liquid soap.
- **Tray storage:** The tray should be kept in the tray case included in the whitening kit.

Home whitening instructions

1. Brush and floss your teeth prior to whitening. The whitening gel is most effective with clean teeth.
2. Load a small drop of whitening gel into the inner front surface of the tray.
3. Insert the loaded tray in the mouth so that the tray firmly seats against the teeth. Wipe off any excess gel with cotton swabs.
4. Wear the tray for at least 2 hours during the daytime or at night during sleep.
5. When treatment has been completed, remove the tray and brush your teeth with a wet tooth brush.
6. After rinsing the tray in running water, dry and store it in the storage case provided.
7. Use the desensitizing gels you have received to treat any sensitivity.
8. If you experience any severe discomfort or sensitivity, please call your dentist or dental staff.

Whitening for your beautiful smile...

Dental Clinic Tel. 00000000

Fig. 3-5 Home whitening instructions.

Fig. 3-6 Initiation phase.

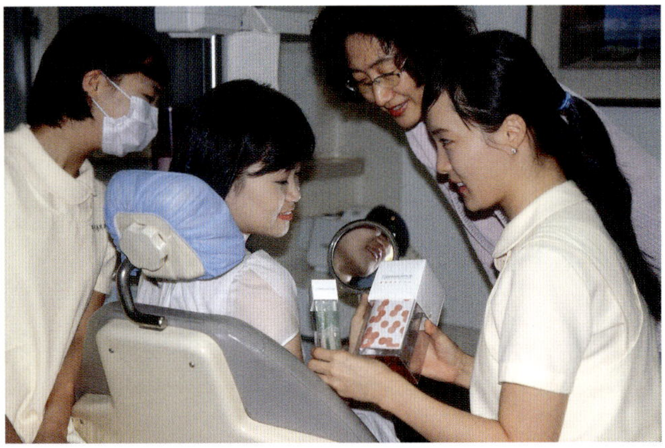

a. Information on the home whitening kit is given to the patient.

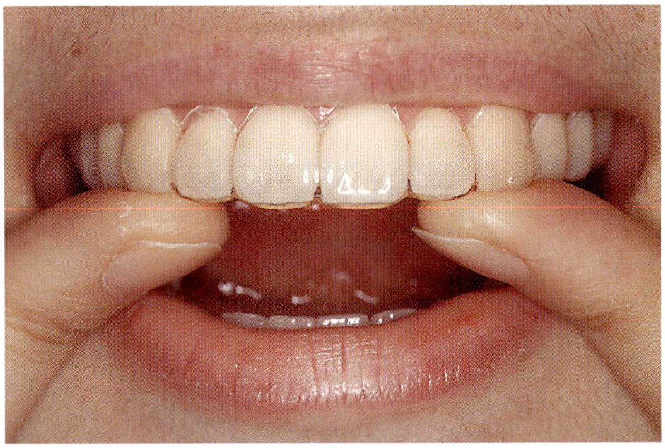

b. Try-in of the tray.

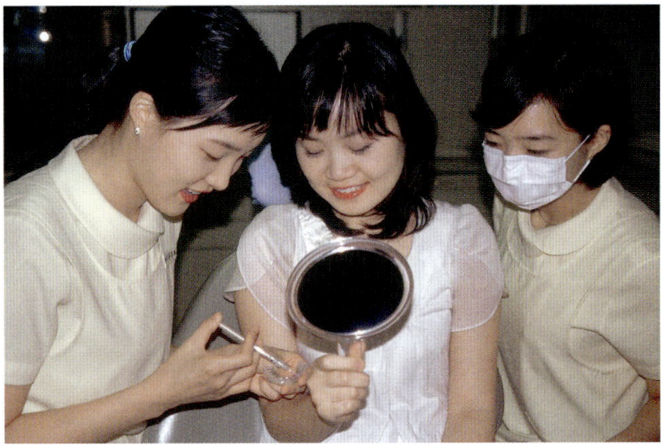

c. Proper tray loading is demonstrated.

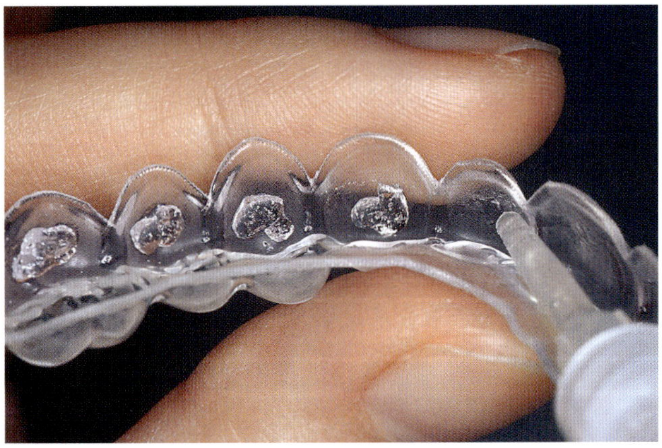

d. Placement of 2 to 3 drops of gel into the labial surface of each tooth in the tray.

Fig. 3-6 Initiation phase, continued.

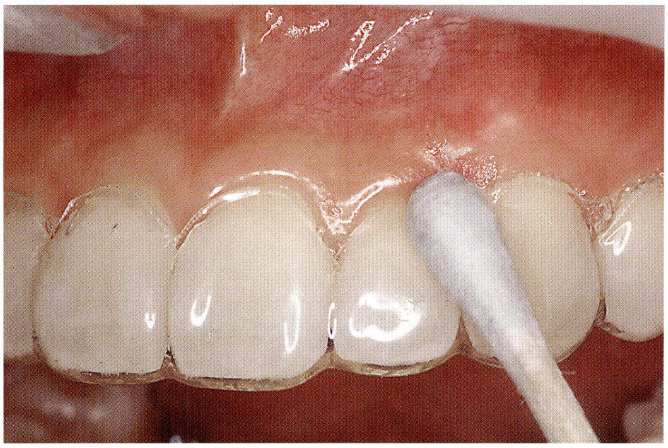

e. Removal of excess whitening material.

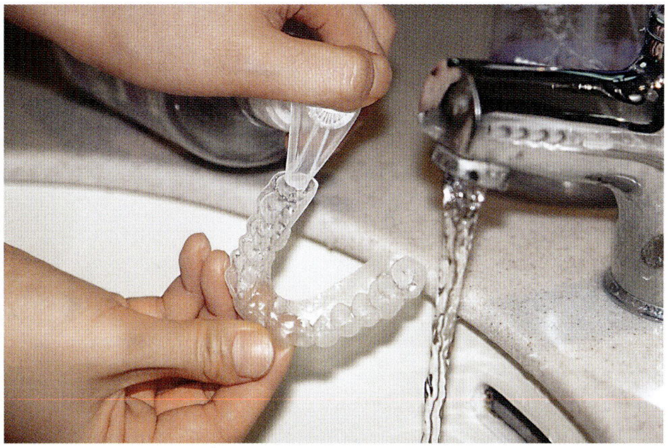

f. Removal of tray and rinsing.

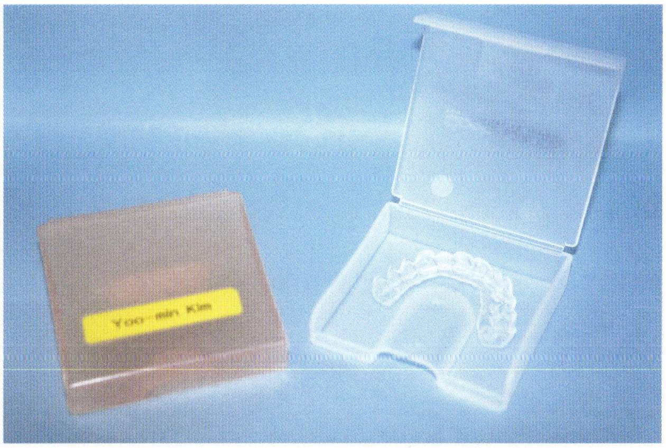

g. The upper tray is given to the patient, whereas the lower tray is kept in the office until completion of the upper arch.

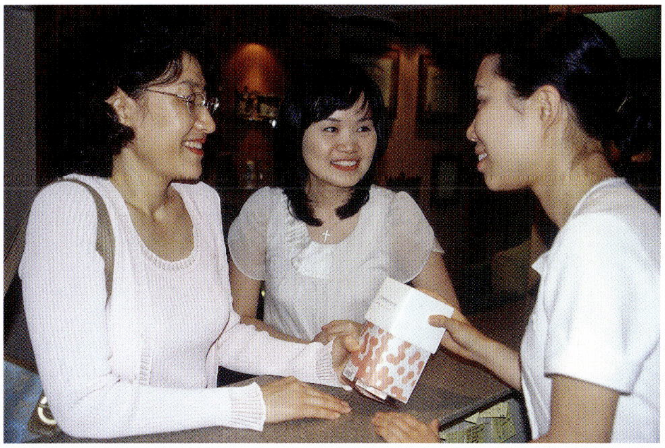

h. Payment is usually completed at the initiation phase.

Information on post-whitening effects

① **Sensitivity:** Patients with existing sensitivity should be advised to undergo pretreatment for sensitivity prior to tooth whitening. Up to 67% of patients experience sensitivity after tooth whitening. If sensitivity is mild, reducing the wearing time will help reduce the sensitivity. If severe, the patient should visit or call the dental office for the prescription of desensitizing agents like fluoride, potassium nitrate and amorphous calcium phosphate.

② **Splotchy stage:** Since some areas in the teeth are more porous than others, a tooth does not lighten homogenously in the beginning. At this stage the tooth has a splotchy appearance, which will gradually resolve as whitening is continued (Fig. 3-7).

③ **Gingival irritation:** Mechanical or chemical irritation may cause a stinging or burning sensation of the gingiva. Mechanical irritation due to a distorted or overextended tray with sharp borders should be instantly checked and corrected. Chemical irritation might be caused by placing too much gel into the tray (Fig. 3-8).

④ **Change of taste:** Though rare, the taste may change during whitening, and patients may experience a metallic taste in the mouth.

⑤ **Discomfort of temporomandibular joint:** Altering a patient's bite may aggravate pain in patients who are susceptible to these problems. Patients experiencing any type of joint pain or muscle spasm should discontinue whitening until the seriousness of the problem has been solved.

⑥ **Susceptibility to stains:** The tooth can be more susceptible to acidic drinks and highly stained food after whitening. Considering the time needed for the reorganization of the pellicle, food and beverages should be avoided for 1 to 2 hours immediately following treatment.

⑦ **Allergy:** Although very rare, there are patients who show hypersensitivity to peroxide, plastic or the preservative in the gel. The reaction may vary from a mild itching sensation to redness, swelling and rashes of the skin. Caution should be taken, and the patient should be advised to stop treatment if an allergic reaction should occur (Fig. 3-9).

⑧ Existing restorations may need to be changed.

Review phase

Patients should be reappointed 1 to 2 weeks after commencing the upper arch whitening. The progress of whitening is then checked and the patient questioned about any side effects and discomfort experienced during the procedure. This review appointment also acts as a strong encouragement that increases the compliance for the treatment. If there is a definite difference between the upper and lower arch and the patient is satisfied with the color, the lower tray can be delivered at this time (Fig. 3-10).

- **Evaluation of discomfort:** The soft tissue is examined for signs of irritation due to overuse of material or irritation from the tray. Any other discomfort experienced during home whitening is evaluated and proper solutions are suggested.
- **Assessment of color change:** A color difference between the upper and lower arch is usually visible at this stage. The degree of color difference is mainly influenced by the nature of the discoloration and the patient's cooperation. If the patient is not satisfied with the color of the upper arch, further motivation should be given to continue whitening of the upper arch.
- **Delivery of the lower tray:** The lower tray can be delivered if the patient is satisfied with the color change of the upper arch.
- **Motivation to proceed with treatment:** The most important purpose of the review appointment is to provide motivation and encouragement to continue the whitening treatment.

Termination phase

Home whitening is performed under the supervision of the dentist following proper diagnosis and treatment planning, and should be terminated once the teeth have reached their maximum whiteness, or when the patient is satisfied with the result. The whitening outcome should be evaluated and recorded in the same manner as prior to whitening.
Finally, instructions on maintenance care should be given to the patient (Fig. 3-11).

- **Assessment of color change:** Color comparison of the upper and lower arch is accomplished visually. The color of the lower teeth should be in harmony with the upper arch. When the patient is pleased with the result, the whitening procedure can be terminated. It often takes longer to whiten the lower arch. This is very common because the lower teeth do not whiten as quickly as the upper teeth and because more sensitivity is experienced due to the smaller size.
- **Photography and shade-taking:** The color change after home whitening is evaluated and recorded in the same manner as prior to whitening by means of shade mapping, photography or shade-taking devices.
- **Before and after smile analysis:** The before-treatment smile analysis is a valuable record that can strongly motivate the patient initiate the whitening treatment. Conversely, the after-treatment smile analysis assures the patient that the treatment has been successfully completed.
- **Maintenance care instructions:** Maintenance care instructions can be given verbally, but it is more effective to give written instructions with before and after photos enclosed.

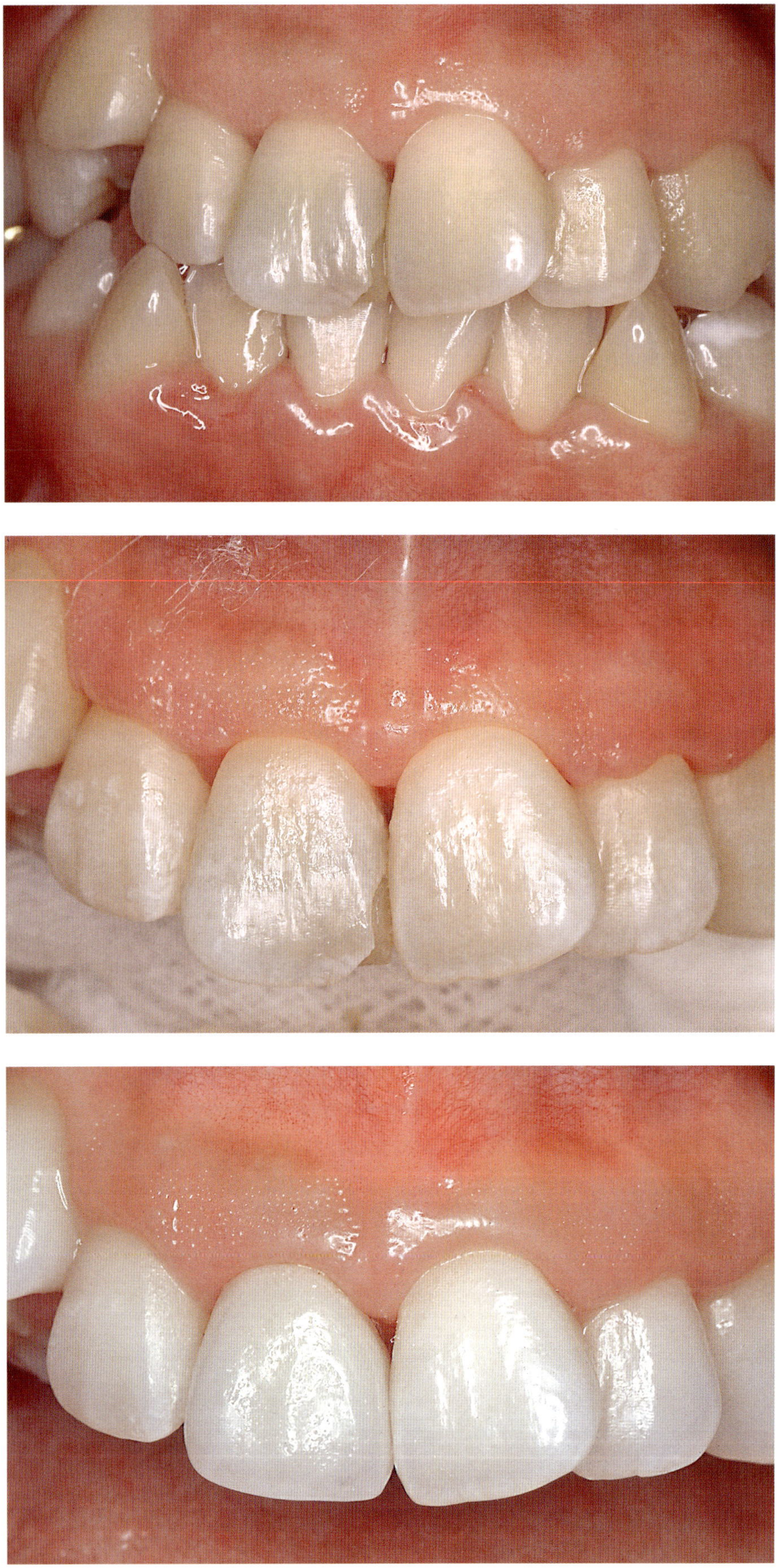

Fig. 3-7 Splotchy stage.

a. Prior to home whitening.

b. Splotchy stage during home whitening.

c. Splotchy stage is naturally resolved as home whitening is continued.

Fig. 3-8 Gingival irritation.

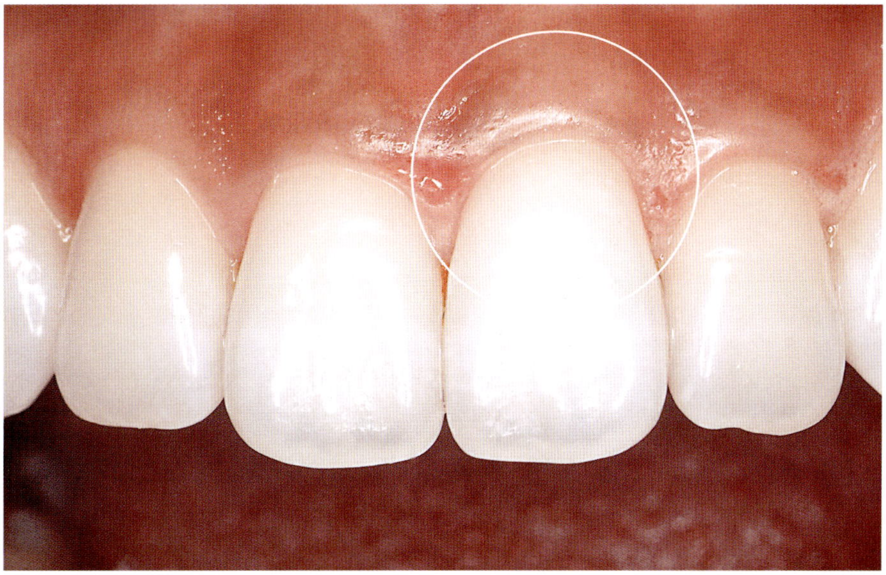

a. Chemical irritation might be caused by placing too much gel in the tray.

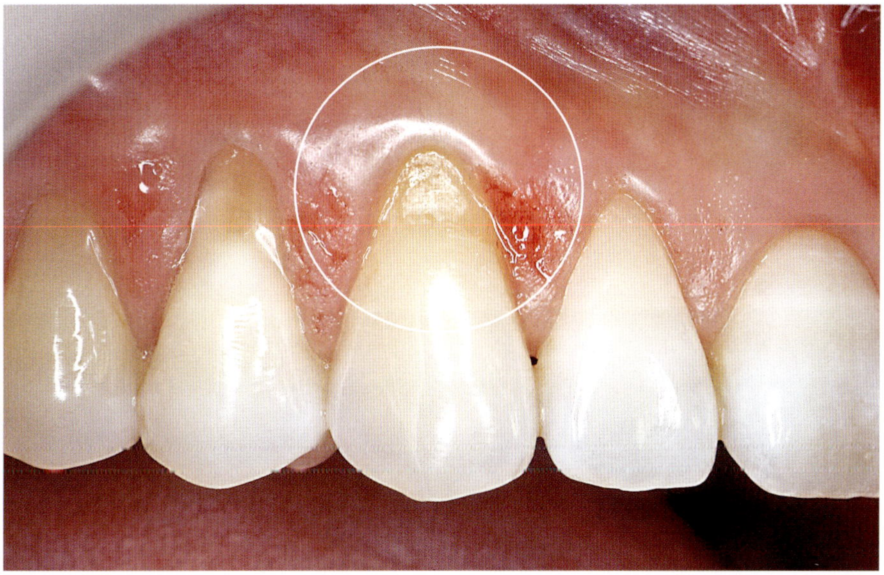

b. Bleeding of the gingiva resulting from excessive irritation from an ill-fitting tray.

Fig. 3-9 Allergy. This patient developed itching and skin rashes after home whitening.

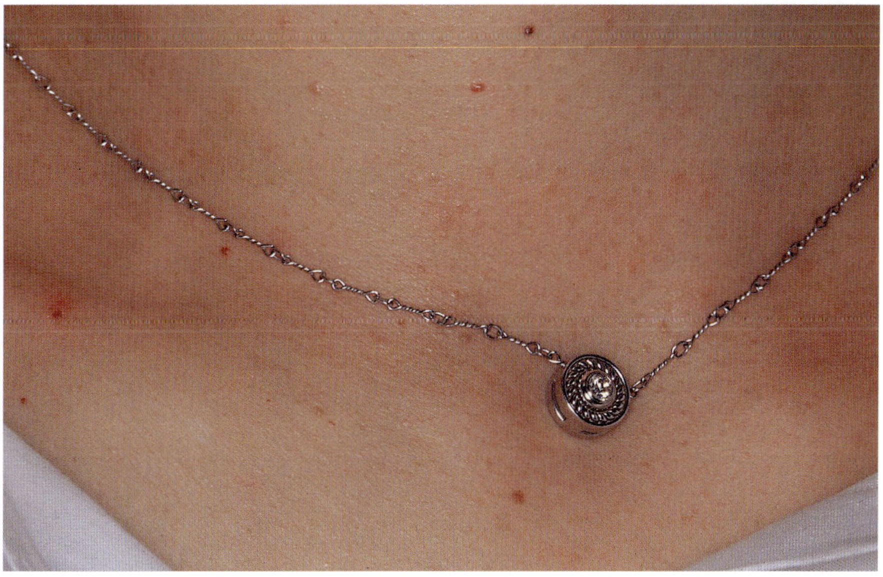

Fig. 3-10 Review phase.

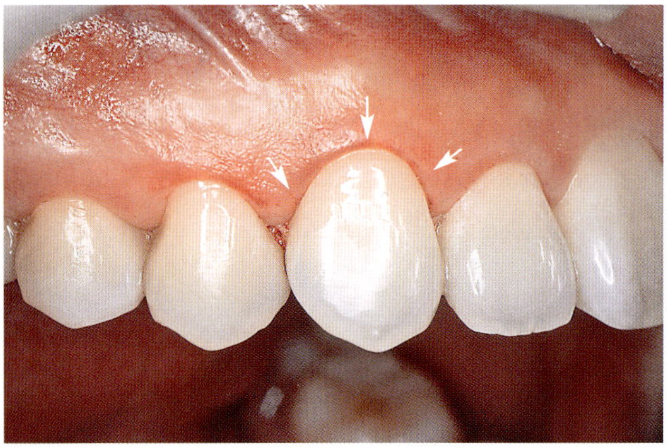

a. Evaluation of discomfort and soft tissue irritation.

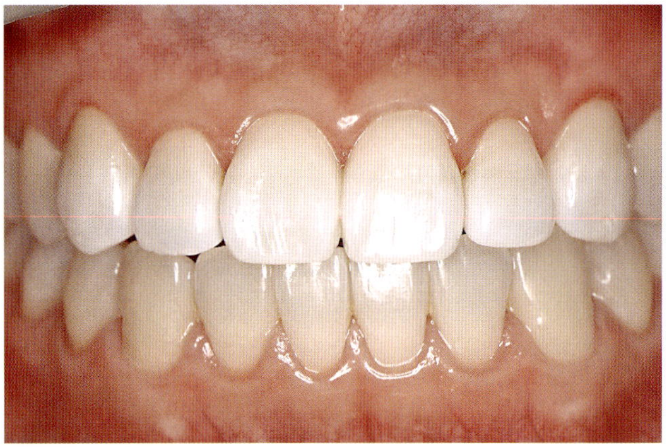

b. Assessment of color change compared to lower arch.

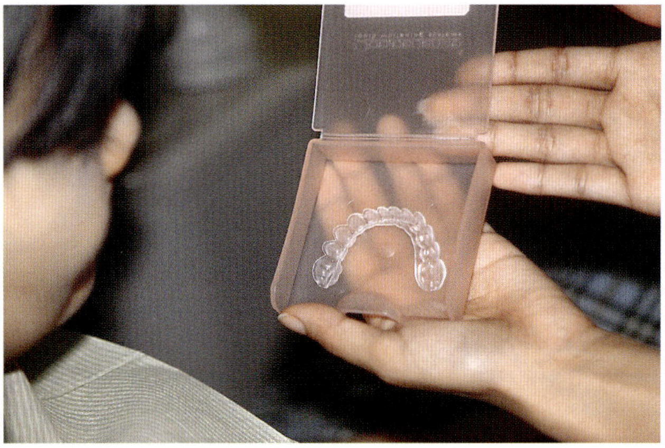

c. Delivery of the lower tray.

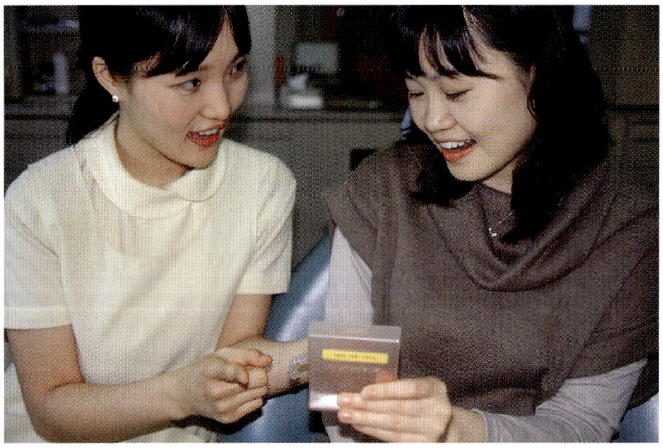

d. Motivation to proceed with treatment.

Fig. 3-11 Termination phase.

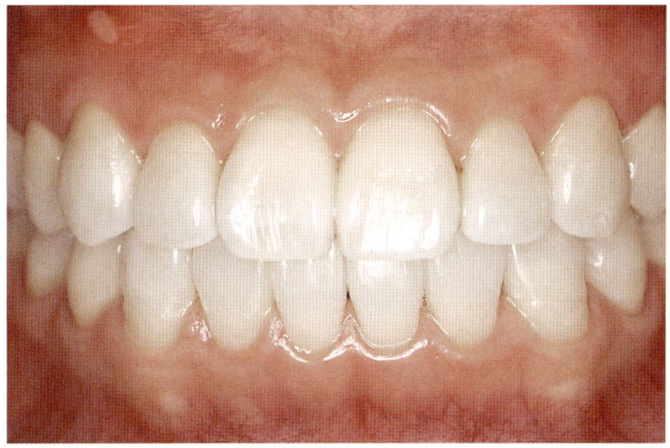

a. Assessment of color change.

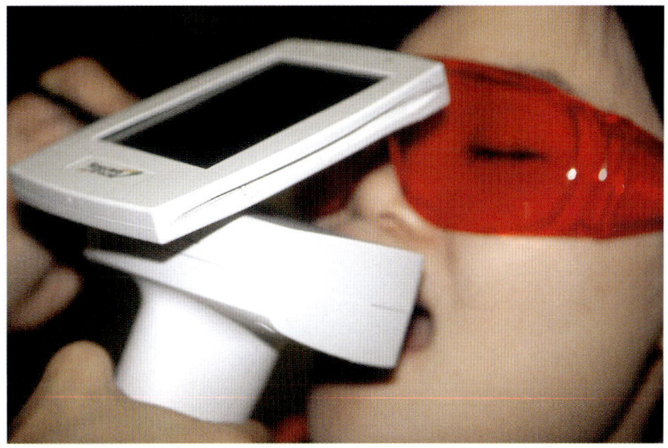

b. Photography and shade-taking.

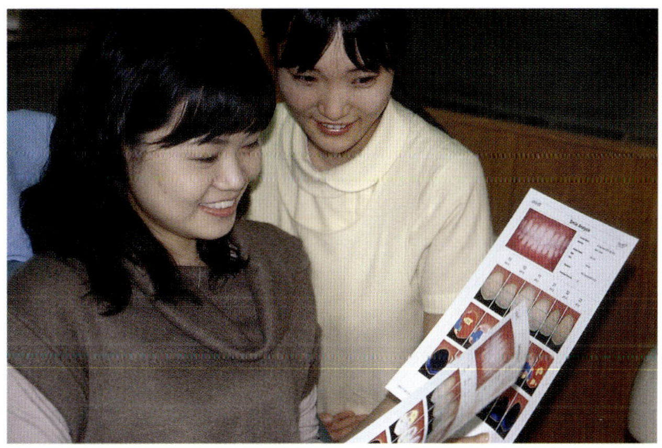

c. Delivery of before and after smile analysis.

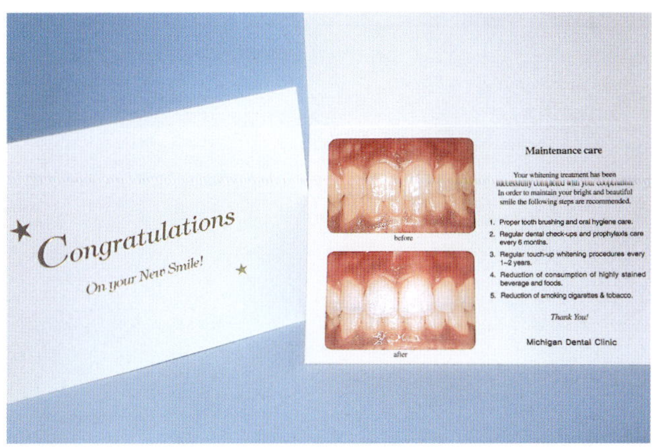

d. Maintenance care instructions.

Fabrication of the trays

Proper design and fabrication of the whitening tray is essential for successful treatment and patient compliance.

Step-by-step procedure (Fig. 3-12 and 3-13)

- **Impression taking:** Select a suitable tray for taking an alginate impression. The impression should be accurate and it should show the entire tooth structure and approximately 1.2cm of tissue surrounding the teeth. If a lingual retainer or severe undercuts are present, proper block-out should be performed prior to impression-taking to prevent any deformation.
- **Model fabrication:** The alginate impression is poured carefully with stone to avoid bubble and void formation. The base can be formed into a smooth horse-shoe shape before the stone is finally set. The set stone model is grossly trimmed with a model trimmer so that the base is flat and parallel to the occlusal plane. If the base is too thick or uneven, the thermo-plasticized sheet will not accurately adapt to the model. If the base is trimmed too excessively, it will weaken and easily fracture. Small bubbles and sharp edges should be removed with a sharp instrument or blade, and the gingival margin should be clearly demarcated. The finished cast should have a flat base that is parallel to the occlusal plane and free of voids and bubbles.
- **Reservoir placement (optional):** A thin layer (≅ 0.5mm) of block-out resin can be placed on the labial surface of the teeth on the model and light-cured. The block-out resin should not cover the whole tooth, but rather should stop 1mm short of the gingival margin and proximal embrasures to ensure a tight-sealing tray. The presence of the reservoir does not seem to affect the whitening result, but it provides space for the whitening gel and prevents excessive flow-out of the gel.
- **Vacuum forming:** A soft, thin sheet is placed into the sandwich holder of the vacuum former, and the finished cast is placed on the vacuum platform. The heater is turned on and the heated plastic sheet is lowered to the cast with the vacuum turned on when the material is lowered about 2cm below the frame. The vacuum remains turned on until the plastic is tightly adapted on the cast. The heater and vacuum are then turned off, and the cast with the adapted plastic sheet is left on the platform to cool down.

- **Trimming the tray:** Bulk trimming of the tray material should be accomplished with large scissors prior to removing the cast to prevent any distortion. The borders of the tray are trimmed with a blade or small and sharp scissors according to the desired pattern. The various tray patterns are described below:
  - *Straight pattern*: The borders of the tray are extended 2 to 3 mm onto the gingiva in a straight and smooth pattern. Although easy to fabricate and very resistant to deformation, it is difficult to remove excess whitening gel from this type of tray, which may lead to gingival irritation.
  - *Scalloped pattern*: The borders of the buccal and lingual side follow the outline of the gingiva in a scalloped pattern.
  - *Combined pattern*: The borders of the buccal side follow the outline of the gingiva in a scalloped pattern, and the borders of the lingual side are extended 2 to 3mm onto the gingiva in a straight smooth pattern.
- **Cleaning and storage of the tray:** The final tray is cleaned and stored in the tray case until delivery to the patient.

Properties of an ideal tray

- Good retention
- Does not irritate soft tissue, gingiva, mucosa, and tongue
- Borders should be smooth and well-polished
- Not easily deformed or distorted during use
- Made of biocompatible materials
- Easily cleaned and dried

Fig. 3-12 Block-out.

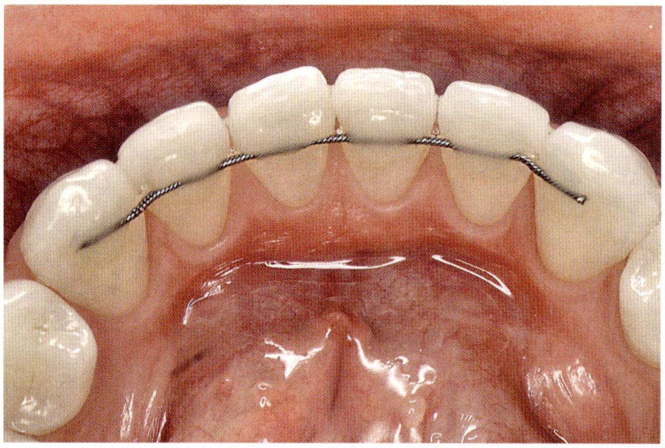

a. Undercuts beneath lingual retainers often cause deformation of the impression.

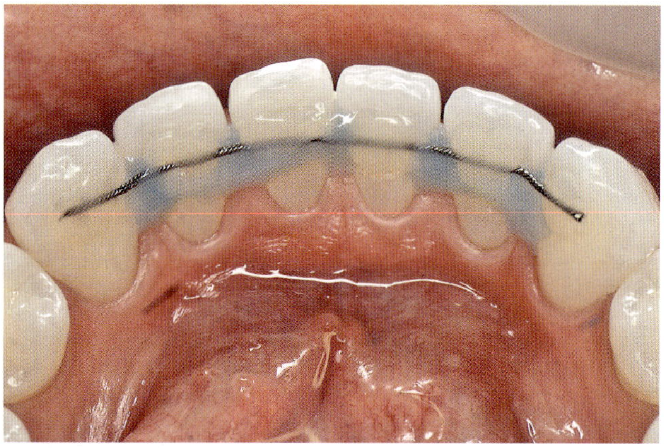

b. Block-out prior to impression-taking.

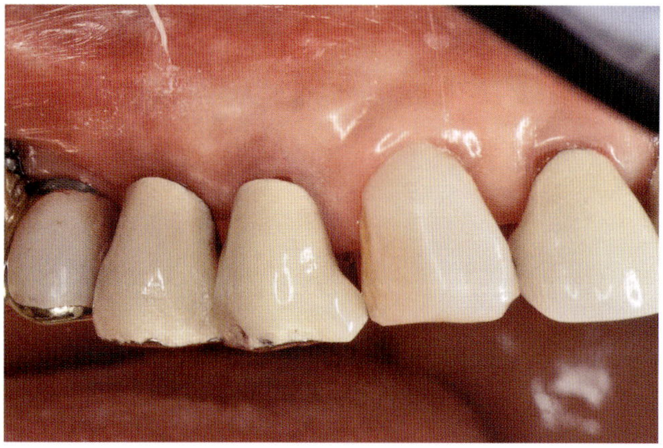

c. Undercuts around the pontic often cause tearing of the impression material.

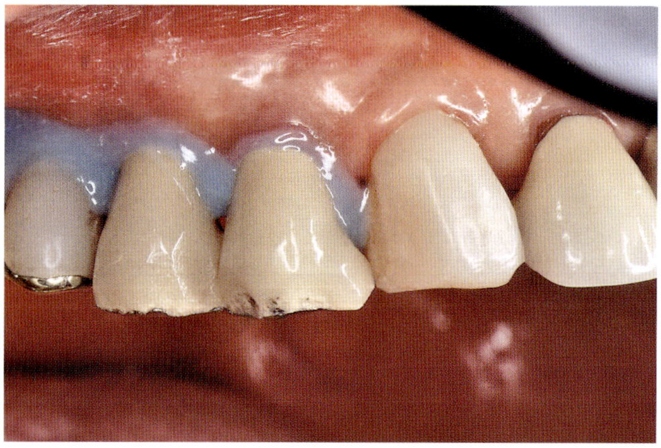

d. Block-out prior to impression taking.

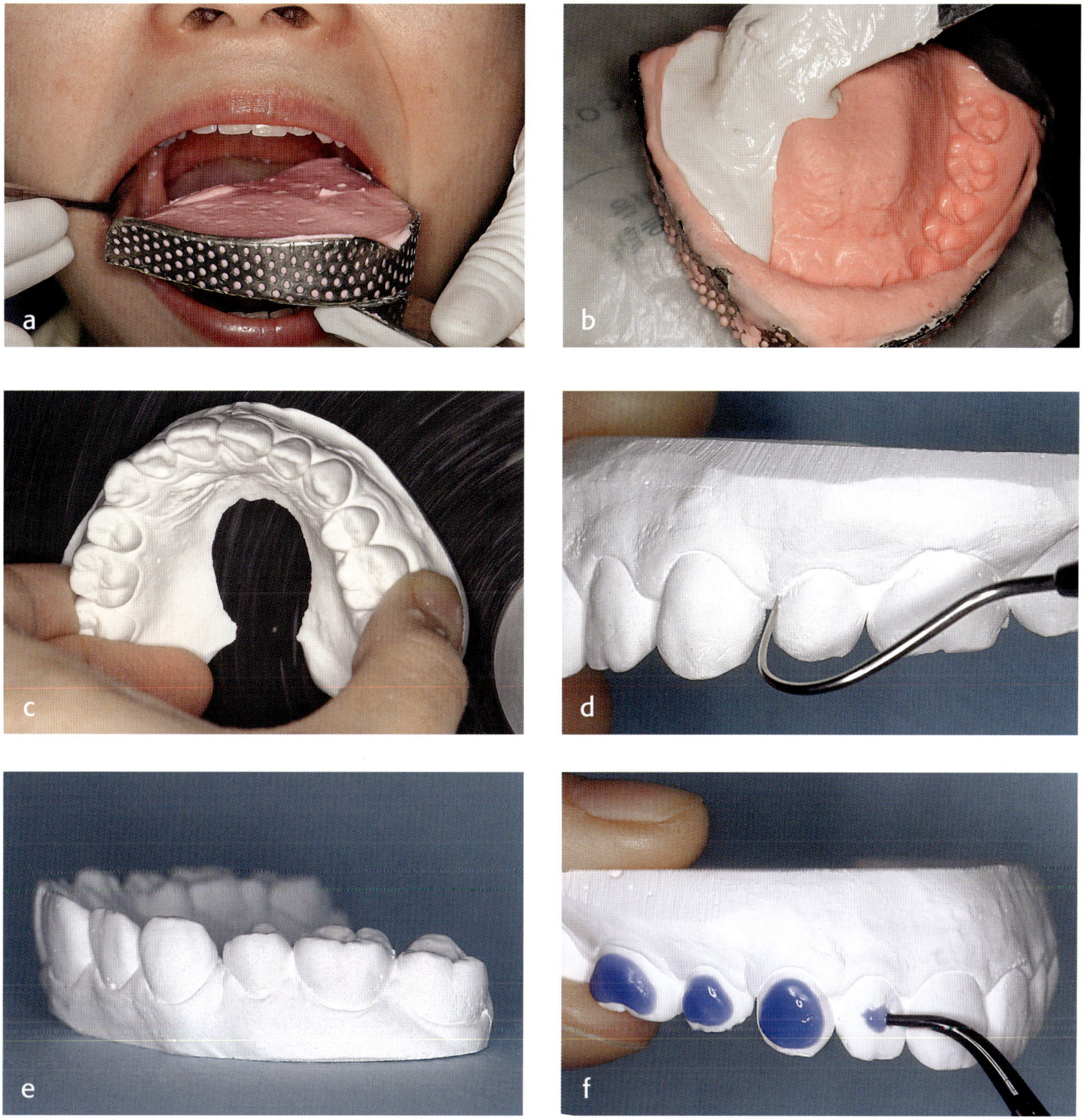

Fig. 3-13 Step-by-step procedure of fabrication of the whitening tray.

a. Alginate impression-taking.
b. The impression is poured carefully with stone to avoid any bubble and void formation.
c. The stone model is trimmed so that the base is flat and parallel to the occlusal plane.
d. Small bubbles and sharp edges are removed.
e. The finished cast should have a flat base that is parallel to the occlusal plane.
f. A thin layer of block-out resin can be placed as a reservoir.

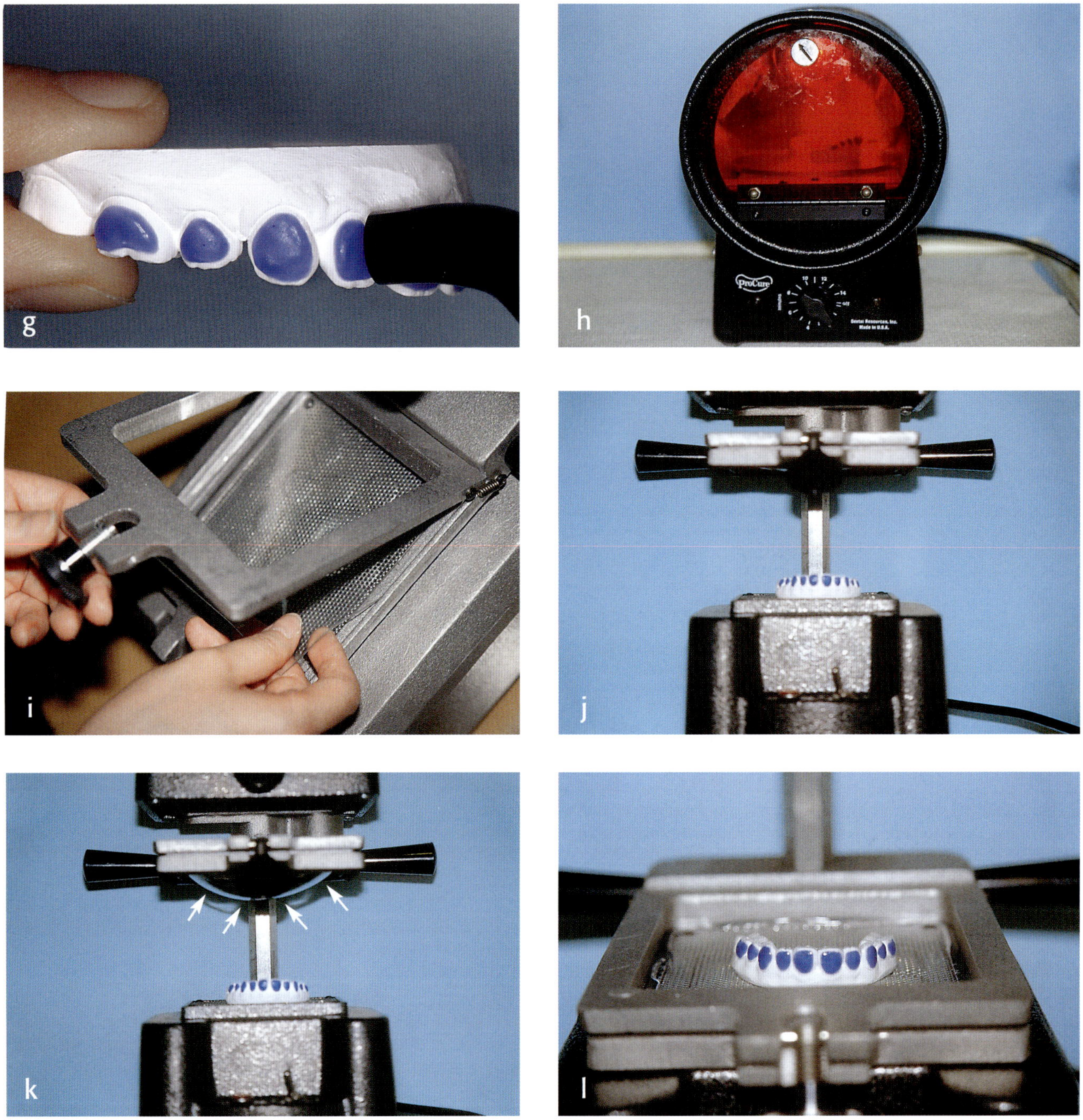

Fig. 3-13 Step-by-step procedure of fabrication of the whitening tray.

g. Light-curing of block-out resin.

h. Light-curing box.

i. A soft, thin sheet is placed into the sandwich holder of the vacuum former.

j. The finished cast is placed on the vacuum platform.

k. The heated plastic sheet is lowered onto the cast when the material has been lowered about 2cm below the frame.

l. The adapted plastic sheet is left on the platform to cool down.

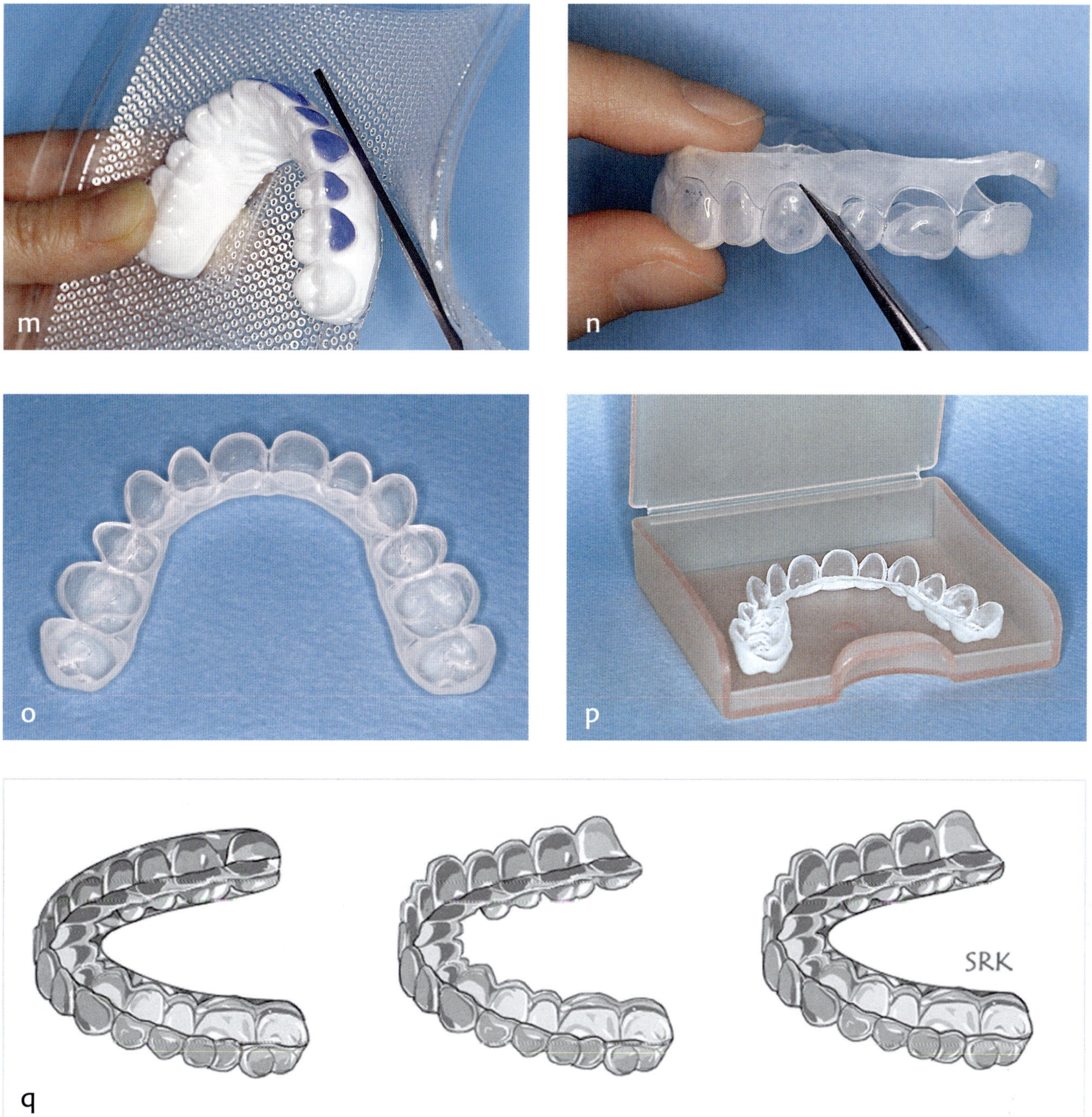

Fig. 3-13 Step-by-step procedure of fabrication of the whitening tray.

m. Bulk trimming is performed with large scissors.

n. The borders of the tray are trimmed with a blade or small and sharp scissors.

o. Finished tray (combined pattern).

p. The finished tray is stored in the tray case until delivery to the patient.

q. Various tray patterns: straight, scalloped and combined.

Patient satisfaction

Since home whitening was first introduced in the literature in 1989, it has been considered to be the simplest and safest method of treating discolored teeth. In 2003, Leonard evaluated patient satisfaction regarding the effect of home whitening, its maintenance, and side effects. Home whitening was effective in 98% of cases of extrinsic and age-related discoloration. In tetracycline discoloration, it was effective in 86% of cases after extending the treatment duration. The side effects of home whitening were mild and mostly transient. The survey showed a high patient satisfaction rate. After 10 years, 43% of patients were satisfied with their tooth color without touch-up treatment. In summary, 96% of the patients were satisfied with home whitening, and 94% would recommend it to their friends (Fig. 3-14).

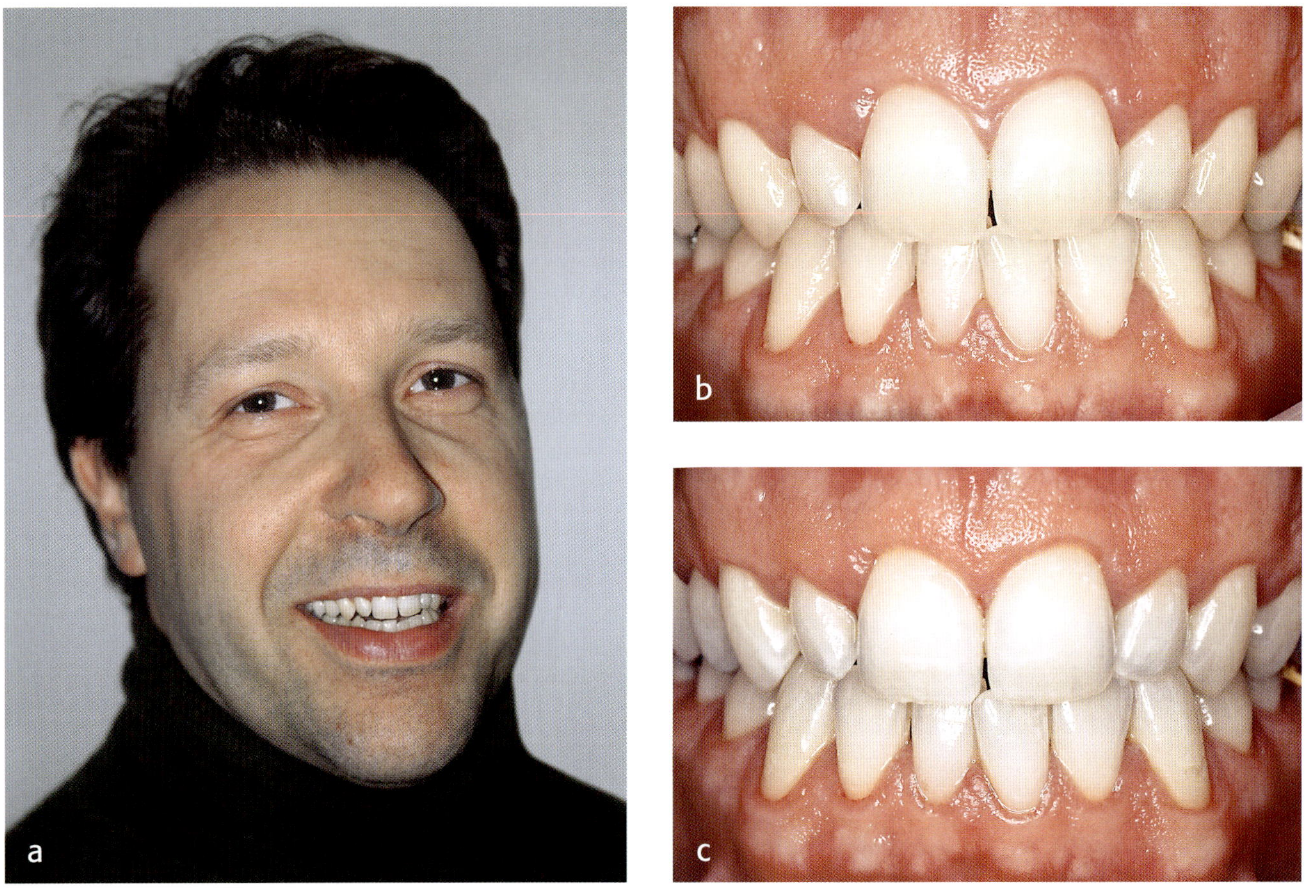

Fig. 3-14 Patient satisfaction.
a. Photo after tooth whitening of a happy patient who was first very skeptical about tooth whitening.
b. Before home whitening.
c. After one week of home whitening of the upper and lower arch.

Feedback letters from patients

Many patients show their appreciation and high satisfaction after whitening treatment by sending a thank-you card or letter to the dentist's office. These feedback items can be displayed in the office to motivate other patients to start whitening treatment (Figs. 3-15 and 16).

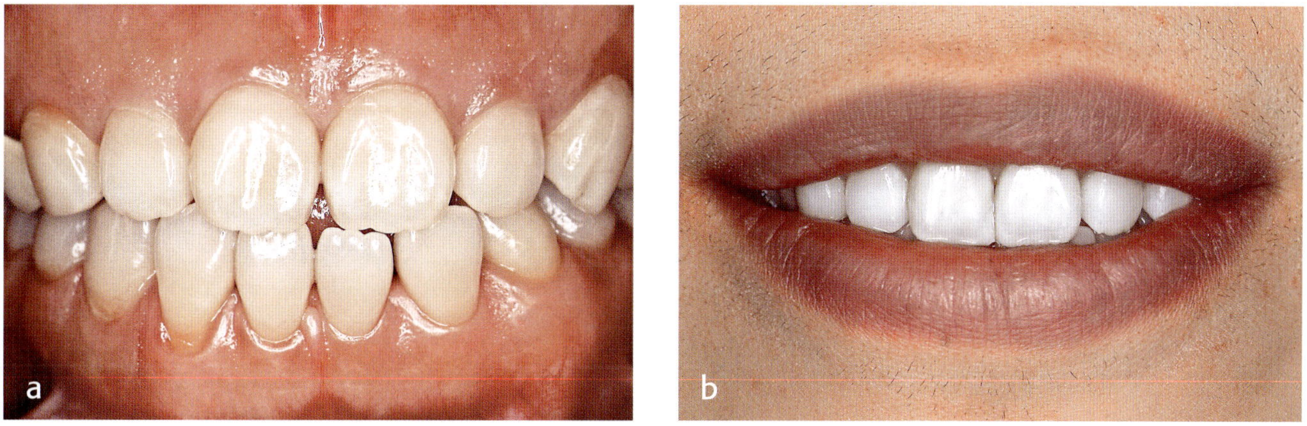

Fig. 3-15 Patient who was reluctant to show her teeth when smiling.
a. Prior to treatment.
b. After home whitening, esthetic trimming and composite resin filling to close the incisal embrasure of the upper central incisors.

My tooth whitening experience

I have always envied friends who had beautiful white smiles. Before whitening, my teeth were yellow and I was reluctant to show my teeth during smiling. I thought that the tooth color was genetically determined so that no change was possible without cutting my teeth for veneers.
I am so happy to have consulted my dentist, who recommended tooth whitening. Now my teeth are white and bright and I am able to proudly show my beautiful smile.
I would like to take this opportunity to thank my dentist, Dr. So-Ran Kwon, and the staff of Michigan Dental Clinic for their expertise in tooth whitening.

Sincerely,
YJ Ko

Fig. 3-16 Feedback letter from a patient.

••• Home whitening is a simple and safe way to whiten teeth provided that all indications and contraindications are carefully considered and the patients comply with the treatment under the supervision of the dentist.

Q&A

Question 1. Are whitening strips effective in tooth whitening?

Answer: Whitening strips contain various concentrations of hydrogen peroxide and are effective in tooth whitening. They are suitable for patients who have evenly shaped teeth with a light tooth shade. However, since the procedure is not supervised by a dentist, abuse and overzealous use might cause problems.

Question 2. Is there any difference between 10% and 15% carbamide peroxide in terms of whitening results?

Answer: Teeth whiten faster with 15% carbamide peroxide gel, but it has been reported that the final whitening results are the same.

Question 3. Why does the cervical part respond to tooth whitening not as well as the middle or incisal part of the tooth?

Answer: The middle and incisal parts, where the enamel is thicker, usually whiten faster and more easily. The cervical part whitens gradually as whitening is continued. However, the patient should always be informed prior to treatment that the cervical region closer to the root may remain somewhat yellow.

Question 4. May I drink water while home whitening?

Answer: It is best to avoid food or beverages during home whitening. However, if you are very thirsty, you may drink water with a straw.

Question 5. Are reservoirs really necessary?

Answer: The presence of the reservoir does not seem to affect the whitening result, but it provides space for the whitening gel and prevents excessive flow-out of the gel. It is best to follow the manufacturers' directions on the necessity of reservoirs for their whitening materials.

Q&A

Question 6. Is tooth whitening possible in young patients?

Answer: Yellow teeth, white spots or mottled teeth are good indications for tooth whitening in young patients. In very young patients who won't comply with home whitening, power whitening can be performed as an alternative with informed consent from their parents (Fig. 3-17).

Fig. 3-17 Whitening in young patients.

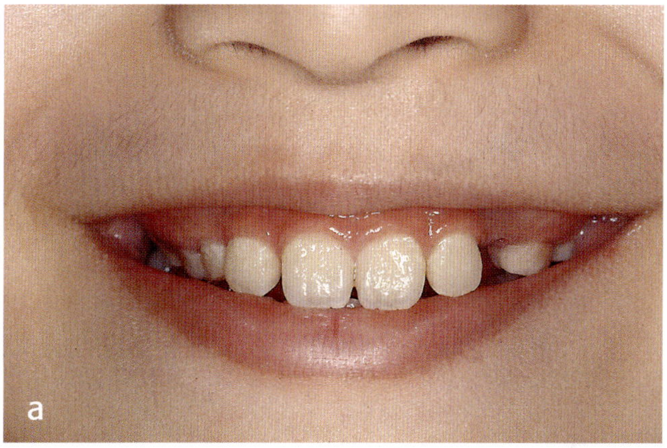

a. Smile prior to whitening.

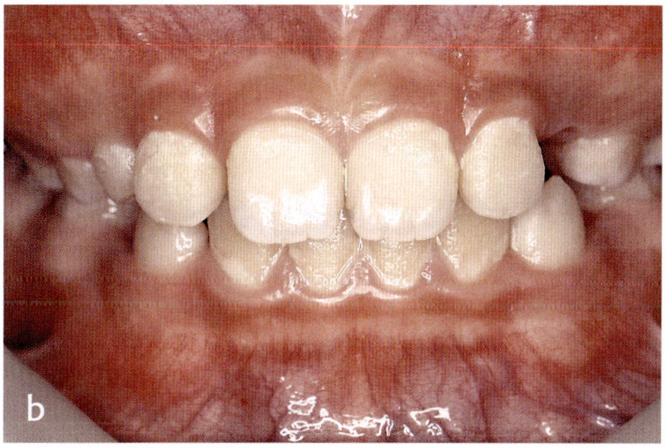

b. In very young patients who won't comply with home whitening, power whitening can be performed as an alternative with informed consent from the parents.

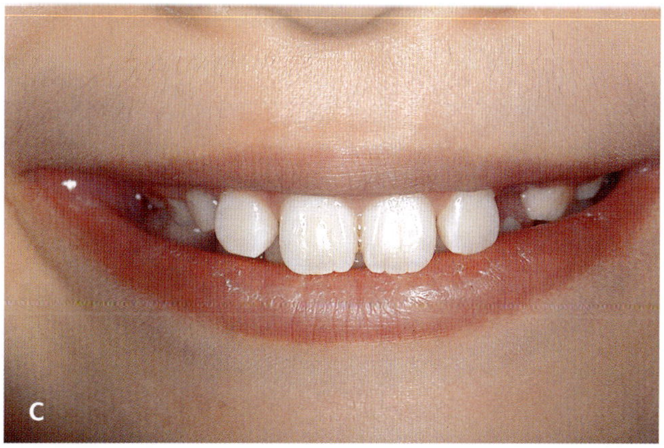

c. Smile after whitening.

References

Albers HF. Dentine and sensitivity. Adept Report 2000; 6:4,10-11.

Donly KJ. Tooth Whitening in children and adolescents. J Esthet Restor Dent 2005; 17(6):380-381.

Dunn JR. Dentist-Prescribed Home Bleaching: Current Status. Compendium 1998; 19(8):760-764.

Goldstein RE, Garber DA. Complete Dental Bleaching, Quintessence Publishing Co, Inc, 1995.

Greenwall LH. Bleaching techniques in restorative dentistry, Martin Dunitz, 2001.

Haywood VB, Heymann HO. Nightguard vital bleaching. Quintessence Int 1989; 20:173-176.

Haywood VB, Heymann HO: Nightguard vital bleaching: How Safe Is It? Quintessence Int 1991; 22:515-523.

Haywood VB. History, safety, and effectiveness of current bleaching techniques and applications of the nightguard vital bleaching technique. Quintessence Int 1992; 23:471-488.

Haywood VB. Nightguard Vital Bleaching: Current Concepts and Research. JADA supplement 1997; 128:19s-25s.

Haywood VB. Overview and Status of Mouthguard Bleaching. J Esthet Dent 1991; 3(5):157-161. Haywood VB: Nightguard Vital Bleaching: Current Information and Research. Esthetic Dentistry Update 1990; 1(2),7-12. Haywood, VB. Achieving, Maintaining, and Recovering Successful Tooth Bleaching. J Esthet Dent 1996; 8(1):31-38.

Haywood, VB. Nightguard Vital Bleaching: Information and Consent Form. Esthetic Dent Update 1995; 6(5):130-132.

Kwon S. Tooth Whitening State of the Art, Dental Publishing Co, Inc, 2004.

Leonard RH: Efficacy, longevity, side effects, and patient perceptions of nightguard vital bleaching, Compend Contin Educ Dent 1998;19:766.

Matis BA. In Vivo Study of Two Carbamide Peroxide Gels with Different Desensitizing Agents. Oper Dent 2007; 32-6:549-555.

McCaslin AJ, Haywood VB, Potter BJ, Dickinson GL, Russell CM. Assessing Dentin Color Changes from Nightguard Vital Bleaching. JADA 1999; 130:1485-1490.

Metz MJ. Clinical Evaluation of 15% Carbamide Peroxide on the Surface Microharness and Shear Bond Strength of Human Enamel. Oper Dent 2007; 32-5:427-436.

chapter 4

Power whitening

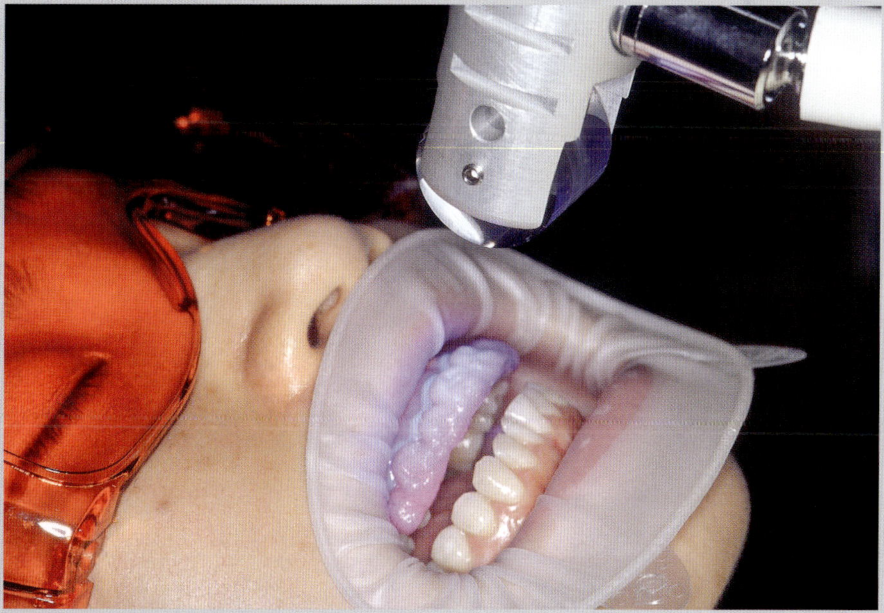

Discolored vital teeth can be successfully whitened with highly concentrated gels at chairside. In-office whitening provides an alternative to home whitening, especially in patients who do not tolerate whitening trays or demonstrate low compliance. In-office whitening is indicated in moderate to severe discoloration, discoloration of a few teeth, and in cases in which speedy treatment is desired. Generally, the whitening effect is noticed immediately after a single session. This can sufficiently motivate the patient to continue treatment. It should be emphasized that a single session of power whitening may not be sufficient to achieve optimal whitening results. This means that, for maximum whitening, several appointments are required and that power whitening should be combined with home whitening, if possible. When the two techniques are combined, faster and whiter results can be achieved than with either technique alone.

Office whitening started as early as 1877, when Chapple reported the use of oxalic acid in vital tooth bleaching. Harlan described the first use of hydrogen peroxide in 1884. Since then, hydrogen peroxide has been the most widely accepted whitening agent for the treatment of discolored teeth in the office. 30 to 35% hydrogen peroxide in liquid form was originally applied to the tooth surface after proper isolation with rubber dam and ligating floss to prevent soft tissue injury. To accelerate the whitening process, a heat source was commonly used (Fig. 4-1).

This concept of power whitening dates back to 1918, when Abbot reported the use of a high-intensity light that generates a rapid rise in the temperature of hydrogen peroxide, which accelerates the chemical process. Since then, discomfort due to the laborious isolation with the rubber dam and ligating floss has been improved by the use of light-cured resin barriers. Furthermore, high concentrations of hydrogen peroxide in a gel or paste form has reduced the incidence of gingival and soft tissue ulceration and irritation. Finally, the high-intensity lights have been developed into more sophisticated units specialized for power whitening.

Equipment

Power whitening materials

A wide variety of power whitening materials are available on the market. Usually, high concentrations of hydrogen peroxide or carbamide peroxide are used in gel form. The gel systems contain water and have the advantage of preventing dehydration during whitening. Many products claim to have a unique catalyst (chemical or photo) that acts as an accelerator to speed up the whitening process. In order to minimize sensitivity, many manufacturers have incorporated desensitizing agents into their systems. The exact mechanism of catalysts and their efficacy in tooth whitening has not been well documented yet. Moreover, further research is required regarding the desensitizing agents incorporated in the whitening systems.

Fig. 4-1 Power whitening using highly concentrated hydrogen peroxide liquid.

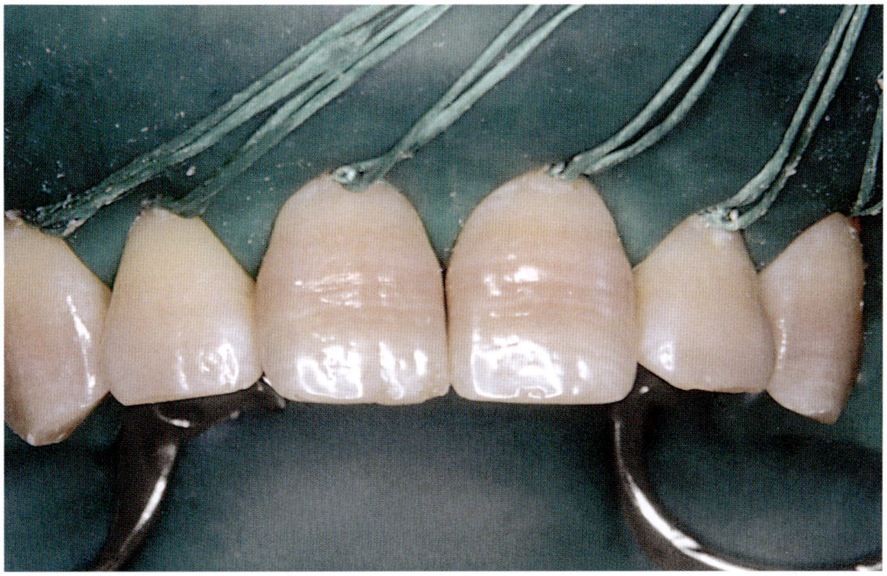

a. The teeth are individually ligated with dental floss after rubber dam placement.

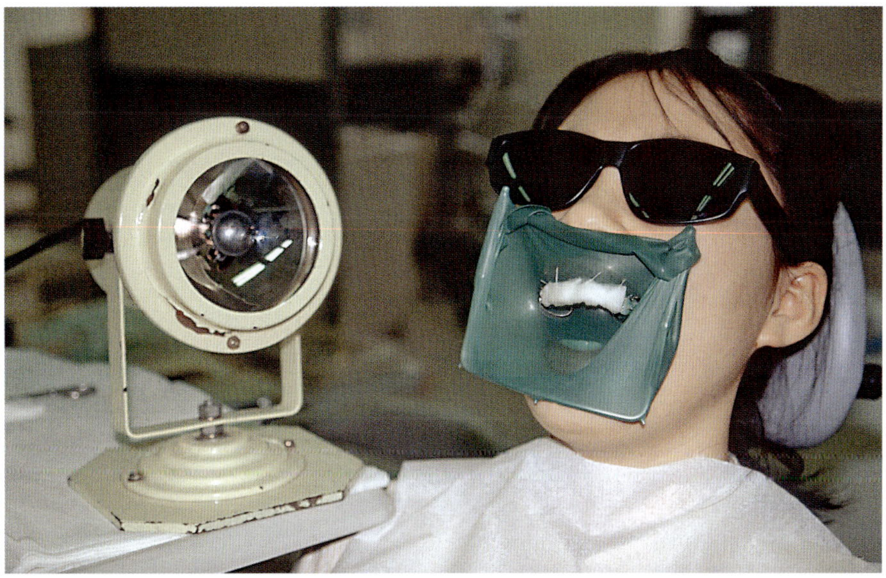

b. A heat source is used to promote the oxidation reaction of hydrogen peroxide.

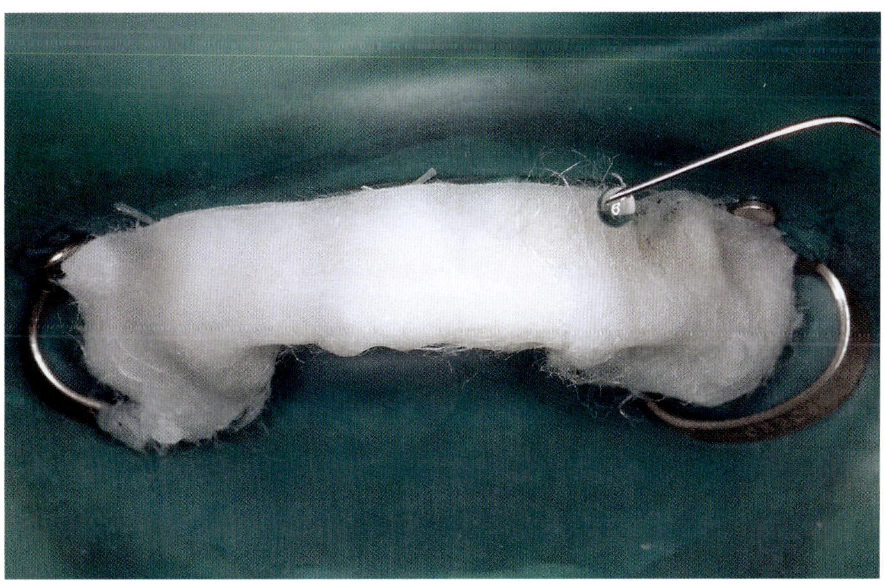

c. Replenishment of the hydrogen peroxide liquid is necessary due to desiccation of the liquid.

Cheek retractor

Proper selection of cheek retractors is important for a comfortable power whitening session. Although all retractors are made of plastic, stiffness and adaptability varies depending on the system. Retractors should be easily placed in the mouth and should retract the lips properly without causing excessive stretching of the tissue. The use of disposable cheek retractors was recently proposed (Fig. 4-2).

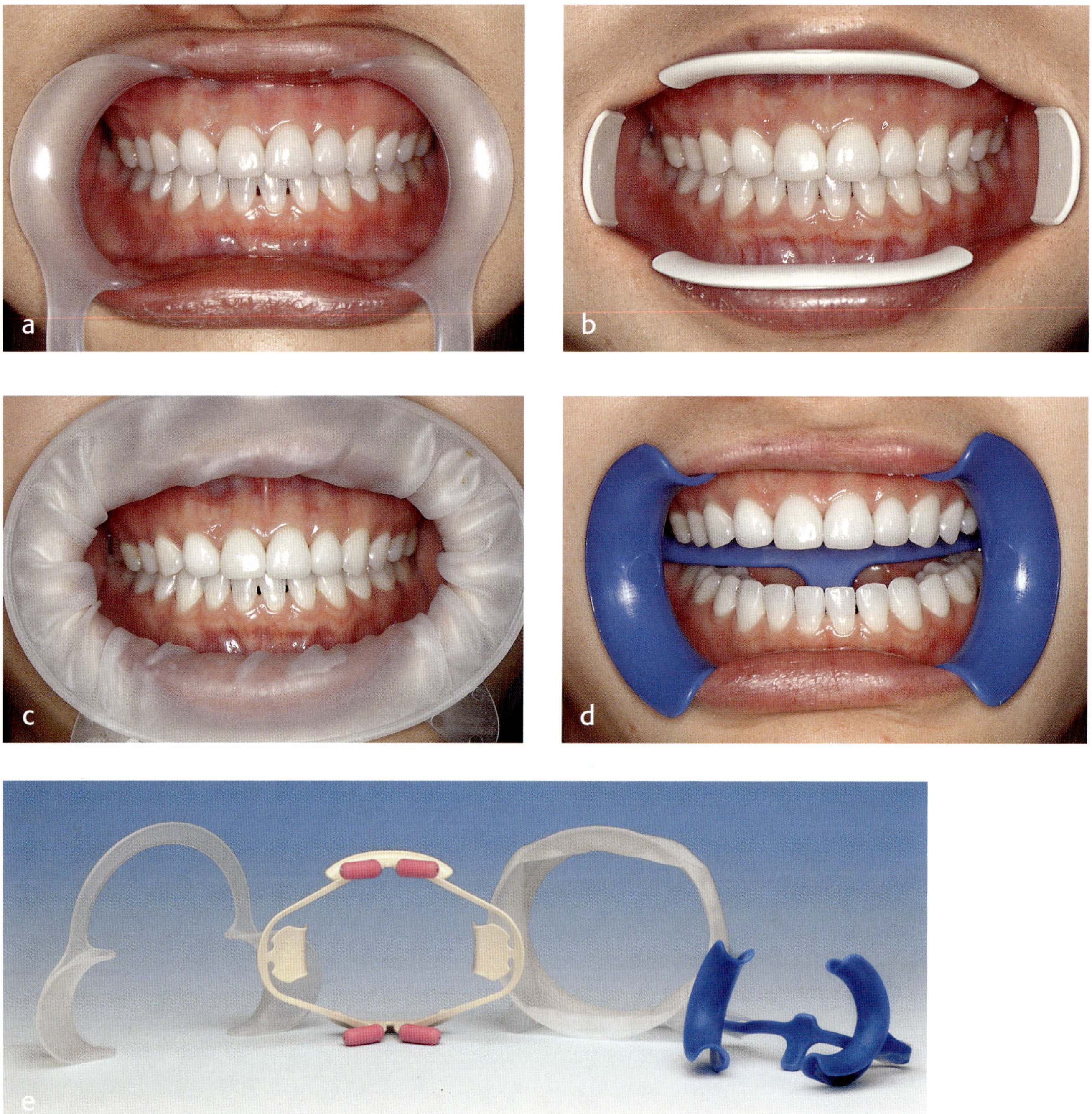

Fig. 4-2 Various types of cheek retractors.
a. Clear retractor, Hanil.
b. Lip and cheek retractor, Hawe.
c. OptraGate, Ivoclar Vivadent.
d. Tongue and lip retractor.
e. Various cheek retractors.

Gingival protector

Isolation and protection of the gingiva with the use of conventional rubber dam, clamp and ligating floss is a safe procedure. The disadvantage, however, is that it is time-consuming and uncomfortable to the patient. Light-cured resin barriers can protect the gingival tissue in a shorter time, without causing any discomfort to the patient. The resin barrier should cover approximately 0.5mm of the tooth and should extend onto the gingiva for about 2 to 3mm (Fig. 4-3).

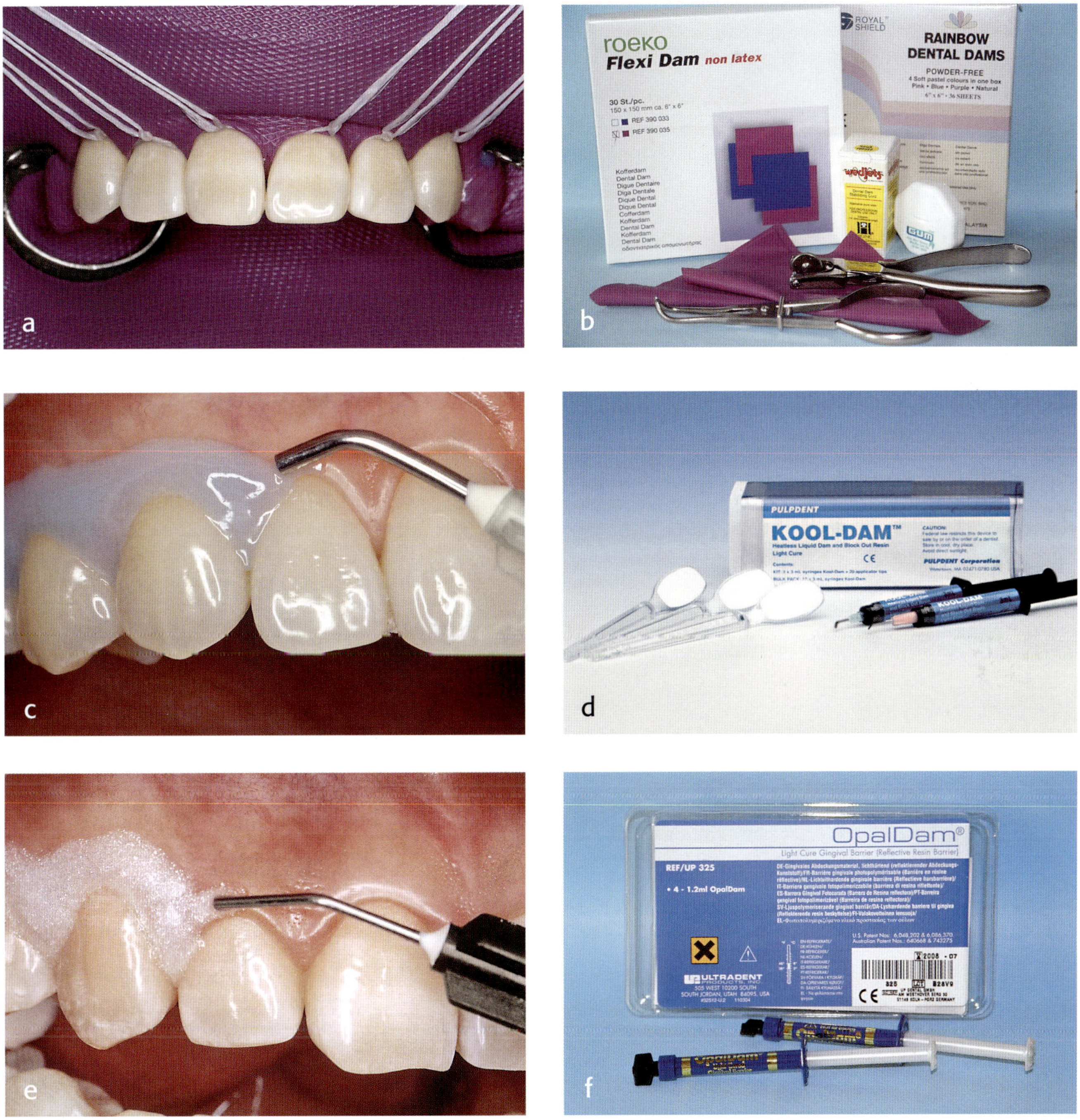

Fig. 4-3 Gingival protector.
a,b. Gingival protection method using rubber dam.
c,d. Resin barrier (Kool Dam, Pulpdent Corporation, USA).
e,f. Resin barrier (Opal Dam, Ultradent Products Inc, Utah, USA).

Light activation units

Halogen lights, plasma arc lamps, light-emitting diodes and laser systems of different wavelengths have been introduced for the activation of power whitening materials. The main difference between these light sources is that lasers emit a well-defined monochromatic light at a specific wavelength, whereas halogen and plasma arc lamps emit a wide range across the visible spectrum (λ=380–750nm), from ultraviolet to infrared (Fig. 4-4). Most lamps used for power whitening were originally conventional resin-curing lights. Due to the limited size of the light tip, each tooth had to be activated separately, making the procedure tedious and laborious. In order to facilitate the activation procedure, most lamps have been modified with a whitening mode and an extra tip to spread the light for illumination of the whole arch. A wide variety of light systems for the specific purpose of power whitening have been designed so that the whole arch can be activated simultaneously without the need for changing the tip. It should be emphasized that all light-activation systems act on the power whitening materials to enhance the whitening process rather than on the tooth substance or tooth stain itself. The virtual increase in efficacy of power whitening materials by light activation and the underlying mechanism have been insufficiently documented. Theoretically, light energy is absorbed by photocatalysts in the whitening gel and transferred to accelerate the decomposition of hydrogen peroxide to free oxygen radicals (Fig. 4-5). Since it is still debatable whether such activation results in superior whitening, application of light-activated systems should be carefully considered. A specific combination of power whitening material and light that demonstrates good color improvement with little temperature elevation should be selected.

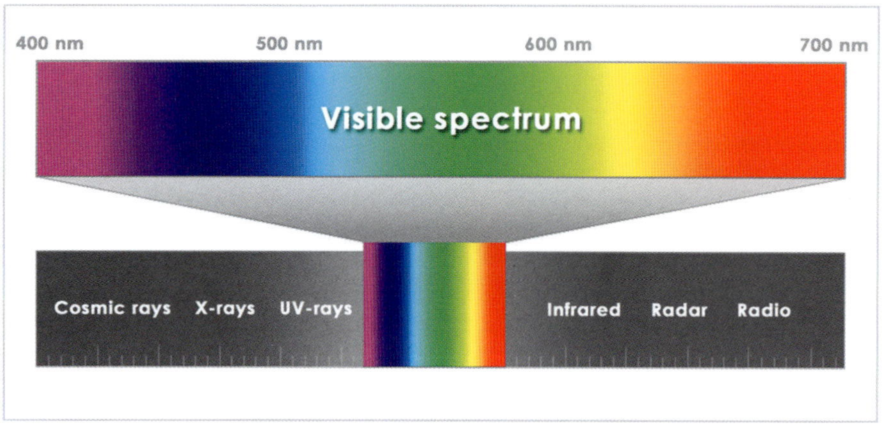

Fig. 4-4 Electromagnetic spectrum.

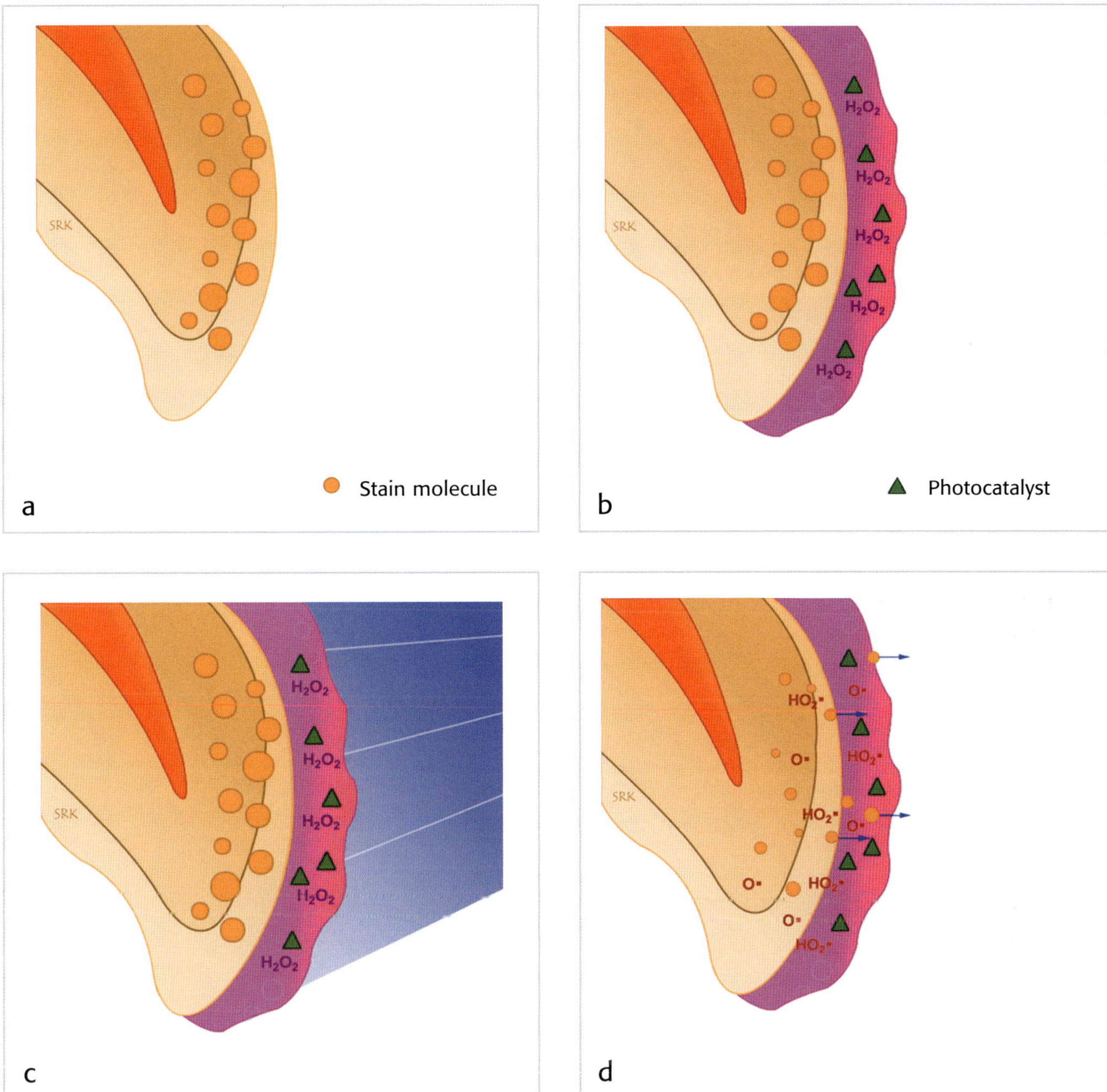

Fig. 4-5 Mechanism of action of bleaching lights in power whitening.

a. Distribution of colorants in the discolored tooth.

b. Application of whitening material containing photocatalysts.

c. Light activation.

d. Light activation of the photocatalysts accelerates the decomposition of hydrogen peroxide into oxygen and perhydroxyl radicals, thus accelerating the whitening process.

Considerations for proper selection of light activation systems (Fig. 4-6)

① The energy absorption characteristics of photocatalysts should match the specific wavelength of the light.
② The wavelength of the light should be within a safe range. If ultraviolet light ($\lambda < 380$ nm) is included, thorough isolation and protection of skin and gingiva is required.
③ Maximum longevity of light intensity.
④ Heat elevation should not exceed the threshold of pulp (41.5 °C)
⑤ Dual mode (curing and whitening) versus whitening mode only.
⑥ Ability to easily move and store.
⑦ Cost-effectiveness.

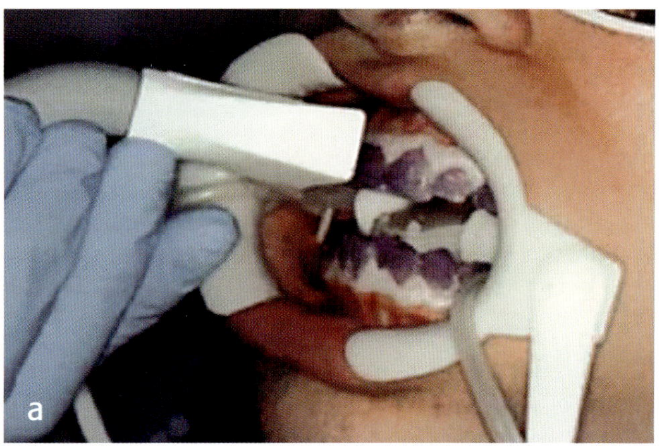

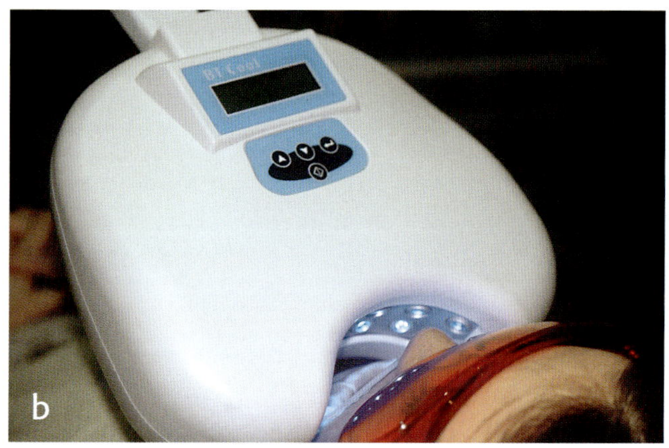

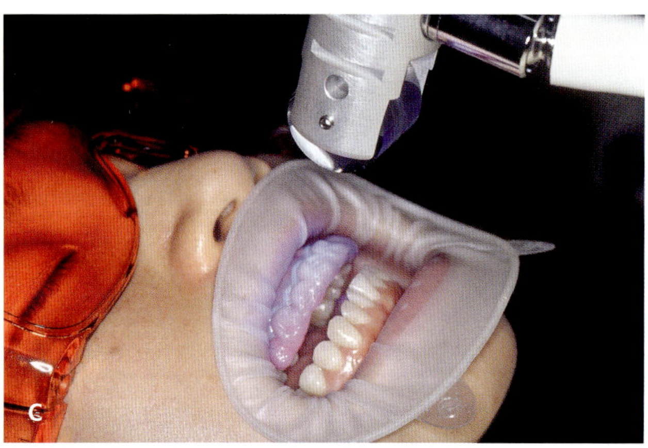

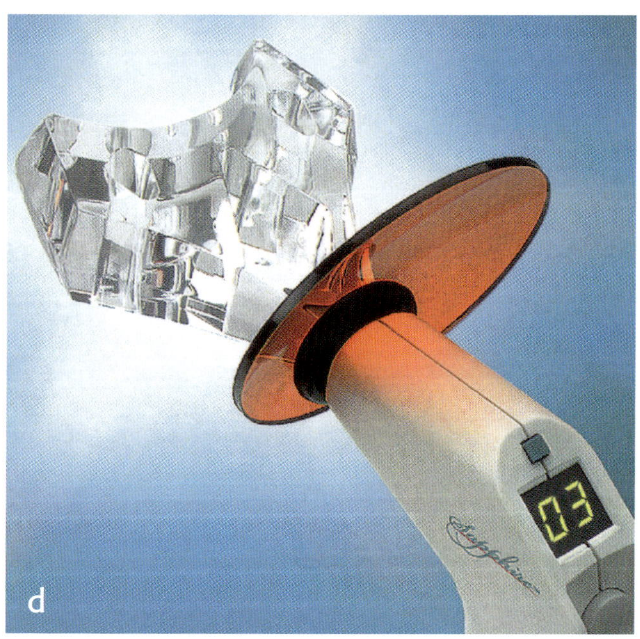

Fig. 4-6 Various types of light activation systems.
a. Lasersmile (Diode Laser). 815±15nm: Whitening mode.
b. BT Cool (LED). 430~490nm: Whitening mode.
c. Flipo White (Plasma Arc): Whitening and curing mode.
d. Sapphire (Plasma Arc): Whitening and curing mode.

Advantages and disadvantages of power whitening

Advantages

- Immediate whitening results
- Less participation needed on the patient's side
- Selective whitening of a few teeth is possible (Fig. 4-7)
- The procedure is performed totally under the control of the dentist

Disadvantages

- Cost
- Frequent visits to the dental office
- Possibility of gingival and soft tissue burns due to leakage
- Possibility of faster relapse of shade
- Higher incidence of post-operative sensitivity

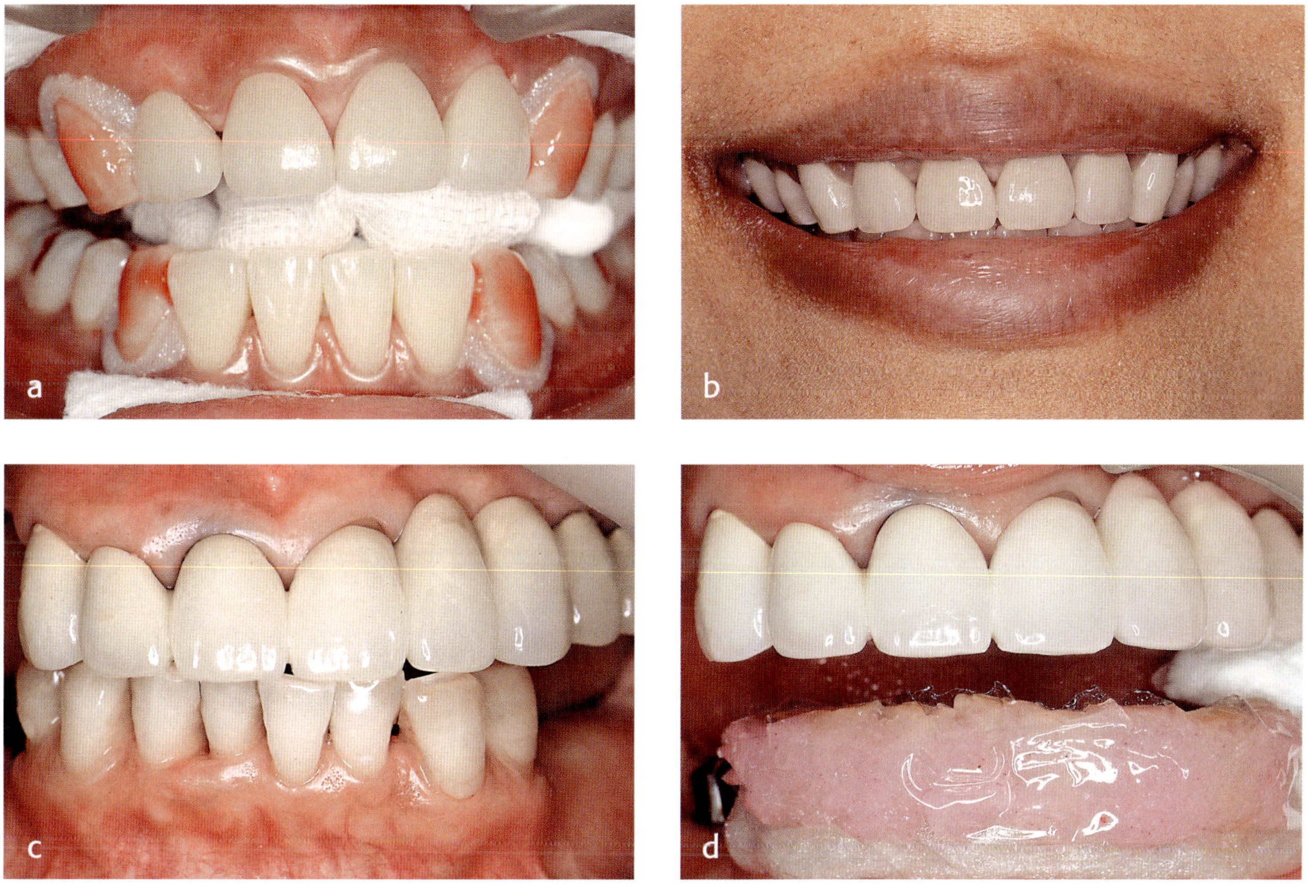

Fig. 4-7 Selective power whitening.
a,b. Selective power whitening of four canines, which were slightly darker than the other teeth.
c,d. Selective power whitening of the remaining lower teeth was performed to match the upper restoration.

Power whitening can be performed with various techniques and materials. Careful diagnosis and treatment planning is of utmost importance to provide the best whitening program, customized for each patient. Although it is best to whiten the upper and lower arch separately, some patients cannot comply with multiple visits to the office, making it necessary to whiten both arches simultaneously. To maximize the whitening efficacy and maintain the whitening result for a long time, power whitening should be combined with home whitening. The dentist should be able to propose several whitening programs with different treatment times and intervals considering the nature of the discoloration and the patient's lifestyle (Fig. 4-8 and 4-9). The patients then can choose a specific program that is best suited for them. The basic power whitening technique is similar in all patients but can be modified considering the factors that affect whitening and according to the manufacturer's specific directions.

Factors that affect whitening

Surface debridement: Thorough scaling and polishing should be performed in order to eliminate all superficial debris.
Hydrogen peroxide concentration: The higher the concentration, the greater the effect of the oxidation process. The highest concentration generally used is 35% hydrogen peroxide.
Note: When gelling agents are added to a 35% solution of hydrogen peroxide, the concentration of H_2O_2 is then reduced to 25%.
Temperature: An increase of 10 °C doubles the rate of the chemical reaction. Generally, if the temperature is elevated to a point at which the patient does not feel discomfort, then the procedure is taking place at a safe range of temperature.
pH: When hydrogen peroxide is stored and shipped, an acidic pH must be maintained to extend shelf life. The optimum pH for hydrogen peroxide intended for oxidation is pH 9.5 to 10.8. This produces a 50% greater result in the same amount of time as at a lower pH.
Time: The effect of the bleach is directly related to the time of exposure. The longer the exposure, the greater the color change.
Sealed environment: Placing the hydrogen peroxide into a sealed environment has been shown to increase its bleaching efficiency.

(Contribution from R.E Goldstein with permission from Quintessence Publishing Inc.)

Fig. 4-8 Two-week program.

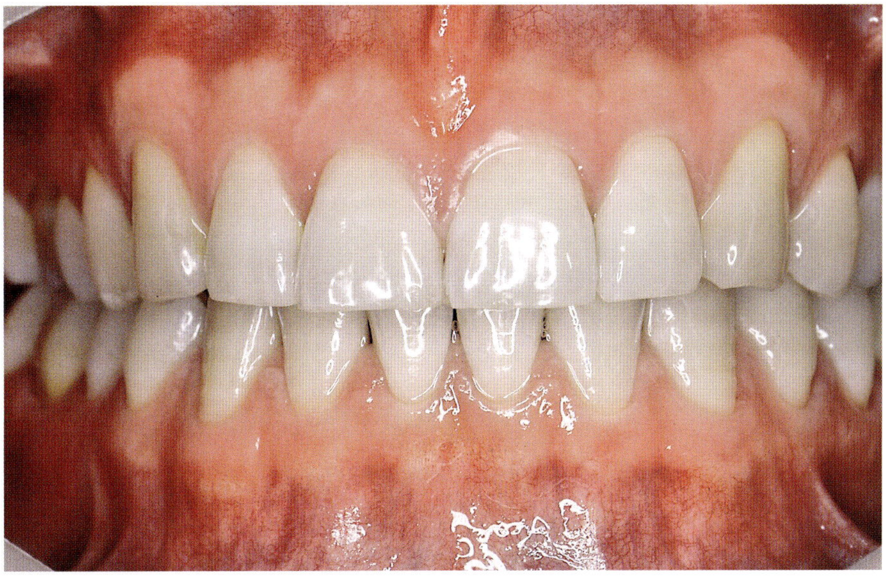

a. Generalized yellow discoloration.

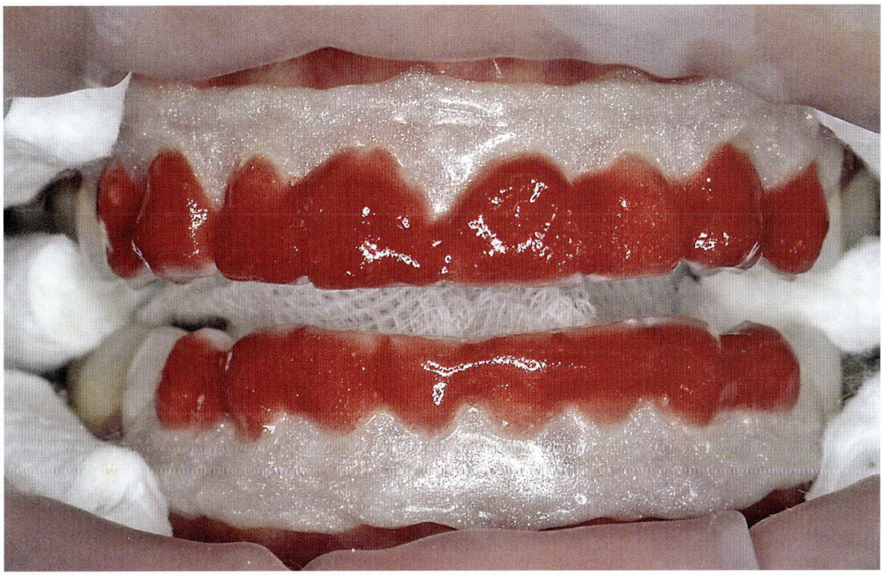

b. Patient insisted on having the upper and lower teeth whitened simultaneously for 2 weeks.

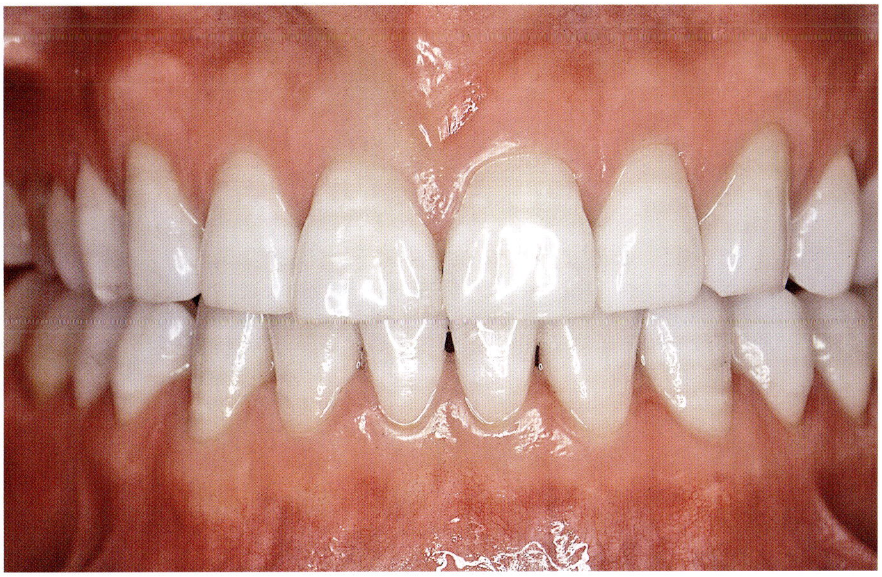

c. Result after three sessions of power whitening every 3 to 4 days combined with home whitening.

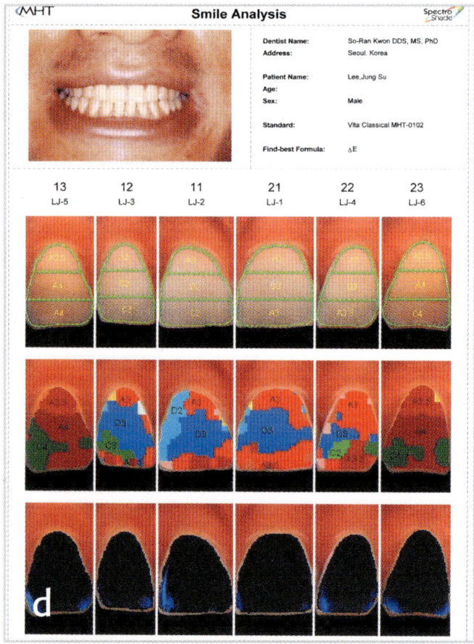

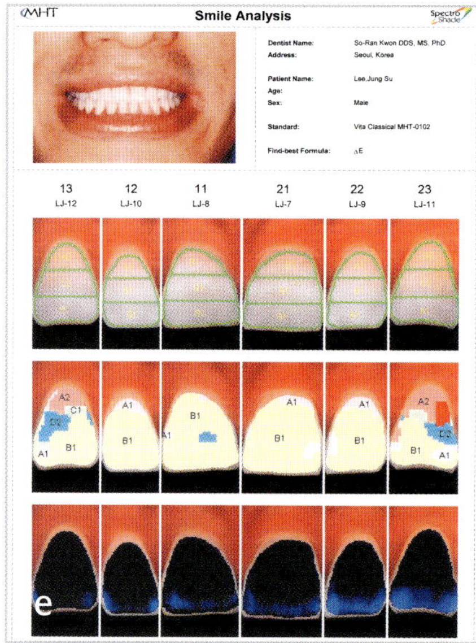

Fig. 4-8 Two-week program.

d. Smile analysis before whitening.

e. Smile analysis after whitening.

f. ΔE values of the upper right central incisor in the cervical, middle and incisal area.

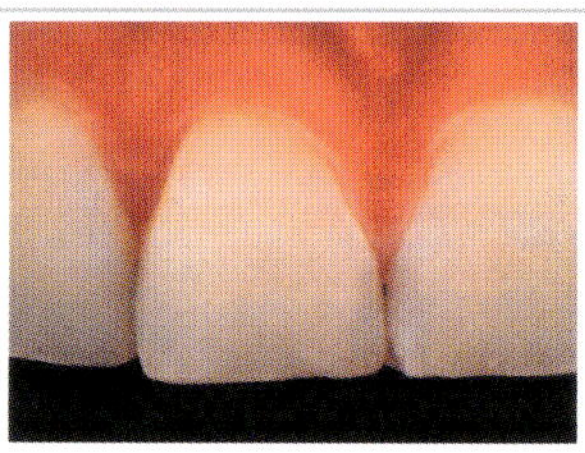

Dentist Name:	So-Ran Kwon DDS, MS, Ph
Address:	Seoul, Korea
Patient Name:	Lee,Jung Su
Age:	
Sex:	Male
Tooth #:	11 / 11
Tooth Label:	LJ-2 / LJ-8
Time:	2007-08-29 12:22:01
Notes:	

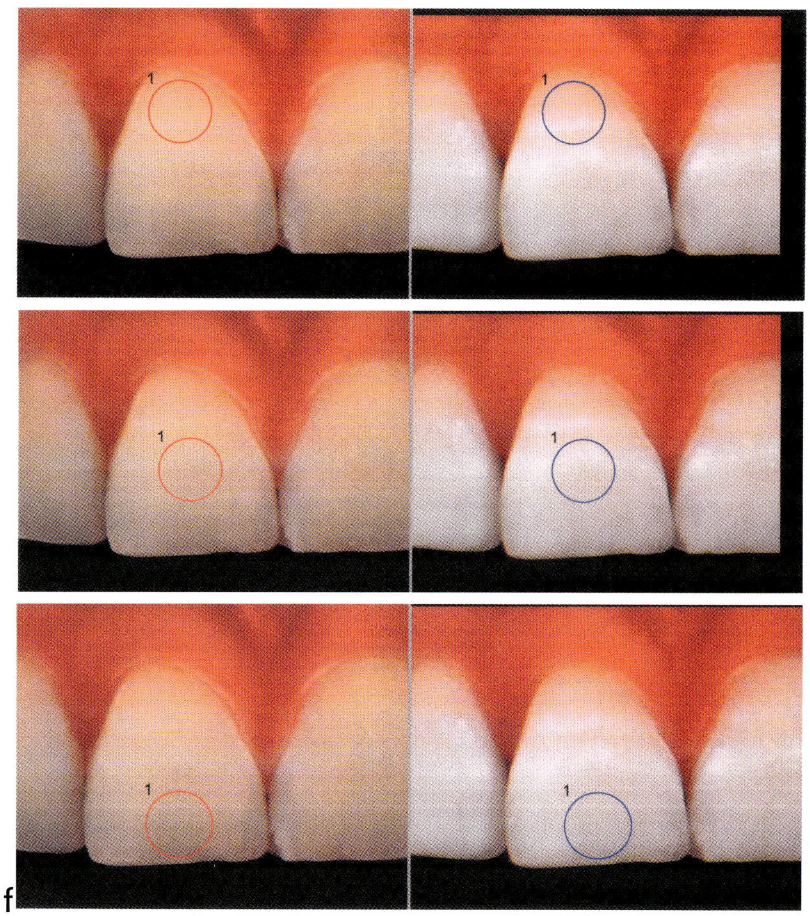

1:	Left:	Right:	Diff.:
L:	71.06	74.27	3.22
a:	8.09	6.92	-1.16
b:	18.75	11.35	-7.39
		ΔE	8.15

1:	Left:	Right:	Diff.:
L:	71.05	75.73	4.68
a:	4.46	2.91	-1.56
b:	17.65	9.58	-8.07
		ΔE	9.46

1:	Left:	Right:	Diff.:
L:	66.37	71.27	4.89
a:	3.11	1.71	-1.40
b:	16.10	7.45	-8.65
		ΔE	10.03

Fig. 4-9 Six-week program.

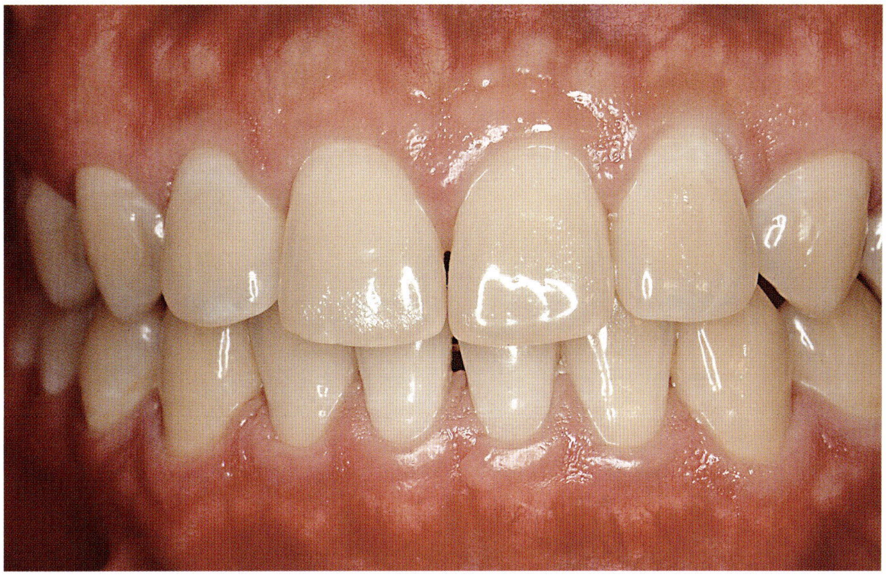

a. Generalized yellow discoloration.

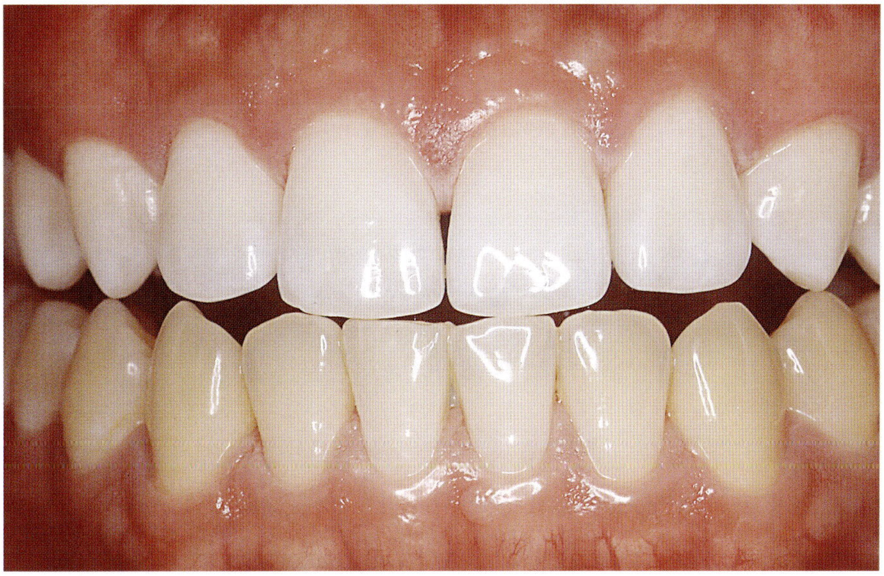

b. Color difference of the upper and lower arch. Three sessions of power whitening combined with home whitening were performed on the upper arch for 3 weeks.

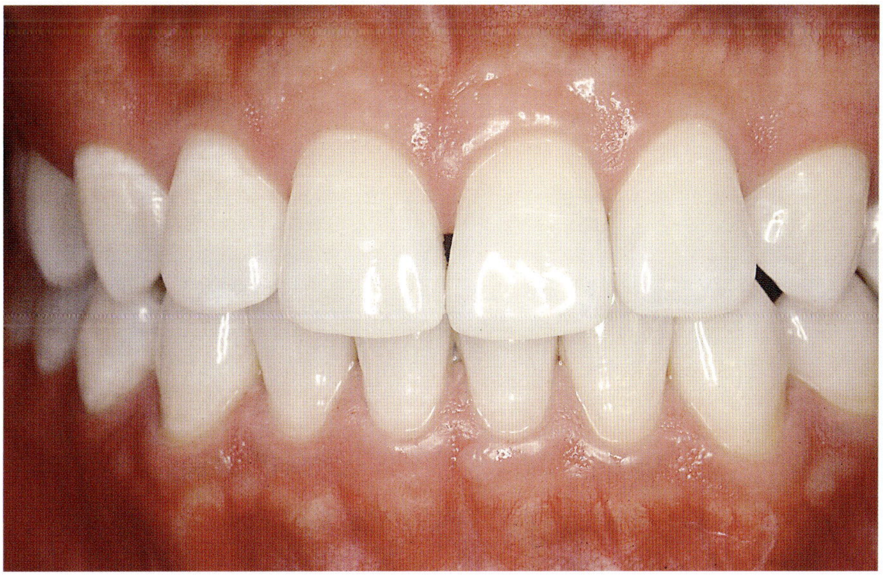

c. Three sessions of power whitening combined with home whitening were performed on the lower arch for 3 weeks. Power whitening was performed once a week.

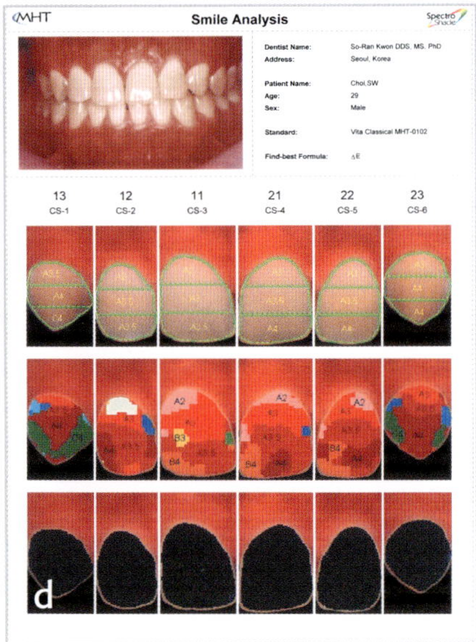

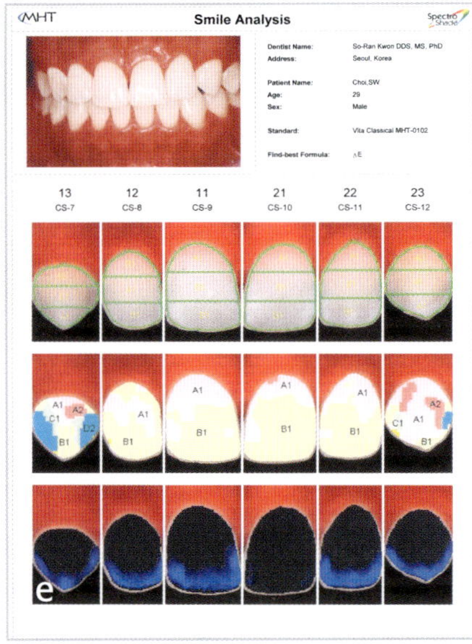

Fig. 4-9 Six-week program.

d. Smile analysis before whitening.

e. Smile analysis after whitening.

f. ΔE values of the upper right central incisor in the cervical, middle and incisal area.

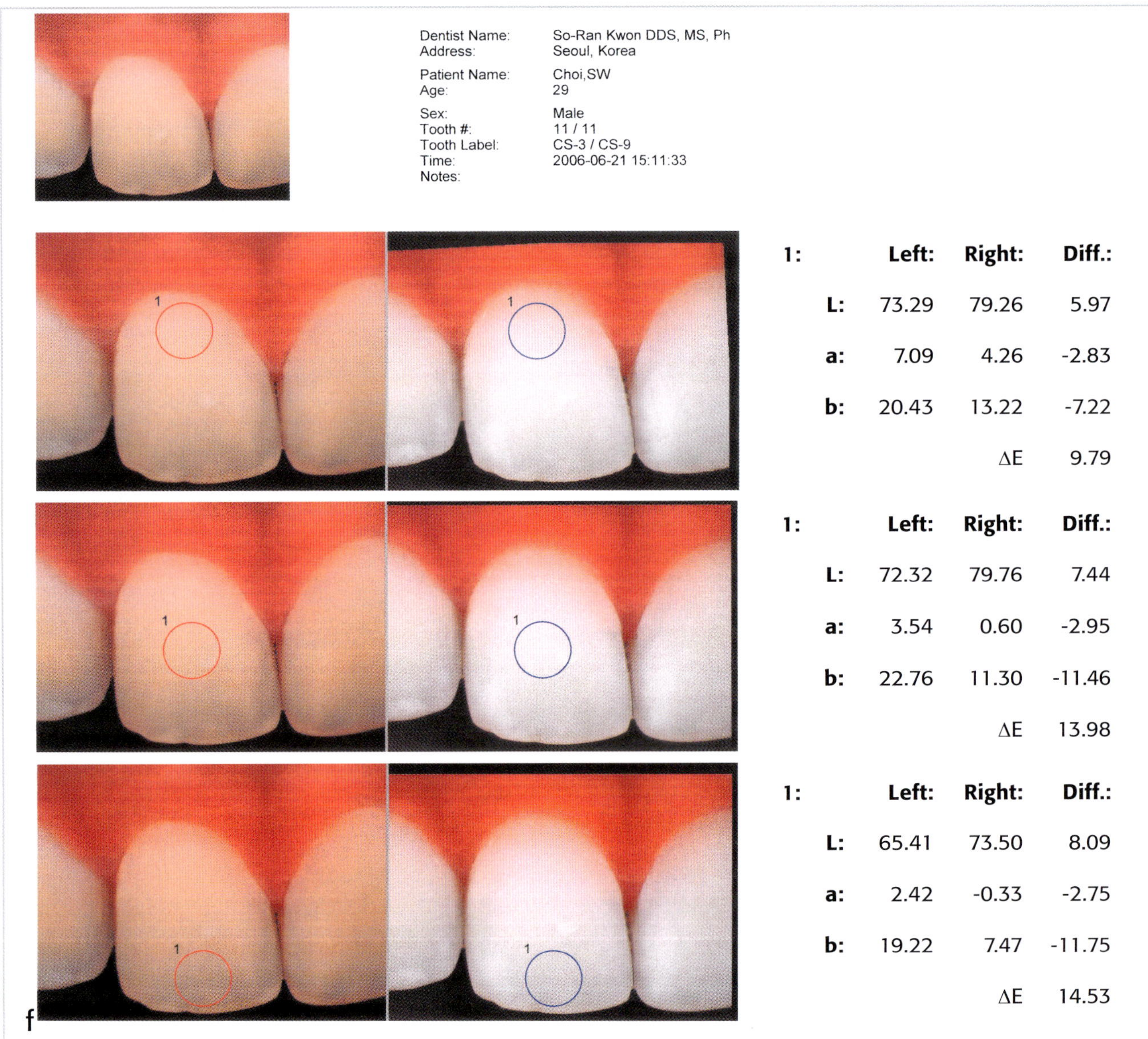

Power whitening technique

(Fig. 4-10)

- **Preparation:** Pretreatment photographs are taken to record the baseline shade. A thorough prophylaxis to remove stains and plaque ensures proper penetration of the whitening material. Special attention should be given to patients who have recently completed orthodontic treatment. Remnants of bonding materials should be completely removed.
- **Tooth isolation:** Proper selection and placement of a cheek retractor is essential to protect the lips and cheeks during the procedure. Dry the mucosa and place a resin barrier to cover approximately 0.5mm of the tooth and 2 to 3mm of the gingiva along the gingival line before light-curing. Proper placement of cotton rolls and gauze will help control saliva. Protective eyewear is placed over the patient's eyes to protect them from the activation light.
- **Application of whitening material:** Apply the power whitening material homogenously onto the teeth.
- **Light activation:** Position the light source as recommended by the manufacturer so that the beam is directed onto the labial surface of the teeth. Periodically remove excess saliva and check for any discomfort or sensitivity.
- **Removal of whitening material:** Depending on the severity of discoloration and the manufacturer's instruction, remove the power whitening material after 30 to 40 minutes and rinse with water.
- **Finishing:** A 2% neutral sodium fluoride gel is applied for 5 to 10 minutes to minimize the sensitivity. Finally, the fluoride gel is rinsed off and the resin barrier removed. Even though the whitening material has been removed from the tooth surface, active oxygen radicals remain on the tooth. Therefore, patients may experience a tingling or sharp sensation after treatment. To minimize sensitivity and maximize patient satisfaction, it is always best to whiten the upper and lower arch separately so that the patient can see the color change and difference.

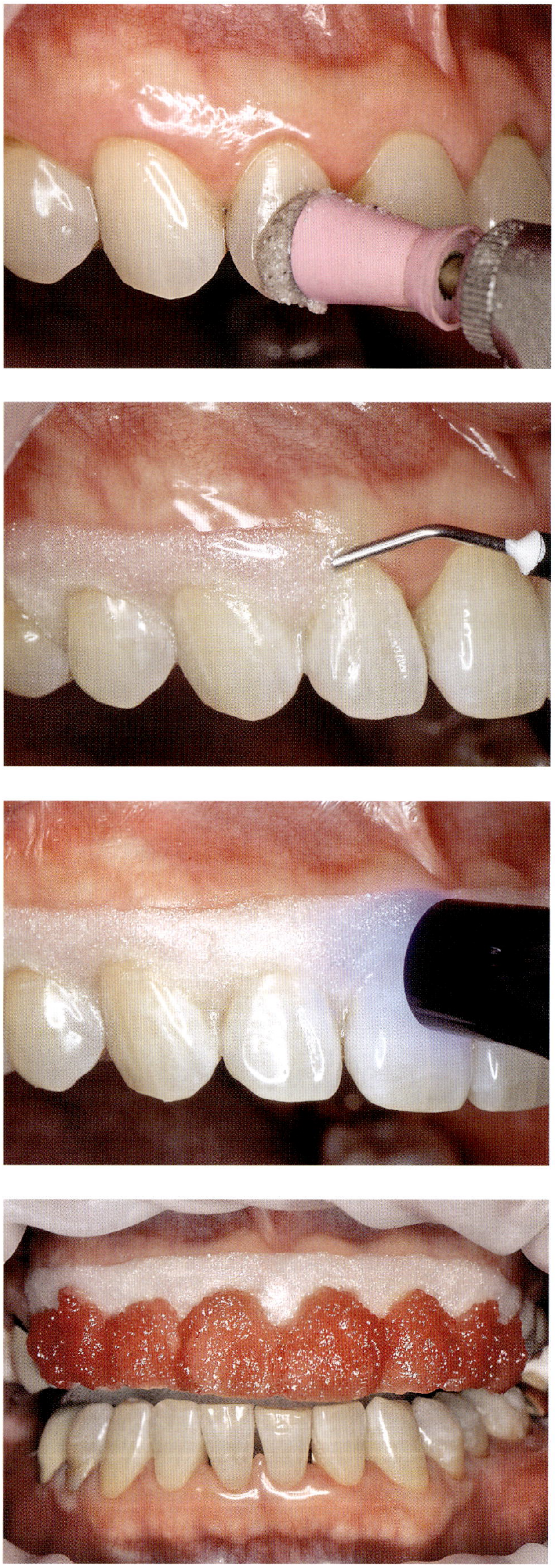

Fig. 4-10 Power whitening technique.

a. Thorough prophylaxis for stain and plaque removal is essential prior to whitening.

b. The resin barrier should cover approximately 0.5mm of the tooth and 2 to 3mm of the gingiva along the gingival line.

c. Light-curing of the resin barrier.

d. Apply the power whitening material homogenously onto the teeth.

Fig. 4-10 Power whitening technique.

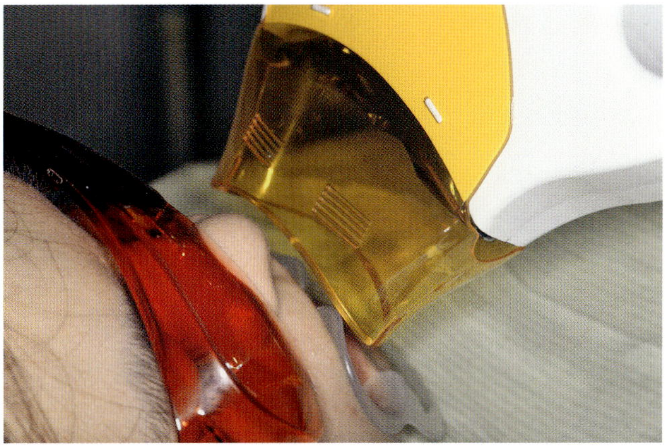

e. Perform light activation (optional).

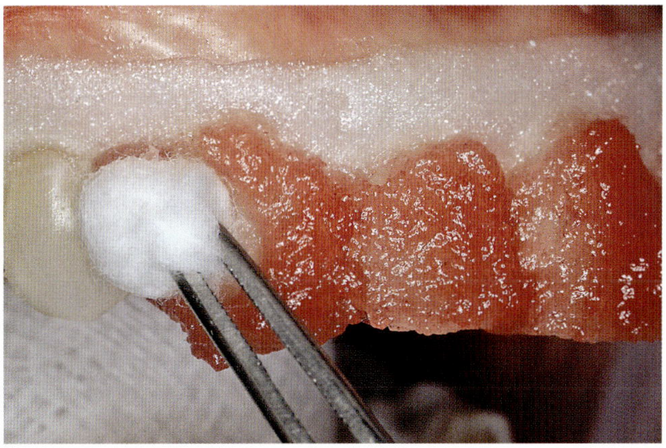

f. Depending on the severity of discoloration and the manufacturer's instruction, remove the power whitening material after 30 to 40 minutes and rinse with water.

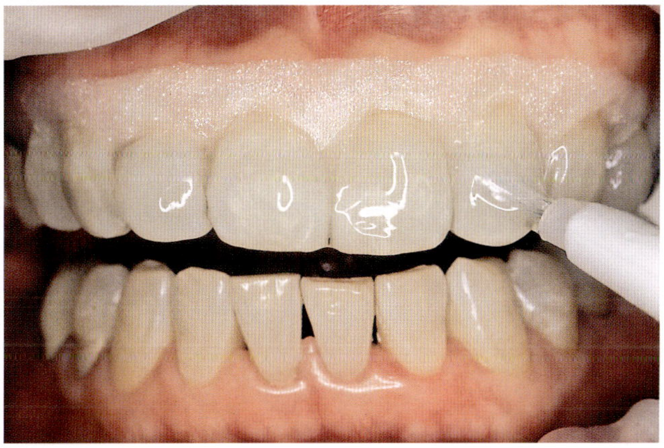

g. Apply a 2% neutral sodium fluoride gel for 5 to 10 minutes.

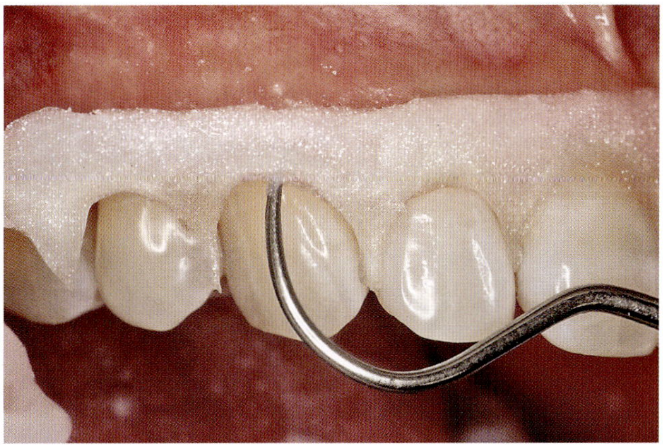

h. Rinse off the fluoride gel and remove the resin barrier.

Power whitening modifications

- Kwon's Sealed Bleaching
- Compressive Bleaching
- Ozone Bleaching

Kwon's Sealed Bleaching

Despite recent improvements of the current power whitening systems, there are still problems to be solved. The predominant problems are multiple visits to the office and false evaluation of the actual shade change due to tooth dehydration. The use of higher concentrations of peroxide may also produce more cases of thermal sensitivity. Since some of its volatile components seem to evaporate, the power whitening material has to be replenished several times during a single session for maximum efficacy. Some patients complain of discomfort and irritation to the nose due to evaporation of the material, and the replenishment of the power whitening material is time-consuming and adds to the expense of the whitening procedure. In 2006, Kwon introduced a new power whitening protocol called the 'Sealed Bleaching Technique', which prevents the evaporation and desiccation of active agents by placing a linear low-density polyethylene (LLDPE) wrap onto the power whitening gel (Fig. 4-11). The mechanism of sealed bleaching is that, by creating a sealed environment, the activated whitening material remains concentrated near the tooth surface so that it is directed into the tooth rather than evaporating into the air. This technique not only improves the efficacy of whitening, but also makes the procedure safer by preventing unintentional exposure. Since the activated whitening material is utilized more effectively, lower concentrations can be used and replenishment is not necessary. This simplifies the procedure and makes it more cost-effective. Another advantage of the technique is that it can be used with any power whitening system regardless of whether light activation is performed. In a study in 2007, Lee showed a greater shade difference after whitening in the sealed bleaching group compared to the conventional bleaching group, demonstrating an improvement of effectiveness through sealing (Fig. 4-12).

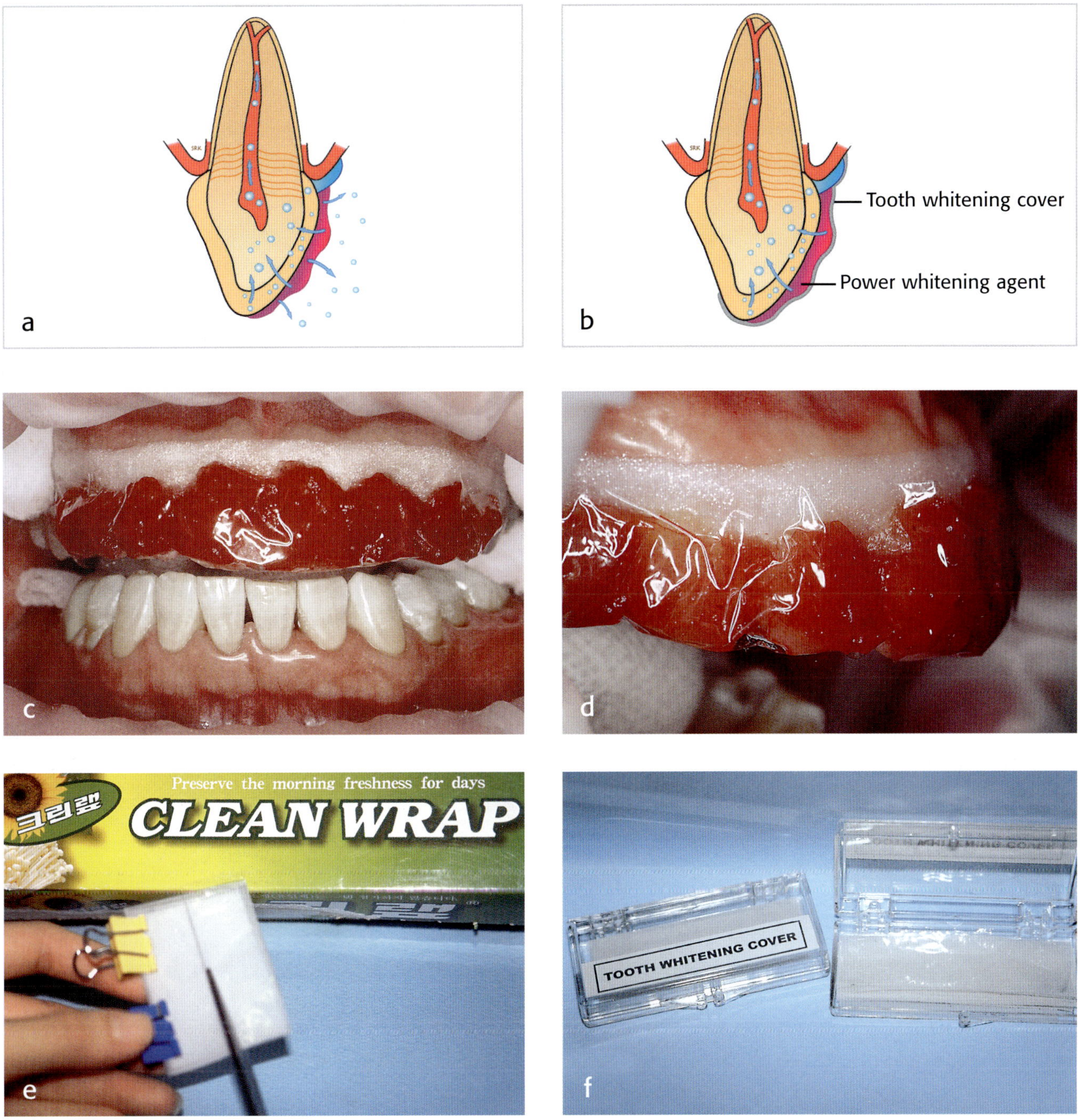

Fig. 4-11 Kwon's sealed bleaching.

a. During conventional power whitening, a portion of the active substances penetrate into the tooth while another evaporates into the air.

b. During sealed bleaching, all activated whitening material is directed into the tooth rather than evaporating into the air.

c. Placement of a linear low density polyethylene (LLDPE) wrap onto the power whitening gel.

d. Lateral view of the wrap in place.

e. Wraps are cut to a size of 2×7 cm.

f. The wraps are kept in a box with oiled paper between them to prevent sticking.

Fig. 4-12 Use of split-arch design to demonstrate the efficacy of sealed bleaching.

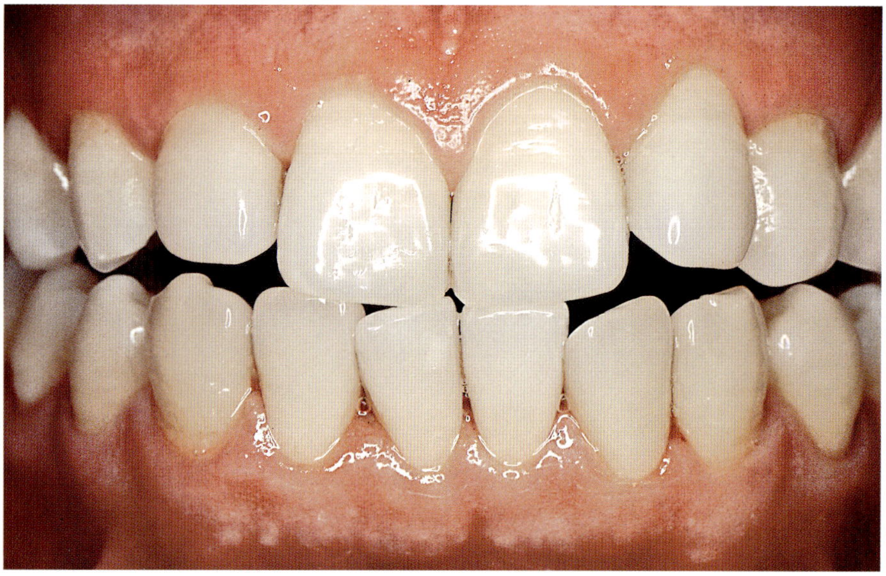

a. Prior to treatment.

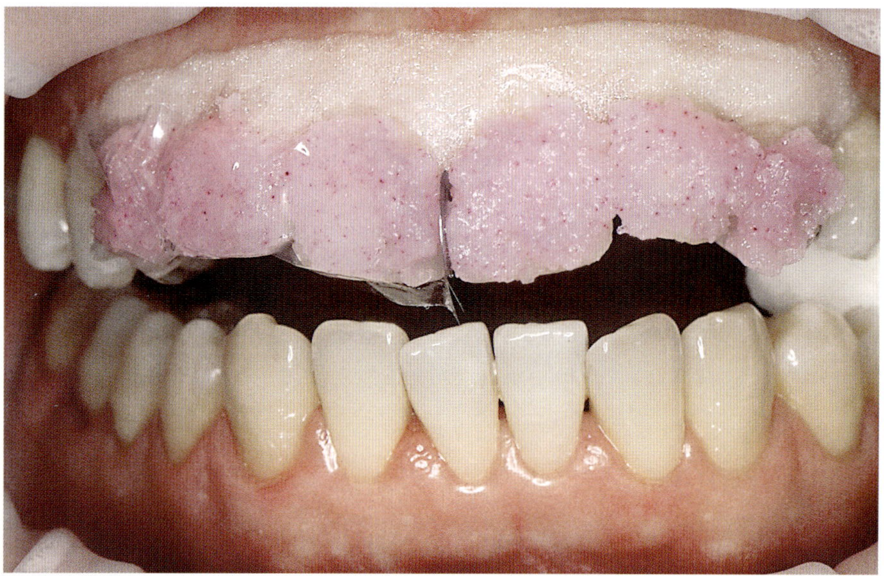

b. Power whitening is performed with a split-arch design. The right side is sealed with a wrap.

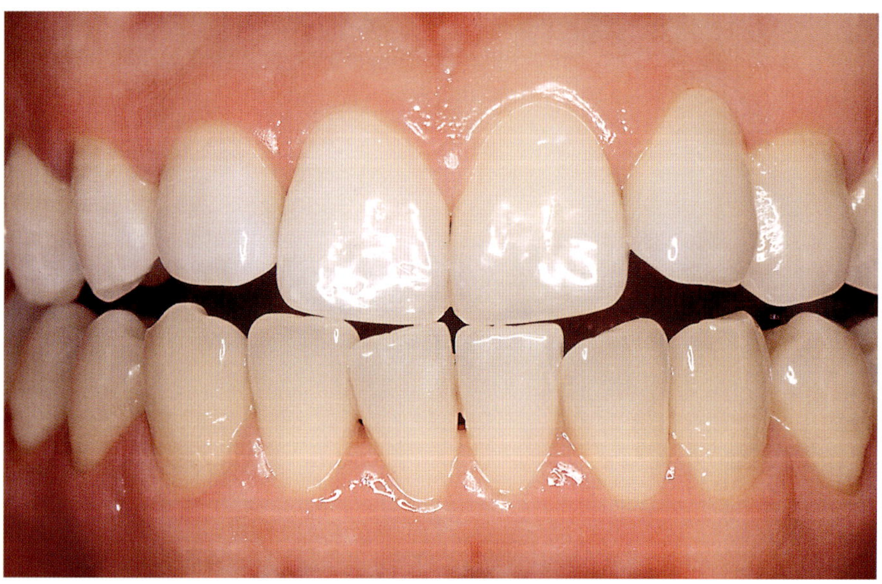

c. After three sessions of power whitening, a slight color difference between the right and left side is visible.

Compressive Bleaching

A similar protocol of creating a sealed environment with claims of increased efficacy was introduced in 2000 by Miara. In this system, called the 'Compressive Bleaching Technique', the whitening tray is filled with power whitening material and placed in the mouth. The borders are finally sealed with a light-cured resin barrier. Power whitening is thought to occur through the permeation of oxygenating perhydroxyl free radicals through enamel micropores along a diffusion gradient into the dentine, where they oxidize stains. It has been suggested that the compressive pressure associated with this leads to a more efficient penetration of oxygen radicals into the enamel (Fig. 4-13).

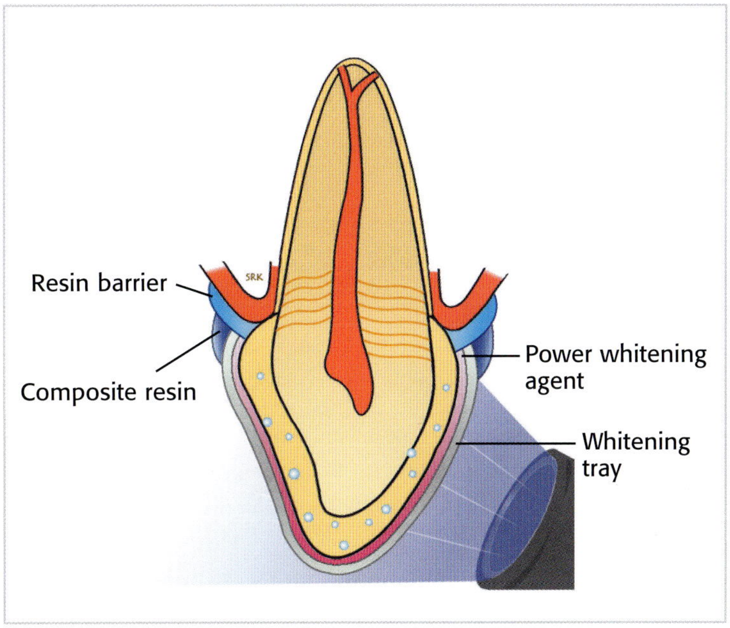

Fig. 4-13 Compressive bleaching technique.

Ozone Bleaching

The recent trend in power whitening shows an increase in the use of activators (photo/chemical) and light systems that allow superior and enhanced whitening with a lower concentration of hydrogen peroxide. In 2005, Holmes and Lynch proposed another modification of power whitening that utilizes an ozone machine to enhance the whitening effect due to the strong oxidizing power of ozone.

Troubleshooting in power whitening

- **Gingival and soft tissue burns:** If the gingiva has not been properly isolated and protected with a resin barrier, leakage of the highly concentrated power whitening material may cause gingival ulceration, irritation and burns. Leakage is evidenced by the formation of small bubbles in the gel or by direct complaints about discomfort and pain from the patient. Gingival burns should be treated immediately by removing the power whitening material and resin barrier, rinsing with a copious amount of water, and applying a topical anesthetic or a cream containing vitamin E (Fig. 4-14). It may be preferable not to use local anesthesia during power whitening so that the patient can immediately inform the dentist about possible leakage and pain.
- **Severe sensitivity and pain during treatment:** If the patient complains about severe pain during treatment, remove the whitening material and switch to a lower concentration or place a desensitizing material onto the teeth depending on the severity of pain.
- **Severe postoperative sensitivity and pain:** Sensitivity and pain usually resolve within 12 to 24 hours. Aspirin, acetaminophen, or non-steroidal anti-inflammatory drugs may be taken for immediate pain relief. Topical desensitizers, such as fluoride, potassium nitrate and amorphous calcium phosphate, can be given to the patient to use at home.

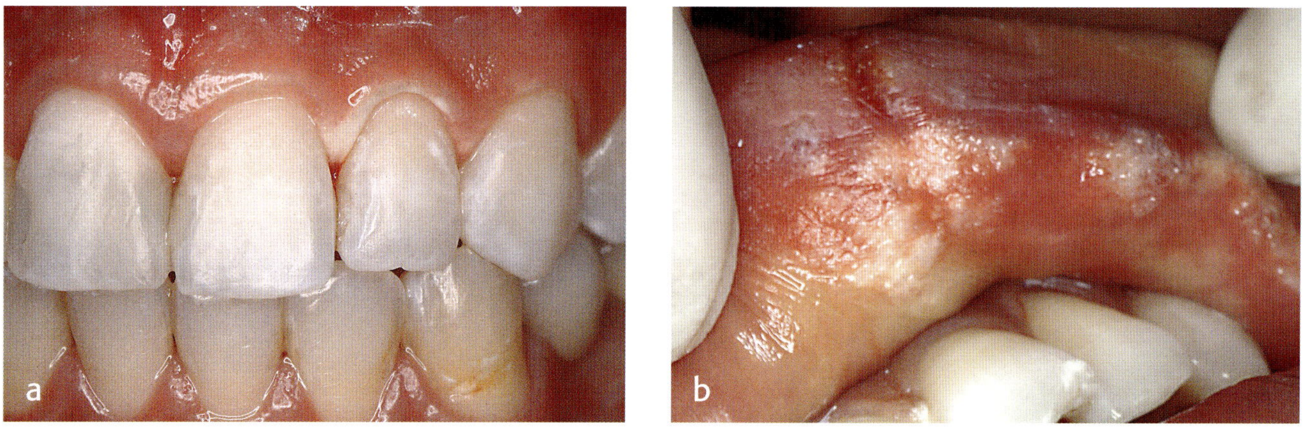

Fig. 4-14 Leakage of power whitening material.
a. Gingival ulceration around the upper left incisor after power whitening.
b. Swelling and burns of the upper lip due to exposure to power whitening material during removal.

••• Power whitening can achieve immediate whitening results. In order to maximize the whitening efficacy and maintain the whitening result for a long time, power whitening should be combined with home whitening.

Q&A

Question 1. Is power whitening more effective than home whitening?

Answer: The whitening result is determined by various factors, such as concentration of whitening material, treatment duration, frequency, etc. However, power whitening uses more highly concentrated materials and achieves immediate results. In order to maintain the result for a long time, it is recommended to combine power whitening with home whitening.

Question 2. Does etching before power whitening improve the whitening result?

Answer: In 1991, Hall reported that acid etching does not have any effect on whitening efficacy.

Question 3. Is it possible to do power whitening without light?

Answer: Since the power whitening material plays the most important role in power whitening, it is not absolutely necessary to use a light.

Question 4. How do you do power whitening when there is cervical abrasion?

Answer: If there is cervical abrasion, protect the area with the resin barrier or temporarily fill the area with a light-cured glass ionomer. After completion of the whitening treatment, the area may be filled with composite resin.

Question 5. How many sessions of power whitening do you recommend?

Answer: Usually, at least 3 sessions are required for a satisfactory result.

Question 6. Why do you combine home whitening with power whitening?

Answer: Though safe and effective, because of its slow rate, patients may often quit home whitening during the course of treatment (drop-out rate: 50%). Therefore, in order to encourage and motivate the patient to complete the treatment, it is best to combine home whitening with power whitening.

References

ADA Council on Scientific Affairs. Laser assisted bleaching: an update. J Am Dent Assoc 1998; 129:1484-7. Barghi NB. Making a clinical decision for vital tooth bleaching: at-home or in-office? Compend Contin Educ Dent Aug, 1998; 19(8):831-8.

Bishara SE, Sulieman AH, Olson M. Effect of enamel bleaching on the bonding strength of orthodontic brackets. Am J Orthod Dentofacial Orthop Nov, 1993; 104(5)444-7.

Bowles WH, Thompson LR. Vital bleaching: the effect of heat and hydrogen peroxide on pulpal enzymes. J Endodont 1986; 12:108-12.

Bowles WH, Ungwuneri Z. Pulp chamber penetration by hydrogen peroxide following vital bleaching procedures. J Endodont 1987; 13:375-7.

Christensen G. New resin curing lights, high intensity vs. multimode intensity. Status Report 2. CRA Newsletter 1999; 23/5: 6.

Christensen G. Tooth bleaching, state-of-the-art. CRA Newsletter 1997; 21/4.

Christensen G. Why resin curing lights do not increase tooth lightening. Status Report. CRA Newsletter 2000; 24/6: 3.

Cohen SC. Human pulpal responses to bleaching procedures in teeth. J Endodont 1979; 5: 134-8.

Dzierzak J. Factors Which Cause Tooth Color Changes…Protocol for In-Office "Power" Bleaching. The Bleaching Report 1991; 3(2):15-20.

Eldeniz Au, Usumez A, Usumez S, Ozturk N. Pulpal temperature rise during light-activated bleaching. J Biomed Mater Res 2005; 72B:254-259.

Gallagher A. Clinical Study to Compare Two In-Office(Chairside) Whitening Systems. J Clin Dent 2002; 13:219-224.

Garber DA. Dentist-monitored bleaching: a discussion of combination and laser bleaching. J Am Dent Assoc Suppl 1997; 128: 26S-30S.

Goldstein RE, Garber DA. Complete Dental Bleaching, Quintessence Publishing Co, Inc, 1995.

Goldstein RE. In-Office bleaching: where we came from, where we are today. J Am Dent Assoc Suppl. 1997; 128:11S-15S.

Hall DA. Should etching be performed as part of a vital bleaching technique. Quintessence Int 1991; 22:679-86.

Holmes J., Lynch E. Uses of ozone in the general dental practice: Integration into general dental practice, Part 2.

Jones AH, Diaz-Arnold AM, Vargas MA, Cobb DS. Colorimetric assessment of laser and home bleaching techniques. J Esthet Dent 1999; 11(2):87-94.

Kwon S. Tooth Whitening State of the Art, Dental Publishing Co, Inc, 2004. Lee, Y. The effectiveness of sealing technique on in-office bleaching. Department of Dentistry, Yonsei University. Master of Science. 2007.

Lu AC. In-Office Bleaching Systems: A Scanning Electron Microscope Study. Compendium 2001; 22(9):798-805.

Luk K, Tam L, Hubert M. Effect of light energy on peroxide tooth bleaching. JADA 2004; 135:194-201.

Matis BA. Eight In-Office Tooth Whitening Systems Evaluated In Vivo: A Pilot Study. Oper Dent 2007; 32-4:322-327.

Miara P. An innovative chairside bleaching protocol for treating stained dentition: initial results. Pract Perio Aesth Dent 2000; 12/7:669-78.

Miller M. (editor) Reality: The information source for esthetic dentistry. Vol. 13. Reality Publishing Company: Houston, Texas, 1999.

Miller M. (editor) Reality: The information source for esthetic dentistry. Vol. 14. Reality Publishing Company: Houston, Texas, 2000.

Papathanasiou A. Clinical Evaluation of a 35% Hydrogen Peroxide In-Office Whitening System. Compendium 2002; 23(4): 335-346.

Reyto R. Laser tooth whitening. Dent Clin North Am 1998; 21(4):755-62.

Ritter AV. In-office Tooth Bleaching. J Esthet Restor Dent 2006; 18(3):168-169.

Rosensteil SF, Gegauff AG, Johnston WM. Duration of tooth colour change after bleaching. J Am Dent Assoc 1991; 123:54-9.

Shethri SA. A Clinical Evaluation of Two In-Office Bleaching Products. Oper Dent 2003; 28-5:488-495.

Tam L. Vital tooth bleaching: review and current status. J Can Dent Assoc 1992; 58(8):654-63.

Wolfgang B., Thomas Attin: External bleaching therapy with activation by heat, light or laser – A systematic review. Dental Materials, 2006.

Zach L, Cohen G. Pulp response to externally applied heat. Oral Surg 1965; 19:515-30.

chapter

5

Microabrasion

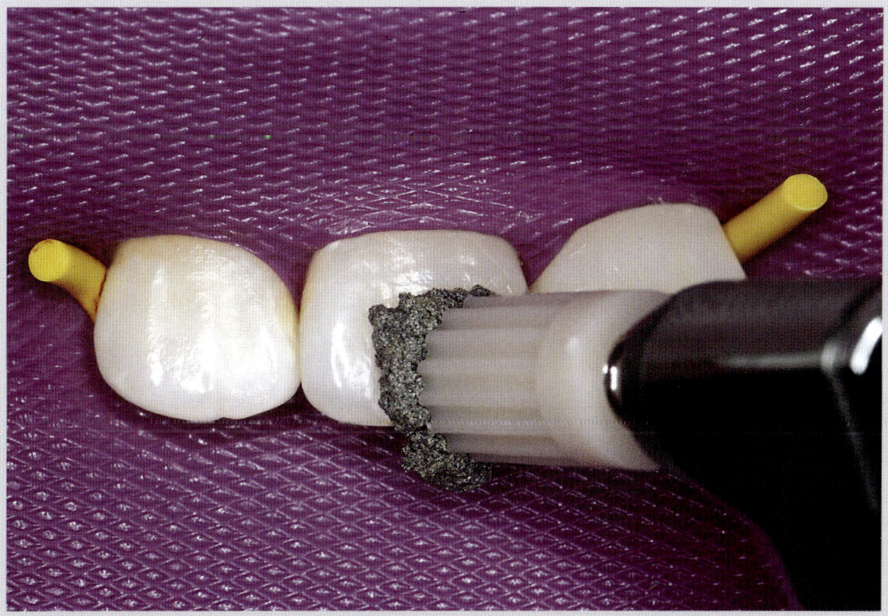

Localized white spots and brown stains on the enamel surface can be alarming to the self-conscious patient. Before the introduction of the microabrasion technique, the best treatment option available was to remove the defect with a handpiece and restore it. However, in localized defects limited to the surface, microabrasion offers a conservative approach to preserve maximum tooth structure. For optimum results, microabrasion can be combined with tooth whitening.

Croll defined enamel microabrasion as a procedure in which a microscopic layer of enamel is simultaneously eroded and abraded with a special compound, leaving a perfectly intact surface behind. The enamel surface layer is restructured to form an amorphous, prismless layer that clinically appears smooth and lustrous. It is used to treat enamel discolorations that may result from hypermineralization, hypomineralization or staining.

Indications and contraindications

Indications	Contraindications
■ Hypermineralized enamel ■ Discoloration limited to the enamel surface ■ Fluorosis ■ White spots ■ Decalcification related to orthodontic bands ■ Tooth with rough surfaces	■ Discoloration related to aging ■ Tetracycline staining ■ Amelogenesis imperfecta ■ Dentinogenesis imperfecta ■ Deep decalcified lesion reaching the dentin ■ Carious lesion subjacent to decalcified lesion

Advantages and disadvantages

Advantages	Disadvantages
■ Simple treatment procedure ■ Conservative and economical ■ Immediate and permanent treatment results ■ No special maintenance required	■ A layer of enamel is removed ■ Prediction of treatment outcome is difficult ■ Strongly erosive materials are used ■ Protection of the patient, assistant and dentist are required

Microabrasion materials

The use of hydrochloric acid to remove stains has been advocated for many years. In the past, McInnes solution – a mixture of 5 parts of 30% hydrogen peroxide, 5 parts of 36% hydrochloric acid, and one part of ether – was used (Fig. 5-1). A cotton pellet was soaked in the solution and applied to the tooth surface. The stain was selectively removed using a disc on a handpiece. Since the use of this solution involved some risk to the patient, assistant and dentist, meticulous protection and caution was required. Recently introduced microabrasion kits including hydrochloric acid in a paste have made the procedure simpler and safer. Prema kit (Premier Dental Products Co., Norris town, PA, Fig. 5-2) contains 10% hydrochloric acid in a preparation of fine grit silicon carbide particles in a water soluble paste; the paste can be applied manually with hand applicators or with a handpiece using specialized synthetic rubber tips. Opalustre (Ultradent Products Inc, Utah, USA, Fig. 5-3) contains 6.6% hydrochloric acid and silicon carbide microparticles in a water-soluble paste, which is packaged in purple syringes. The paste is applied and used with specialized rubber cups with bristles.

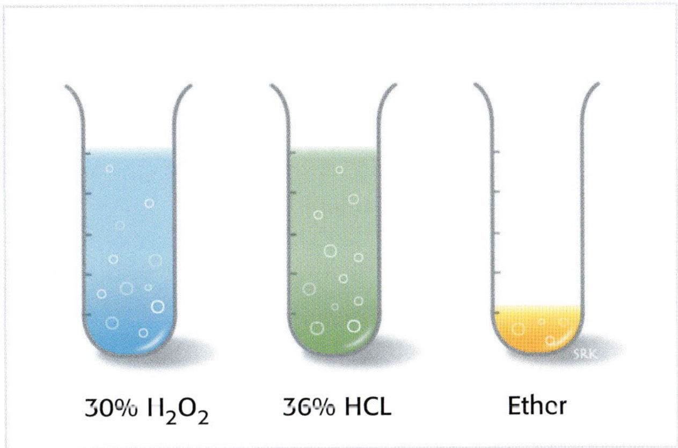

Fig. 5-1 McInnes solution.

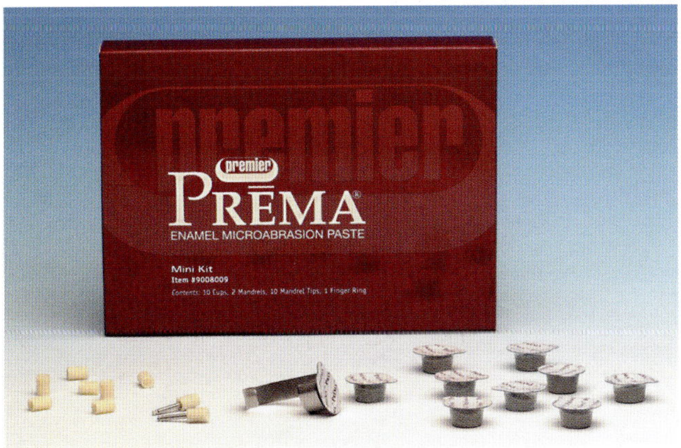

Fig. 5-2 Prema (Premier Dental Products Co., Norris Town, PA).

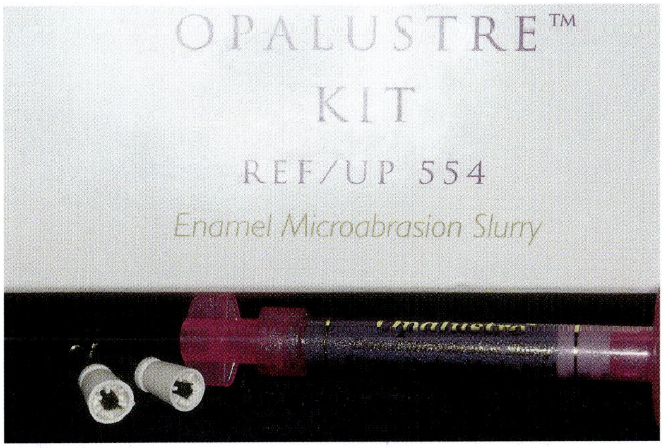

Fig. 5-3 Opalustre (Ultradent Products Inc, Utah, USA).

Microabrasion technique

Enamel microabrasion cannot solve all tooth discoloration problems. Many times, it is difficult to predict the prognosis of the procedure because the exact depth of the lesion is difficult to determine. Therefore, patients should be fully informed about the situation and understand that, after attempting microabrasion, a restorative treatment such as composite resin filling or laminate veneers may be required for optimum results. In order to evaluate the depth of the white spot or hypomineralized area, inspection of the incisal surface using a dental mirror to observe the penetration in the labio-lingual direction is recommended. The following steps cover the basic procedures for microabrasion.

- **Tooth isolation:** Isolate the teeth to be treated with a rubber dam. Clamps or 'Wedjets' (Hygienic Corporation, USA) may be used to stabilize the rubber dam. Evaluate the labio-lingual thickness of the tooth to be treated to evaluate the amount of enamel reduction possible.
- **Fine removal of lesion:** To shorten the treatment time, the lesion may be initially removed with a fine grit diamond or tungsten carbide bur.
- **Placement of microabrasion paste:** Place the microabrasion paste onto the treatment area, and abrade the area with light pressure using a special rubber cup for 30 to 60 seconds. Generally, 22 to 27 μm of enamel is removed per application. Use a gear reduction (10:1) handpiece to prevent the paste from splattering. Intermittent observation and rehydration may be required, and the procedure may be repeated, if necessary.
- **Polishing:** Polish the tooth surface with a prophy paste containing fluoride.
- **Neutral sodium fluoride gel:** Place a neutral sodium fluoride gel for 5 to 10 minutes.
- **Check up:** Recall the patient in 1 to 2 weeks and evaluate the result. Repeat the procedure, if necessary (Fig. 5-4).

Precautions

Immediately after microabrasion, the tooth surface may look unnatural due to small areas of decalcification remaining. However, in most cases at the 2 month or 6 month follow-up, the enamel surface is remineralized, creating a shiny clean surface.

Fig. 5-4 Microabrasion technique.

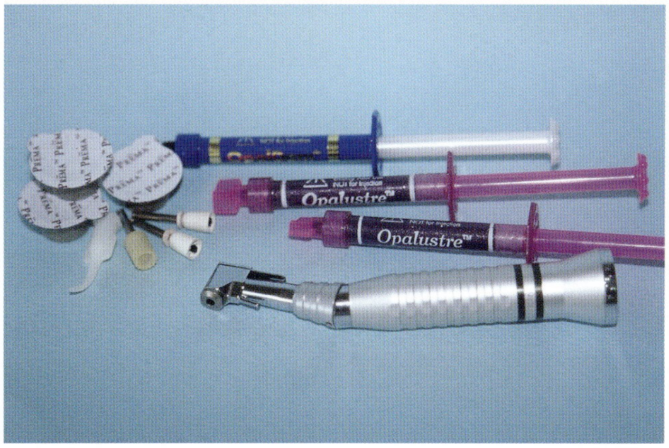

a. Microabrasion materials.

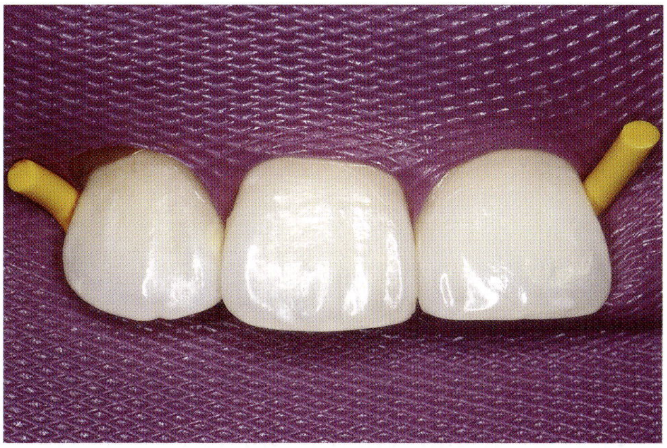

b. Isolation of tooth to be treated.

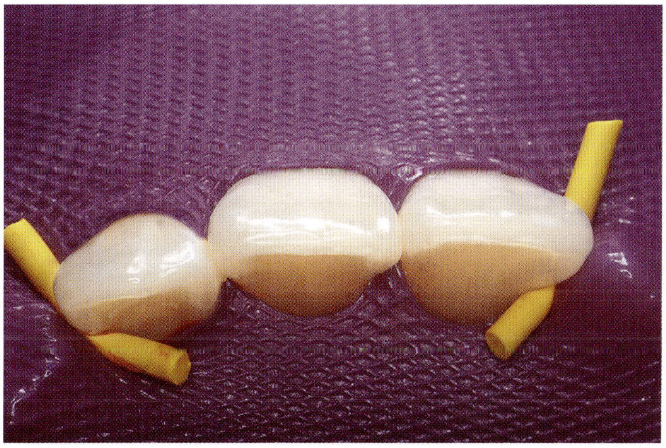

c. Evaluation of labio-lingual thickness of enamel.

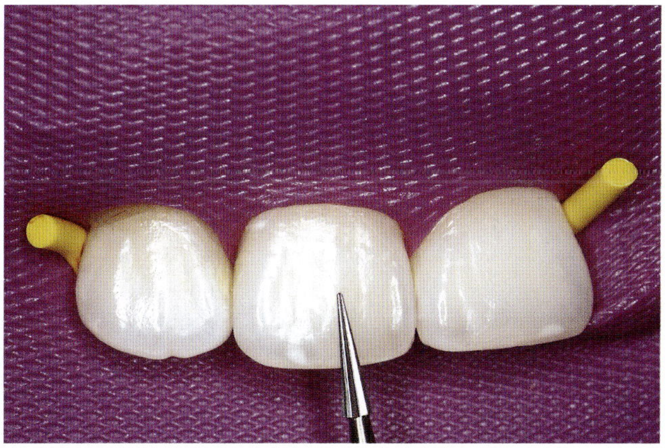

d. Use of fine-grit diamond or tungsten carbide bur to shorten treatment time.

Fig. 5-4 Microabrasion technique.

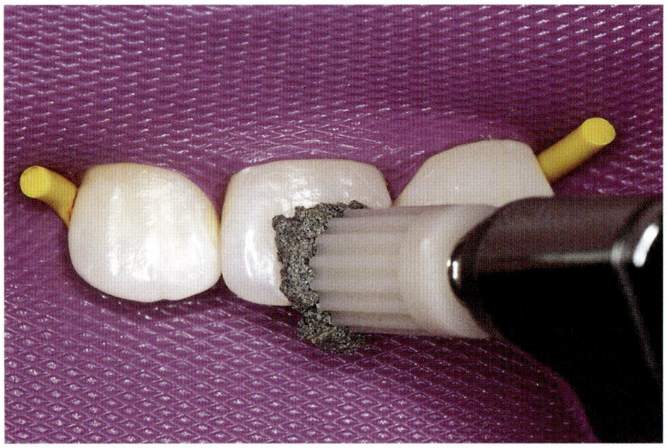

e. Microabrasion using light pressure and a special rubber cup.

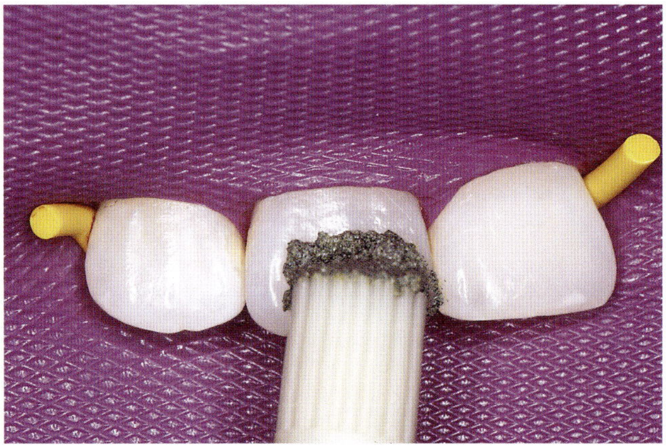

f. The position and direction of the rubber cup may be changed.

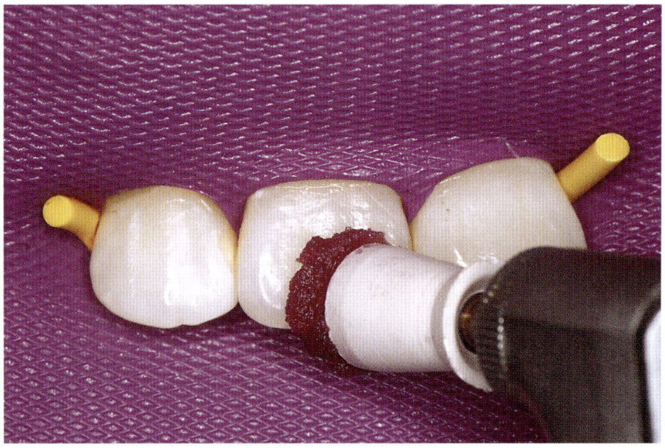

g. Polishing with a prophy paste containing fluoride.

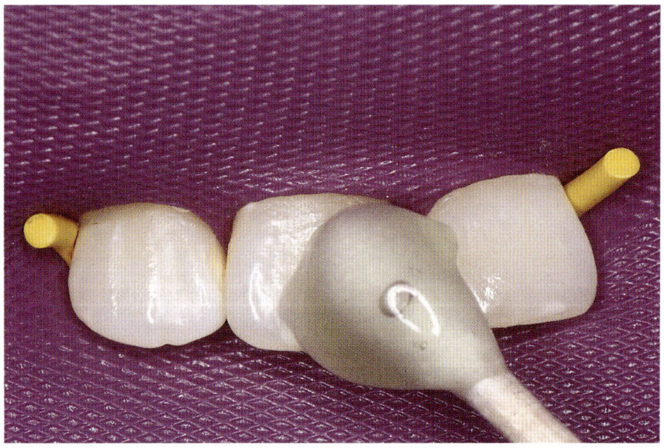

h. Application of neutral sodium fluoride gel for 5 to 10 minutes.

Microabrasion and other treatments

Microabrasion can be used prior to whitening to remove white and brown spots that are difficult to treat with whitening alone. In cases of tooth whitening after orthodontic treatment, microabrasion might be especially indicated to remove the decalcified areas around the brackets and smooth the rough tooth surface (Fig. 5-5 and 5-6). Superficial white spots can be successfully removed with microabrasion. If an attempted microabrasion has failed because the depth of the lesion was greater than 0.2mm, a restorative treatment like composite resin fillings or veneers may be required (Fig. 5-7). In some cases, white spots that were slightly visible on the tooth before whitening can become even more noticeable after whitening, making microabrasion or other esthetic bonded restorations necessary (Fig. 5-8).

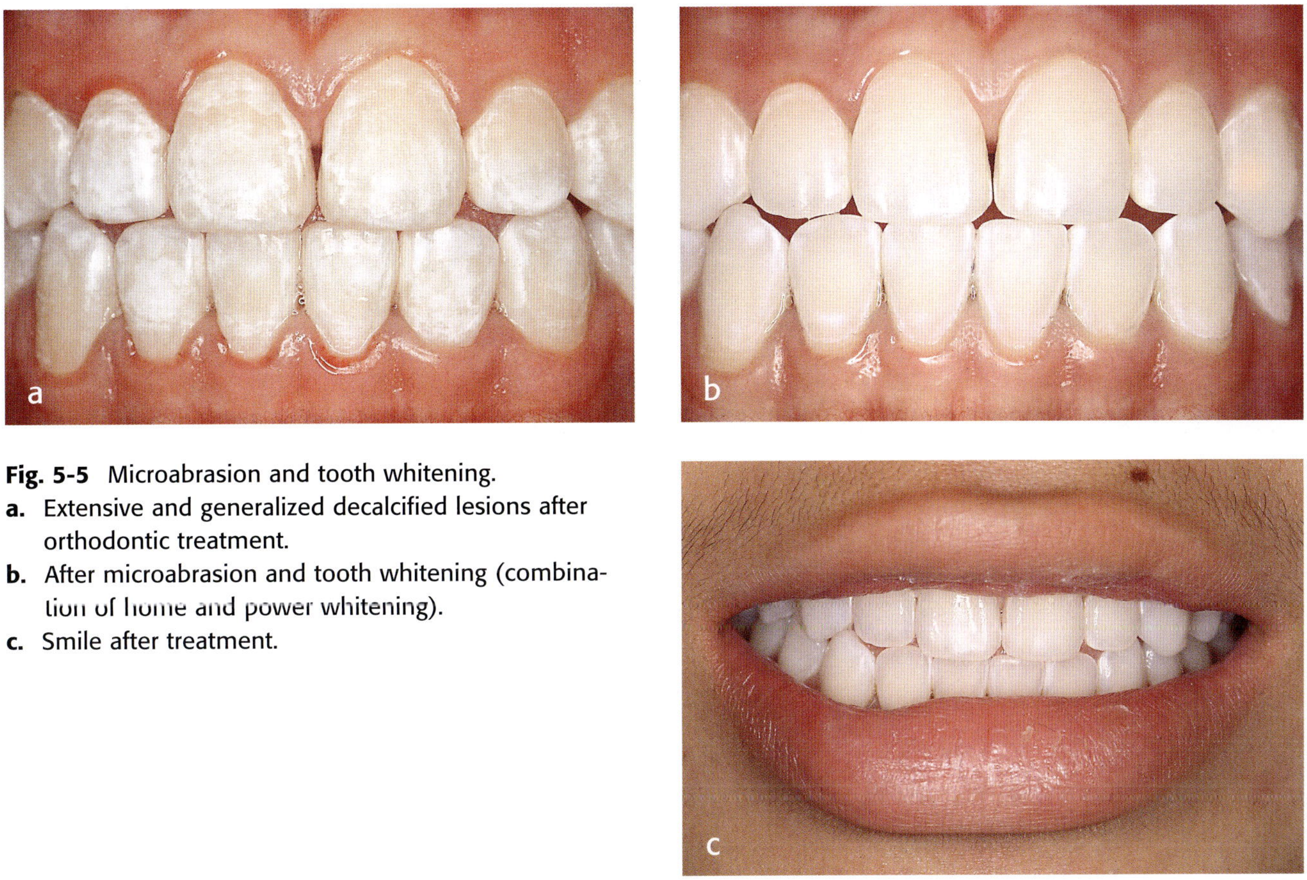

Fig. 5-5 Microabrasion and tooth whitening.
a. Extensive and generalized decalcified lesions after orthodontic treatment.
b. After microabrasion and tooth whitening (combination of home and power whitening).
c. Smile after treatment.

••• **During microabrasion, a microscopic layer of enamel is uniformly eroded and abraded with a special compound, leaving an undamaged enamel surface behind. The results are permanent.**

Fig. 5-6 Microabrasion and tooth whitening.

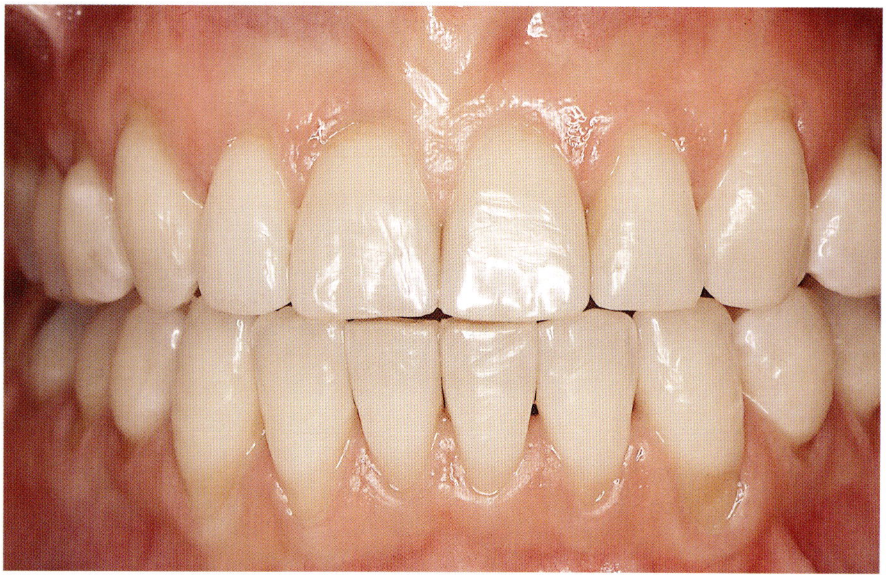

a. Generalized yellow discoloration with rough tooth surfaces after orthodontic treatment.

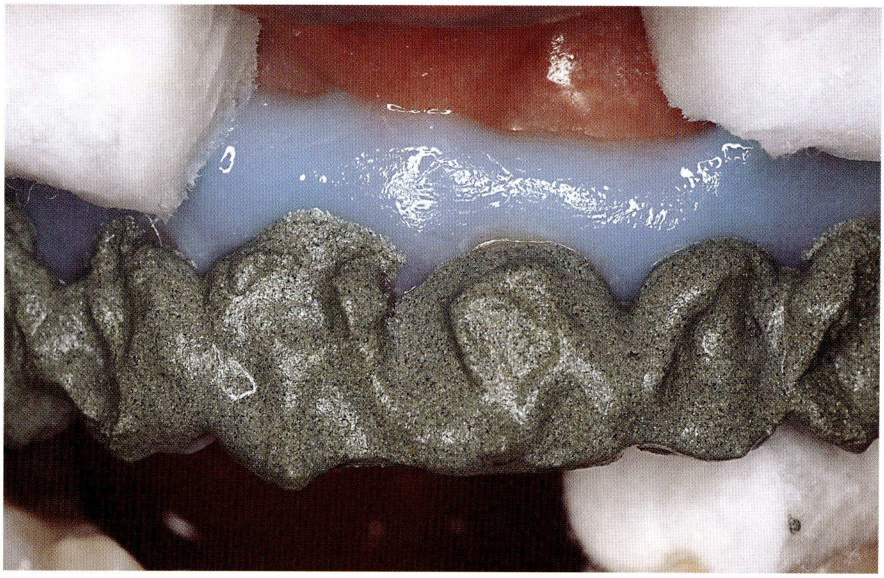

b. Placement of microabrasion slurry.

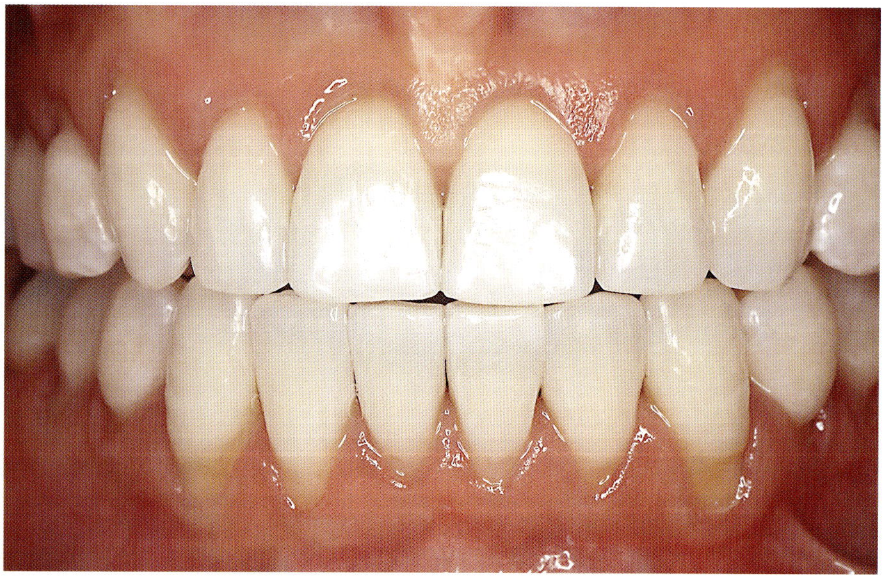

c. After power whitening and microabrasion, the rough tooth surface has become smooth and bright.

Fig. 5-7 Microabrasion and restorative treatment.

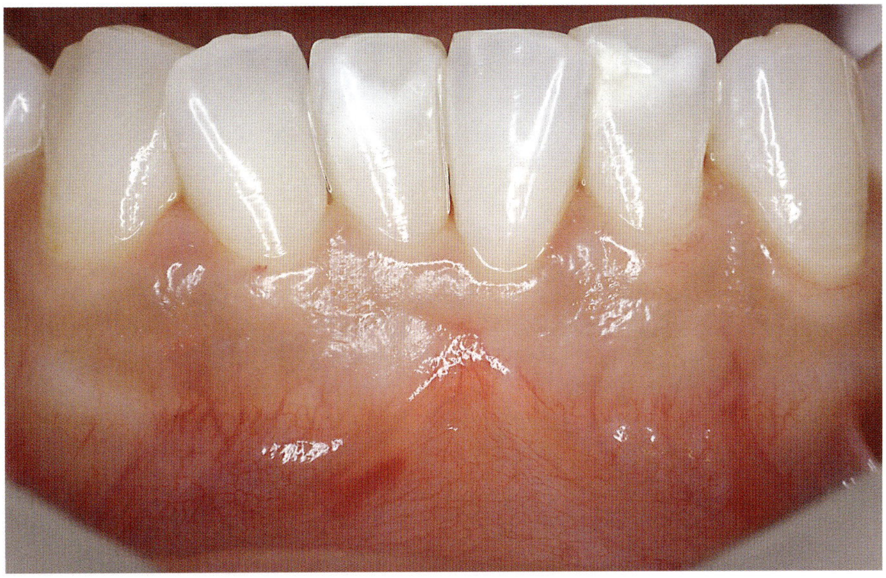

a. Attempts at microabrasion failed to remove the white spots.

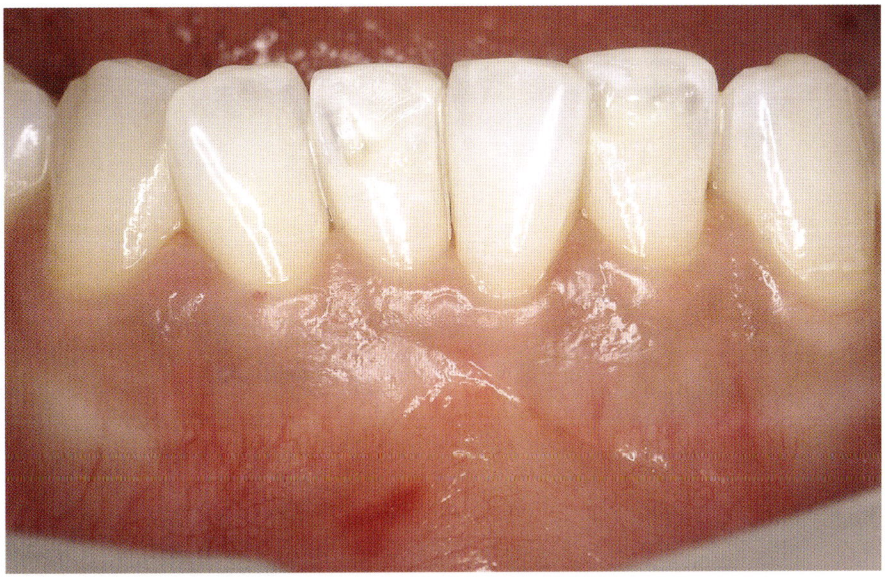

b. Removal of white spots with carbide burs.

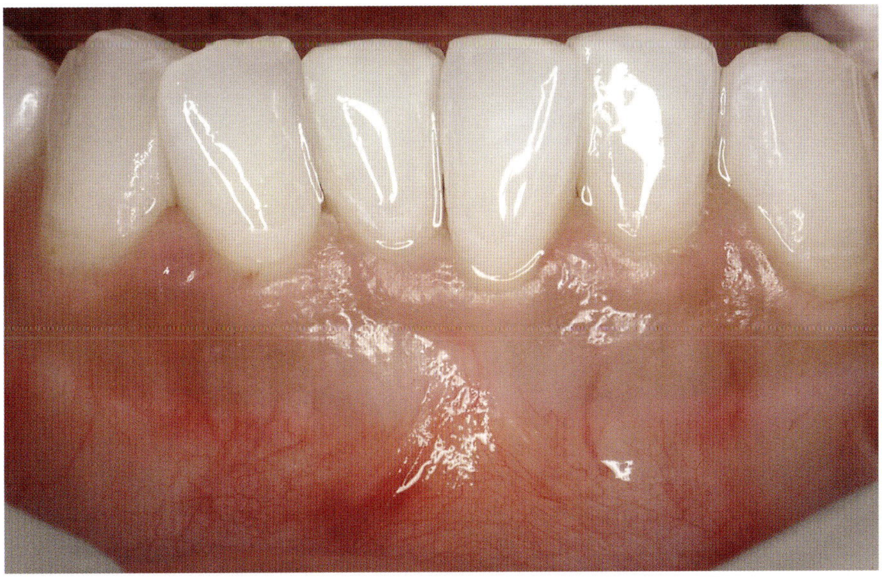

c. After composite resin filling of the lesion.

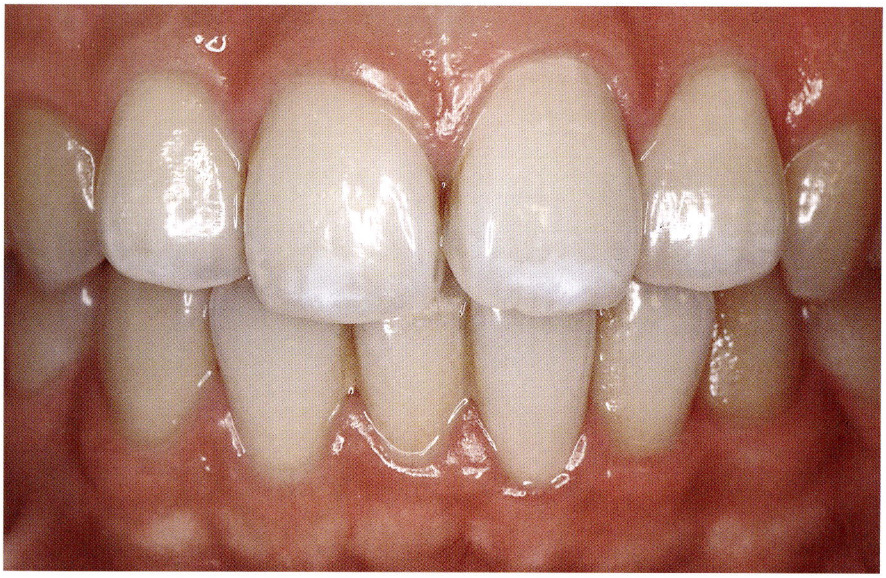

Fig. 5-8 Tooth whitening, microabrasion and restorative treatment.

a. Prior to tooth whitening, there was generalized yellow discoloration with white spots on the upper central incisors.

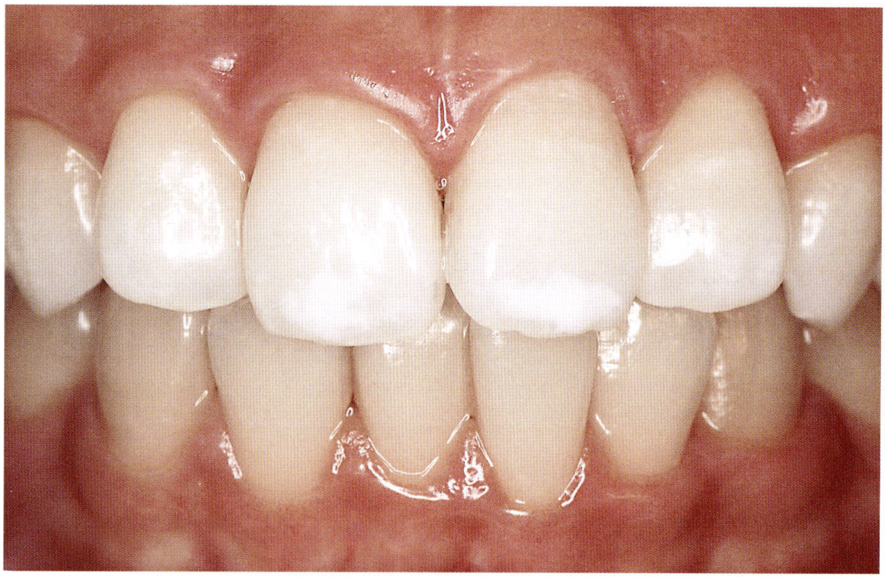

b. The white spots became even more noticeable after whitening of the upper arch.

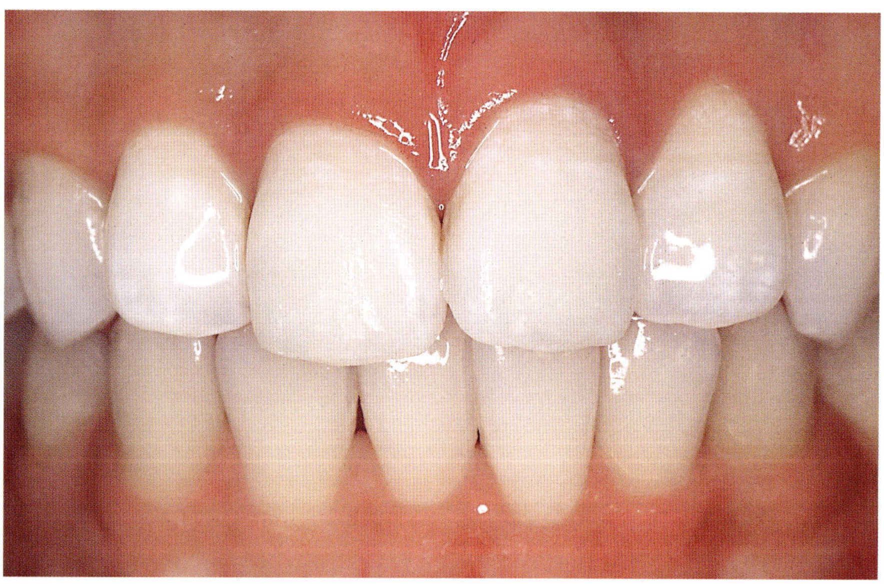

c. Microabrasion was initially attempted. However, the depth of the lesion required restorative treatment with composite resin.

Q&A

Question 1. How do you predict the depth of a lesion before treatment?

Answer: It is very difficult to predict the depth of the lesion. However, the incisal surface should be observed with a dental mirror or a loupe. This way, it is possible to evaluate how deep the decalcification has penetrated labio-lingually. During the microabrasion procedure, the teeth should be inspected from this aspect periodically.

Question 2. Do patients experience sensitivity after microabrasion?

Answer: When performed properly, microabrasion usually does not cause any sensitivity. However, if the enamel surface is removed excessively, the patient may experience sensitivity, and composite resin fillings may be required.

Question 3. Is the final result of microabrasion permanent?

Answer: One of the greatest advantages of microabrasion is that the result is usually permanent.

Question 4. Does the age of the patient need to be considered for microabrasion?

Answer: The age of the patient doesn't affect microabrasion. The most important factor is whether there is enough enamel thickness remaining.

References

Baumgartner JC, Reid DE, Pickett AB: Human pulpal reaction to the modified McInnes bleaching technique. J Endodont 1983; 9:527-529.

Croll TP. Enamel Microabrasion, Quintessence Publishing Co, Inc, 1991.

Goldstein RE, Garber DA. Complete Dental Bleaching, Quintessence Publishing Co, Inc, 1995.

Greenwall LH. Bleaching techniques in restorative dentistry, Martin Dunitz, 2001.

Kwon S. Tooth Whitening State of the Art, Dental Publishing Co, Inc, 2004.

Mcevoy SA. Removing Intrinsic Stains from Vital Teeth by Microabrasion and Bleaching. J Esthet Dent 1995; 7:104-109.

Ritter AV. Microabrasion. J Esthet Restor Dent 2005; 17:384.

Sundfeld RH. Enamel Microabrasion Followed by Dental Bleaching for Patients after Orthodontic Treatment-Case Reports. Oper Dent 2007; 19:71-78.

Suzuki M. Esthetic Improvement of "White Spot" Enamel Stains. J Esthet Dent 1991; 3:34-36.

chapter 6

Gingival bleaching

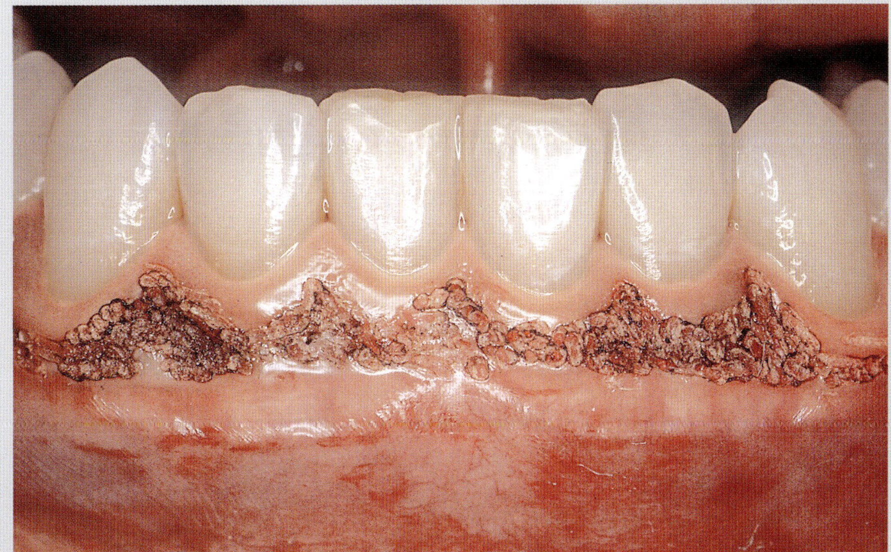

It is not uncommon to see beautifully aligned bright teeth with unsightly dark gingiva, which can be very annoying to patients. Staining of the gingiva can be seen in the upper and lower anterior labial attached gingiva, and may be classified into extrinsic and intrinsic discoloration. Causes of intrinsic discoloration include melanin, melanoid, oxyhemoglobin, reduced hemoglobin and carotin. The most common intrinsic cause is melanin, which is produced by melanocytes located at the basal layer of the epithelium. Smoking, poor oral hygiene, and oral contraceptives stimulate melanocytes to produce large amounts of melanin, leading to its accumulation. Extrinsic causes include amalgam, iron, etc. Pigments are usually distributed in the basal layer of the epithelium and may be removed surgically, chemically, or by laser ablation.

Surgical removal of discolored gingiva

Surgical removal of superficial stained attached gingiva with a high-speed carbide bur or a #15 blade scalpel can be easily accomplished under anesthesia (Fig. 6-1).

- Administer local anesthesia after topical anesthesia.
- Remove the superficial stained attached gingiva using high-speed carbide bur. Removal can also be performed with a #15 blade scalpel.
- Achieve hemostasis by applying pressure with a piece of gauze for 5 minutes.
- Instruct the patient of the possibility of pain and edema, and prescribe analgesics for pain control.

Chemical removal of discolored gingiva

The phenol-alcohol method of chemical removal was introduced by Hirschfeld in 1951. It works by detaching the epithelium along with the melanin pigments by causing rapid coagulation and necrosis of the epithelium (Fig. 6-2).

- Apply topical anesthesia.
- Soak a cotton swab in phenol solution and apply it to the stained surface for 30 seconds.
- Apply ethanol for 30 seconds to neutralize the phenol.
- Rinse with a copious amount of water.
- Detachment of the epithelium layer occurs within 3 days, followed by healing of the epithelium in 5 to 7 days.
- Regeneration of the gingiva is completed in 2 to 3 weeks.
- The regeneration state of the gingiva is checked after 20 to 25 days, and the procedure is repeated, if necessary.

Laser treatment of discolored gingiva

A laser is a monochromatic light beam that delivers concentrated energy to the irradiated site. The amount of energy absorbed is determined by the wavelength of the laser beam (nm), the energy output, and the optical characteristics of the treated area. The diode laser is especially useful for the removal of stained gingiva. Diode lasers have a wavelength of 812–980 nm; which coincides with the absorption pattern of melanin (Fig. 6-3).

- Apply topical anesthesia.
- Protect the eyes of the dentist, assistant, and the patient with protective eyewear.
- Using the pulse mode rather than the continuous mode, irradiate the area with the tip of the diode laser in 0.5 second intervals.
- Rinse with water and finish.
- Detachment of the epithelial layer occurs within 3 days, followed by healing of the epithelium in 5 to 7 days.
- Regeneration of the gingiva is completed in 2 to 3 weeks.

Advantages of laser treatment for gingival bleaching

- Accurate removal of melanin pigments with immediate hemostasis is possible.
- Less damage to adjacent tissue.
- Minimal postoperative swelling and pain.
- Less chance of postoperative infection.

••• Gingiva with severe melanin accumulation may be treated surgically, chemically, or by laser.

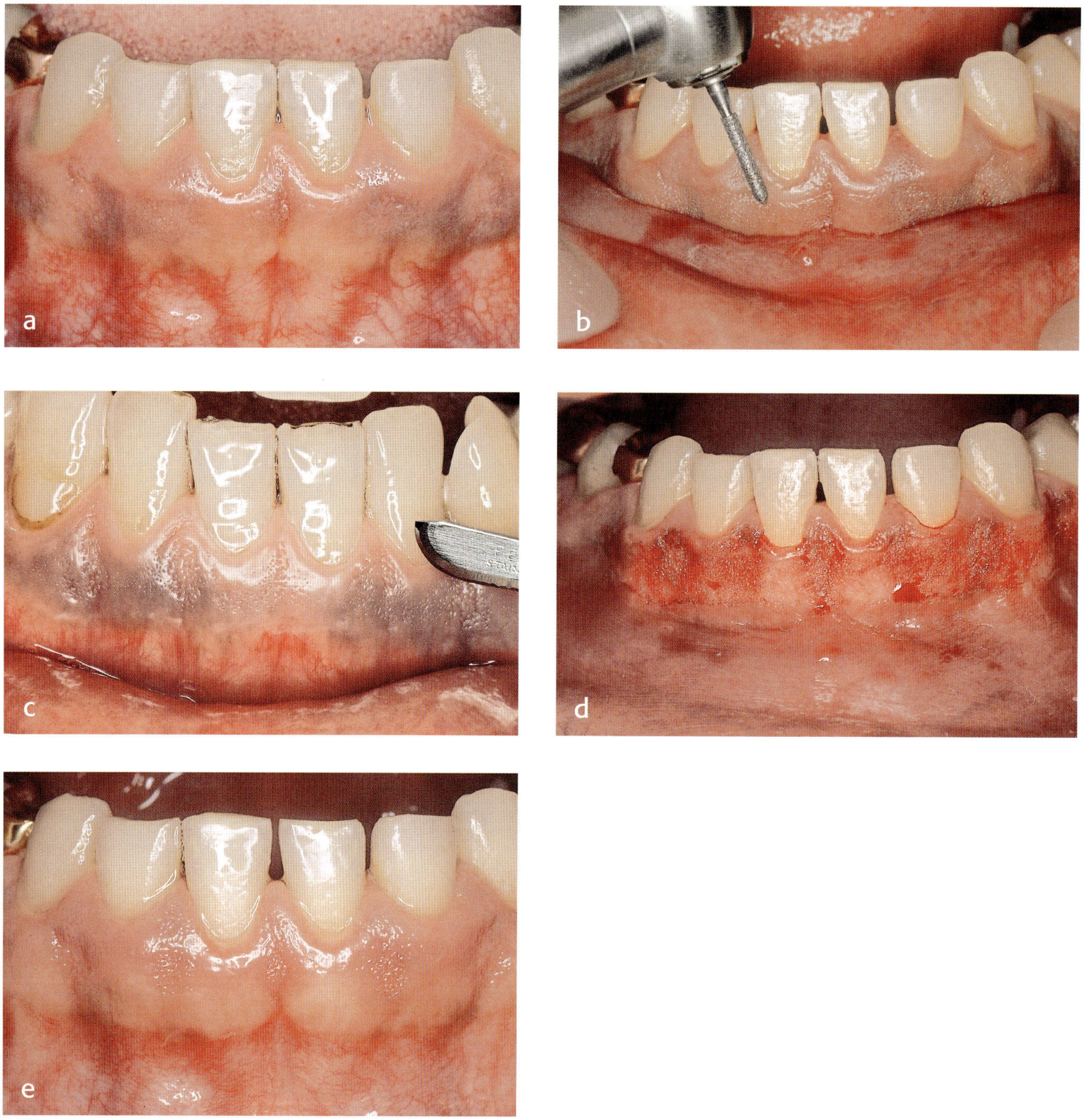

Fig. 6-1 Surgical removal.

a. Melanin pigmentation on the attached gingiva of the lower anterior teeth.
b. The surface of the attached gingiva was removed with high-speed carbide bur.
c. It can also be scraped off with a #15 blade scalpel.
d. Immediately after melanin pigmentation removal.
e. Follow-up after one year shows little relapse.

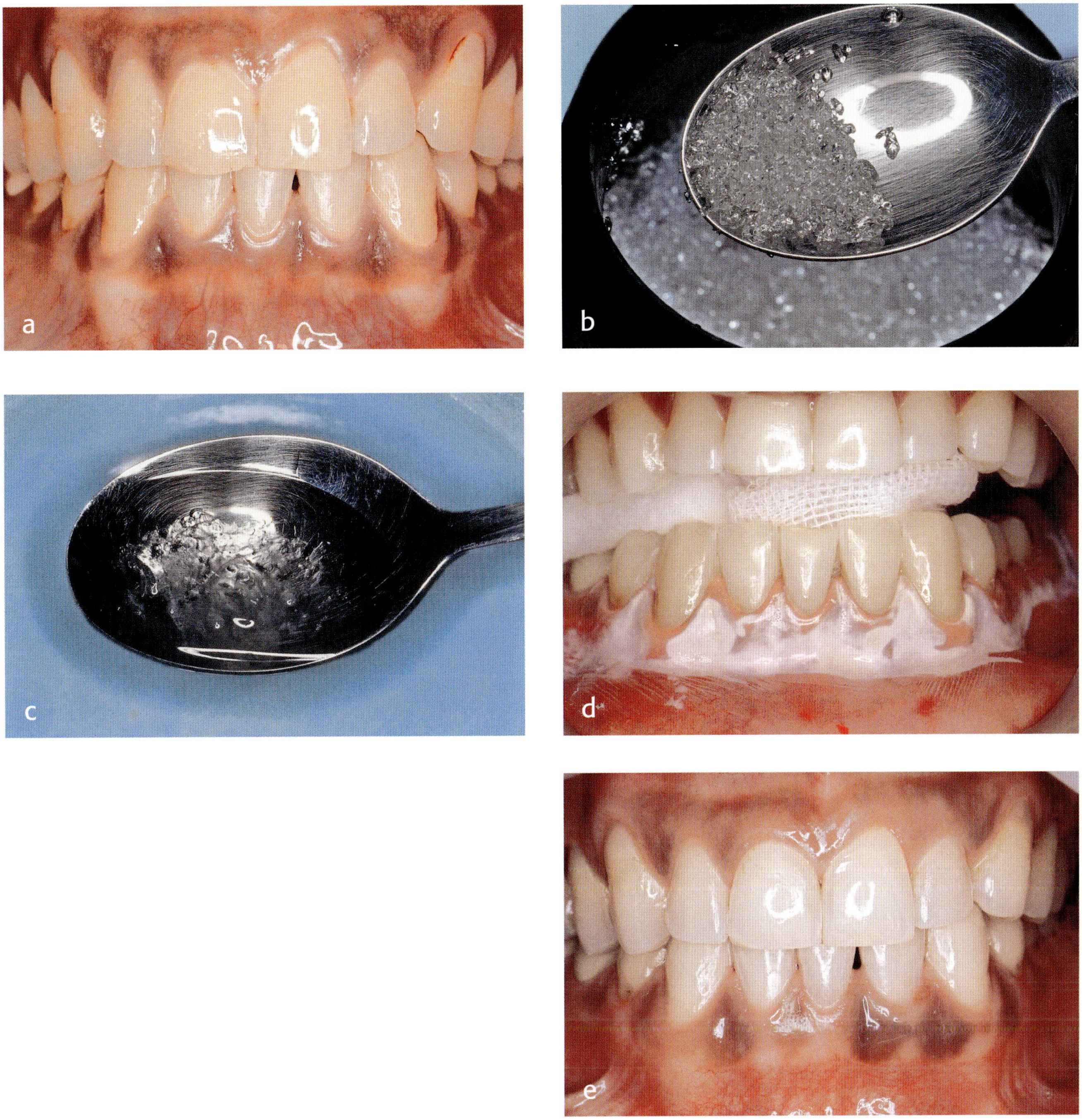

Fig. 6-2 Chemical removal.

a. Prior to gingival bleaching.

b. Phenol particles are placed on a spoon and melted with warm water.

c. The phenol particles melt into liquid form.

d. The phenol is applied to the attached gingiva with cotton swabs.

e. The 5 year follow-up photo shows a noticeable relapse of melanin pigmentation.

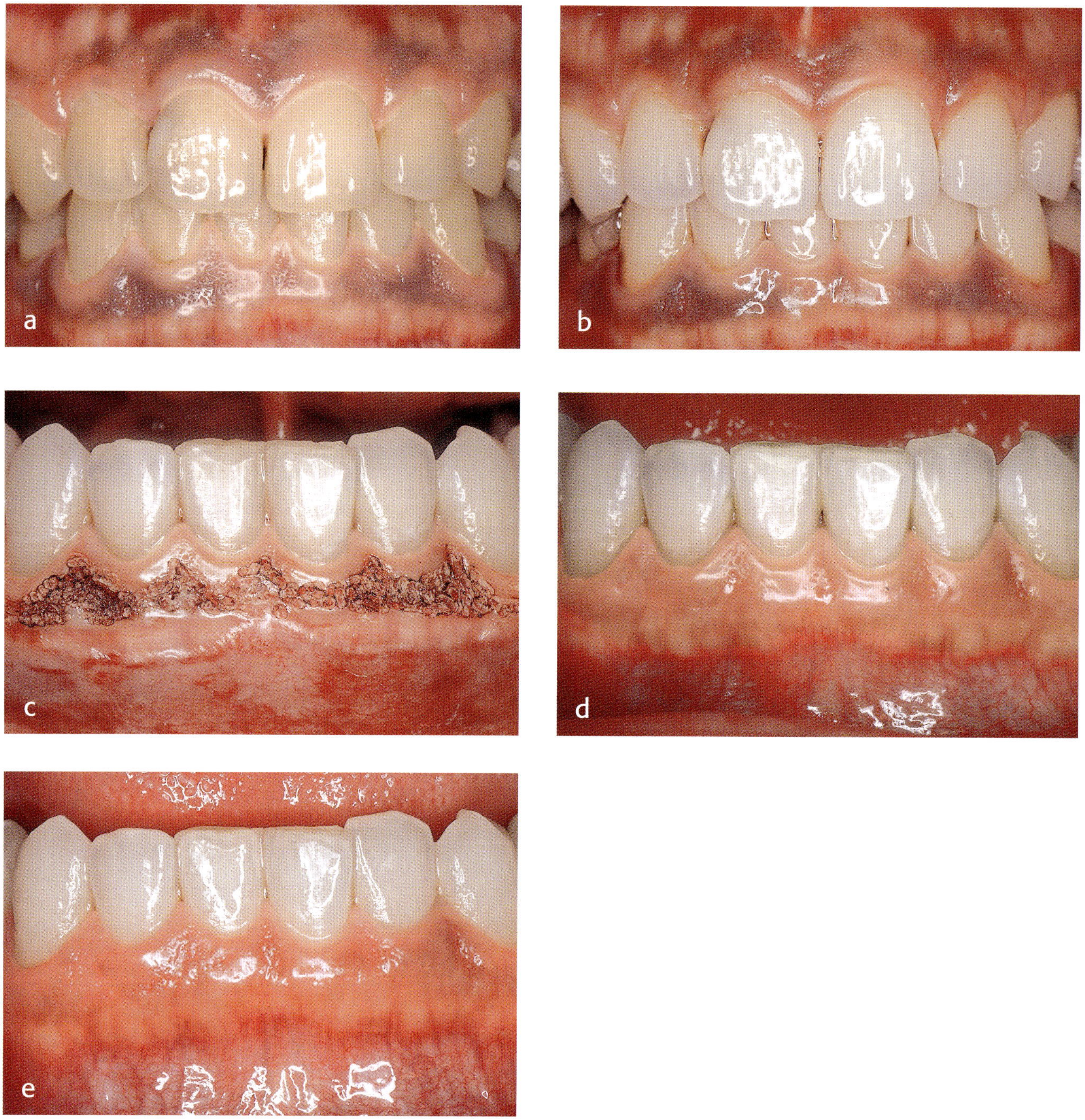

Fig. 6-3 Laser treatment.

a. Prior to tooth and gingival bleaching.

b. After tooth whitening, the whiteness of the teeth makes the melanin pigmentation on the gingiva even more noticeable.

c. The melanin pigmentation on the attached gingiva was removed with a diode laser.

d. After gingival healing.

e. Good maintenance was noted at the 2-year follow-up.

Q&A

Question 1. How long does the effect of gingival bleaching last?
Answer: It varies depending on the cause of melanin pigmentation and the method of treatment. Relapse tends to be faster in smokers.

Question 2. Should a perio pack be applied after gingival bleaching?
Answer: A perio pack is not necessary after gingival bleaching. However, verify that the bleeding has stopped (especially after surgical removal) and prescribe ice packs and analgesics.

Question 3. Is anesthesia necessary for gingival bleaching?
Answer: For surgical removal, topical anesthesia followed by local anesthesia is needed. For chemical and laser removal, only topical anesthesia is recommended.

References

長谷川明, 岡本秀生. Phenol-Alcohol 法による歯肉部メラニン色素除去法, 42(5), 673–676, 1973.
Hisamitsu H, Toko T. Tooth Whitening basics and clinical techniques. Quintessence Japan, 2004.
Kwon S. Tooth Whitening State of the Art, Dental Publishing Co, Inc, 2004.

chapter

7

Tooth whitening in esthetic dentistry

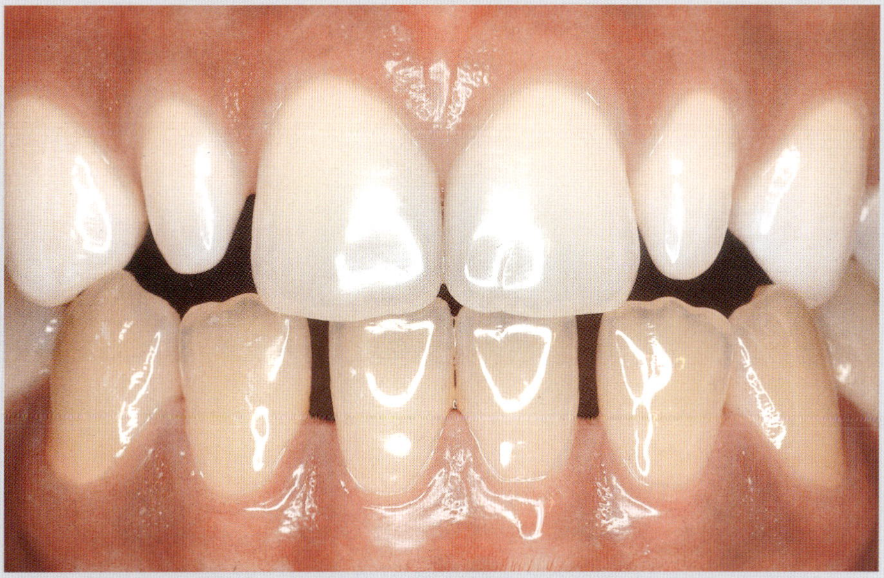

Clinical classification of tooth whitening

Proper consultation is the key factor to success in tooth whitening. Consultation should vary according to the severity of the discoloration and the extent and complexity of the total treatment. Kwon classifies all whitening cases as basic, moderate or advanced bleaching cases to provide a systematic approach to whitening and to facilitate consultation (Table 7-1). This approach makes it possible for the clinician to include tooth whitening more actively into daily practice.

Basic bleaching case (BBC)

Patients who only desire whitening of their teeth and require no further dental treatment belong to a basic bleaching case category. Consultation should focus on the various whitening programs available so that the patients can choose the specific program that is best suited for them. Treatment should be specifically designed to achieve maximum whiteness according to the patient's wishes (Fig. 7-1).

Moderate bleaching case (MBC)

In some cases, tooth whitening must be combined with simple composite resin bondings, laminate veneers or all-ceramic crowns to meet the expectations of the patient regarding a beautiful smile. In these moderate bleaching cases treatment should be aimed at achieving an esthetic result with minimum tooth reduction. Therefore, a conservative approach combining tooth whitening with bonded restorations can be proposed to the patient. Consultation on special maintenance care of the whitened teeth and the bonded restorations is needed (Figs. 7-2 to 7-4).

Advanced bleaching case (ABC)

Tooth whitening can be proposed as part of a very comprehensive treatment including various treatment procedures to improve the total esthetic outcome. In advanced bleaching cases, tooth whitening is usually performed selectively on the remaining natural teeth. Treatment should be aimed at recovering function and esthetics with minimal pain and discomfort. Since advanced bleaching cases with an extended treatment time can be very exhausting to patients, consultation on proper sequencing of every procedure is of utmost importance (Figs. 7-5 and 6).

Table 7-1 Classification of tooth whitening cases.

Basic Bleaching Case	Moderate Bleaching Case	Advanced Bleaching Case
Chief complaint: Discoloration of teeth.	More beautiful smile.	Recovery of function and esthetics.
Treatment sequence: Oral prophylaxis followed by tooth whitening. Home, power or both combined.	Oral prophylaxis followed by tooth whitening. Home, power or both combined. Bonded esthetic restorations should be placed 2 weeks after whitening to allow for color stability and recovery of bonding strength of enamel.	Pain control and recovery of function should be of first priority. Oral surgery, periodontal surgery and orthodontic treatment are performed prior to tooth whitening. In some cases, tooth whitening can be used as a starter treatment or scheduled during the healing or retention phase.
Treatment duration: 2–6 weeks.	2–3 months.	3 months to several years.
Special considerations: Various whitening programs should be available to the patient. Treatment should be aimed at achieving whiteness according to the patient's expectations. Since the bulk of the treatment is performed by staff members, proper role assignment is important.	Treatment should be aimed to achieve a esthetic result with minimum tooth reduction. Meticulous care is required to match the color of the esthetic bonded restoration to the whitened teeth.	Treatment should be aimed to recover function and esthetics with minimal pain and discomfort. Extended treatment times can be very exhausting to the patient. Therefore, continuous motivation and encouragement should be provided.
Maintenance care: Regular prophylaxis every 6 months and touch-up whitening, as needed.	Regular prophylaxis every 6 months and touch-up whitening, as needed. Special attention should be given to proper maintenance of the bonded restorations.	Regular prophylaxis every 6 months and touch-up whitening, as needed. Special attention should be given to proper maintenance of the complex treatment.

Fig. 7-1 Basic bleaching case.

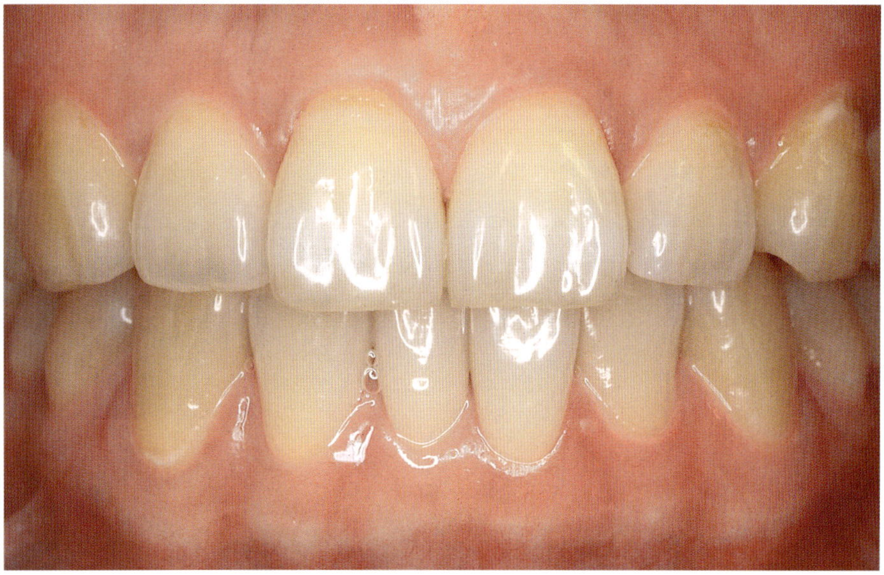

a. Generalized yellow discoloration.

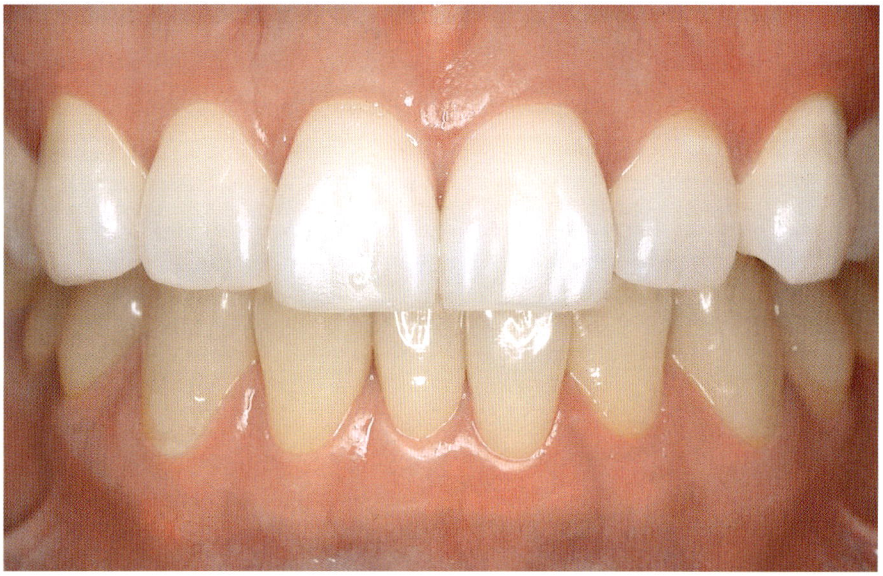

b. Color difference after 3 weeks of home and power whitening of the upper arch.

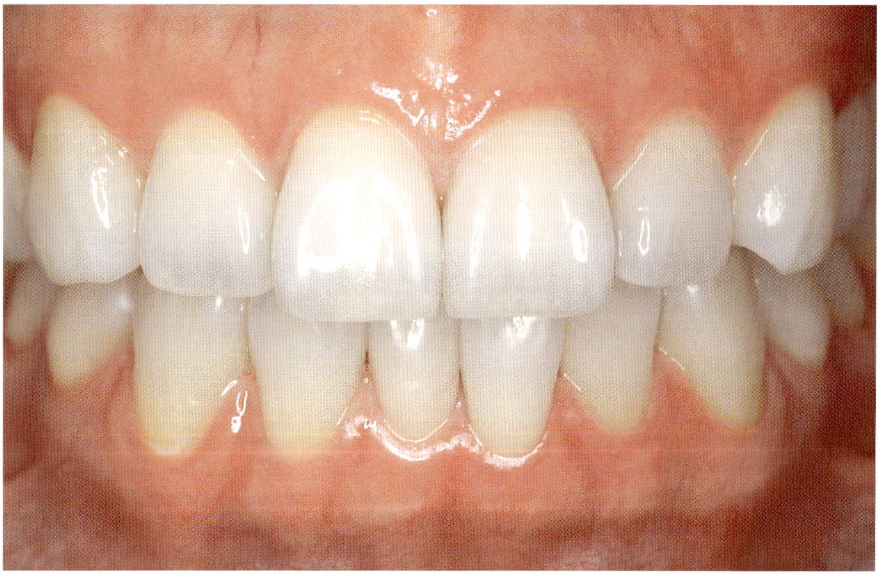

c. According to patient's wishes, the patient had extremely white teeth after whitening treatment.

Fig. 7-2 Moderate bleaching case.

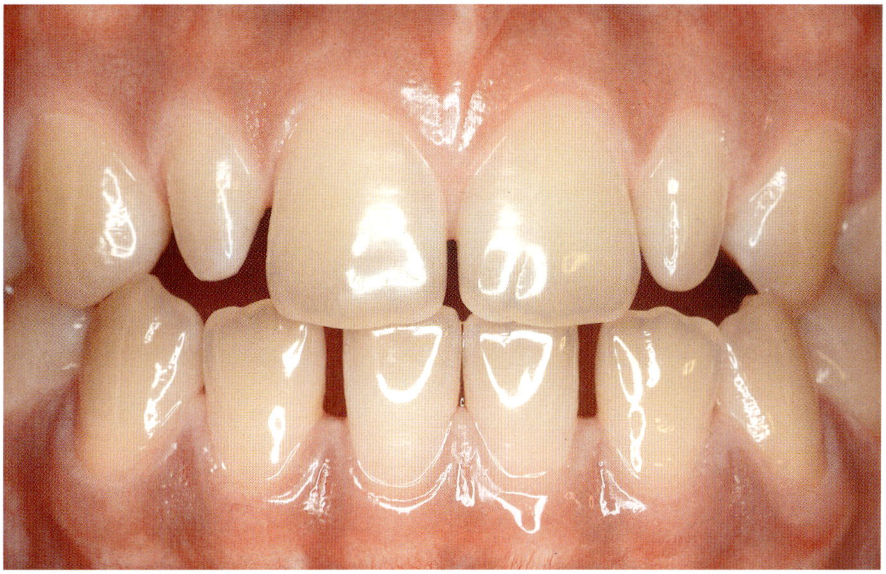

a. Generalized yellow discoloration with spacing.

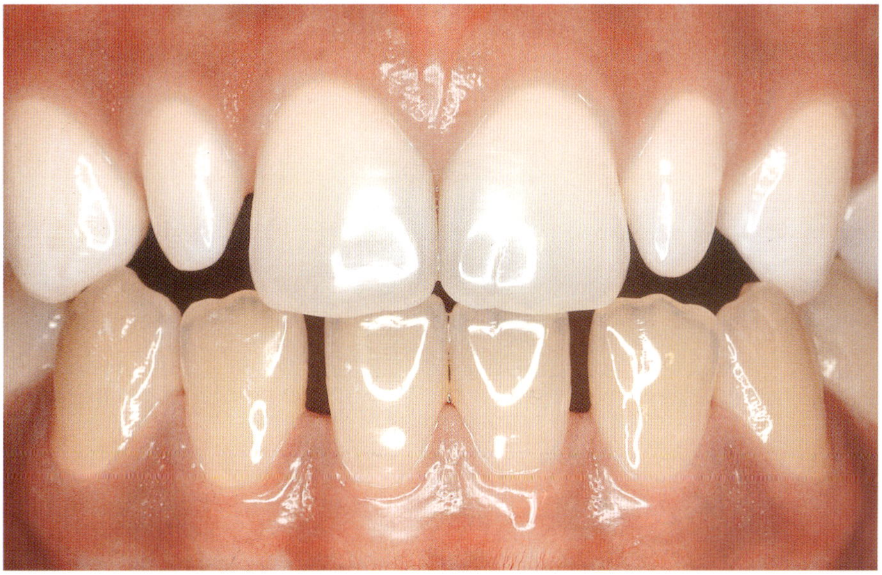

b. Minor tooth movement of the upper central incisors with a clear retainer, followed by tooth whitening of the upper arch.

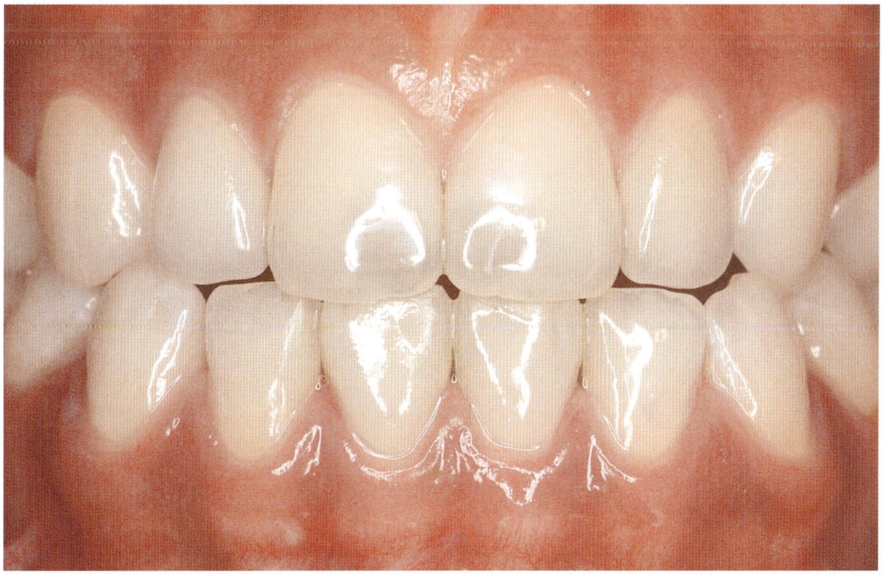

c. Treatment was completed with porcelain laminate veneers on the upper lateral incisors and composite resin bonding on the lower central incisors.

Fig. 7-3 Moderate bleaching case.

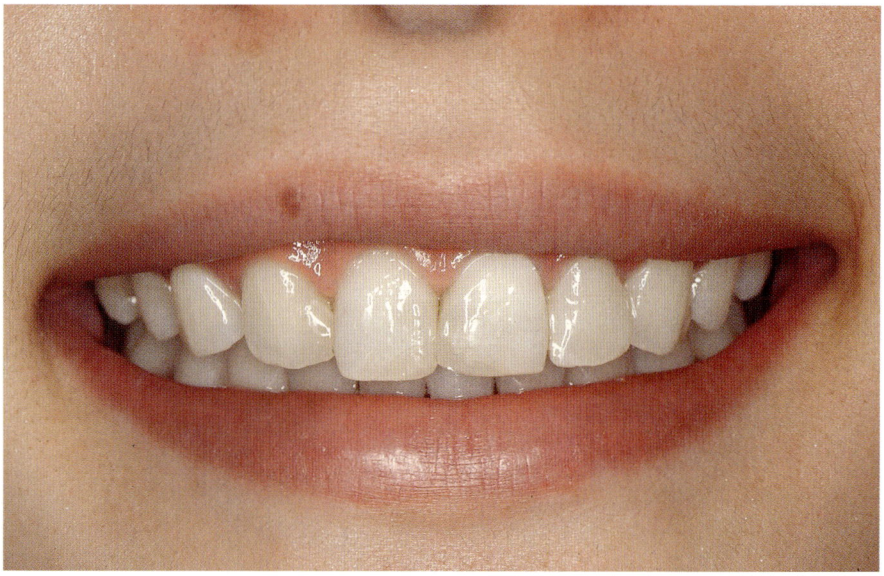

a. Generalized yellow discoloration with extensive composite restorations due to former traumatic injury to the four upper incisors.

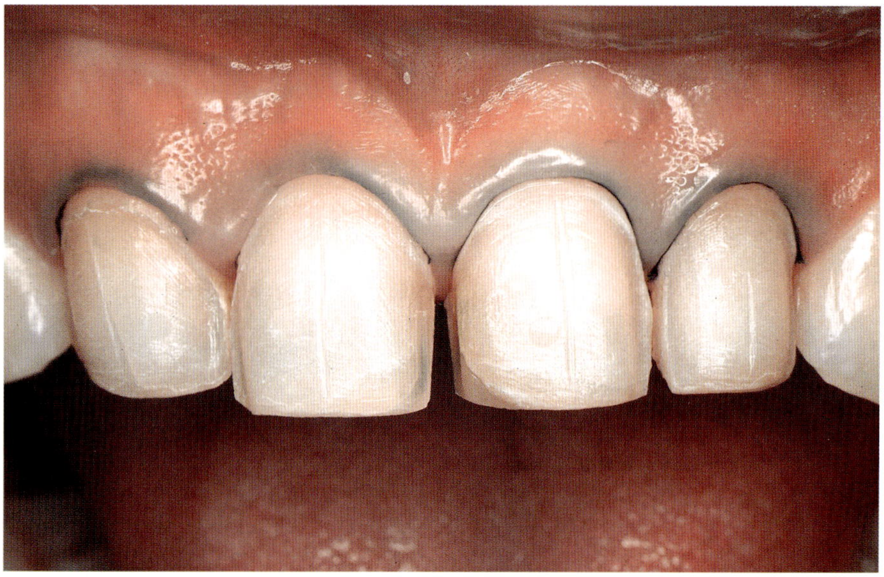

b. Home and power whitening were followed by placement of four porcelain laminate veneers on the upper incisors.

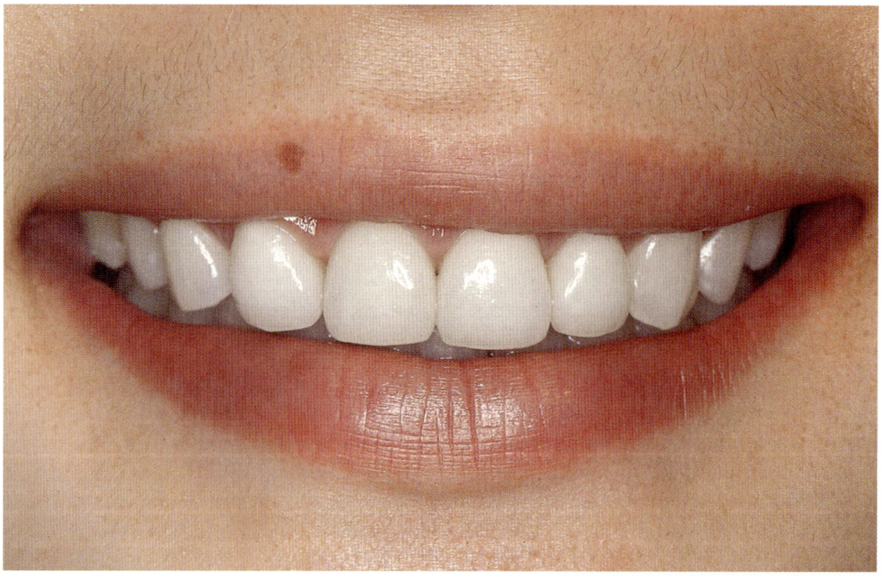

c. Smile after treatment.

Fig. 7-4 Moderate bleaching case.

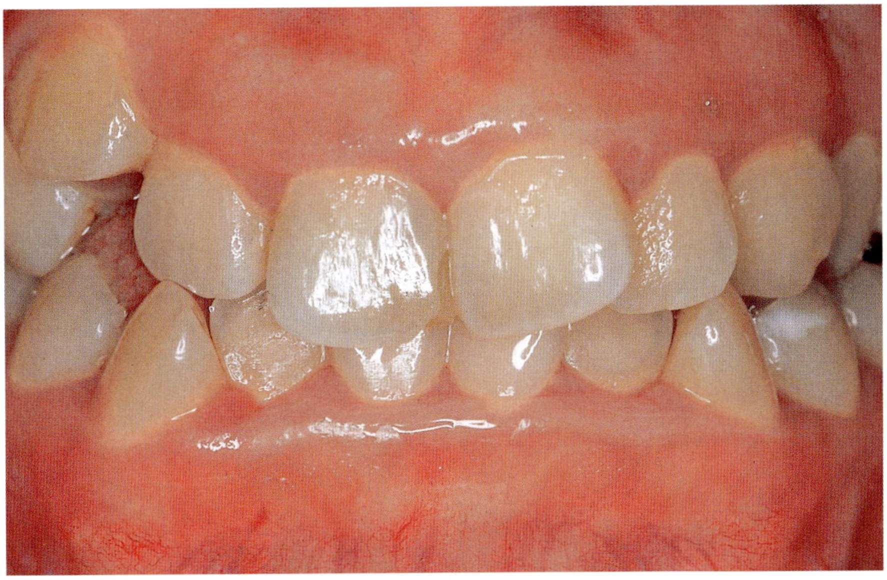

a. Generalized yellow discoloration with short clinical crowns.

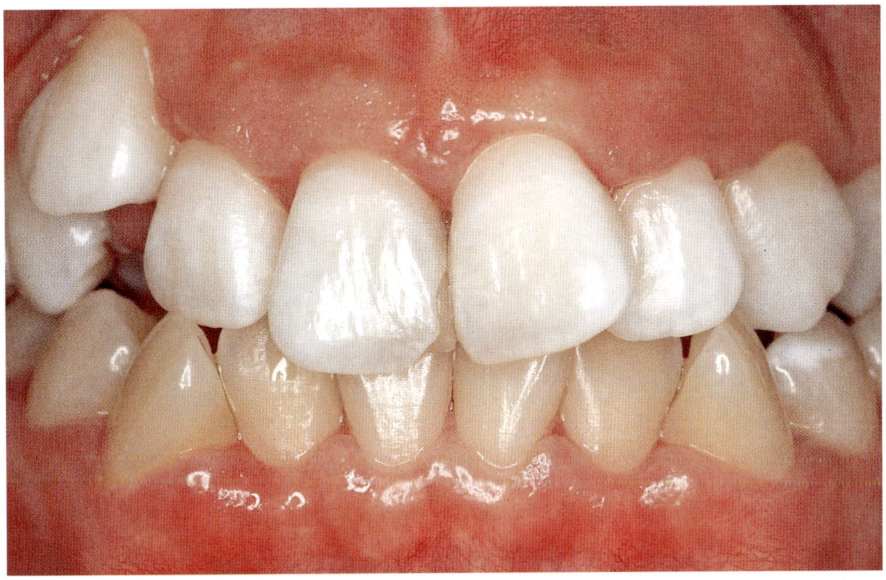

b. Crown lengthening procedure followed by home and power whitening of the upper arch.

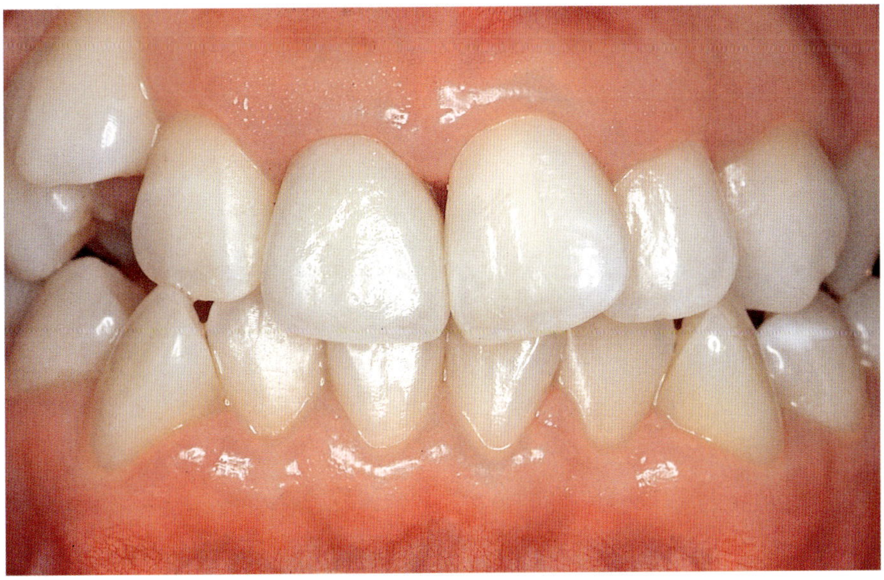

c. Treatment was completed with placement of an Empress crown on the upper right central incisor.

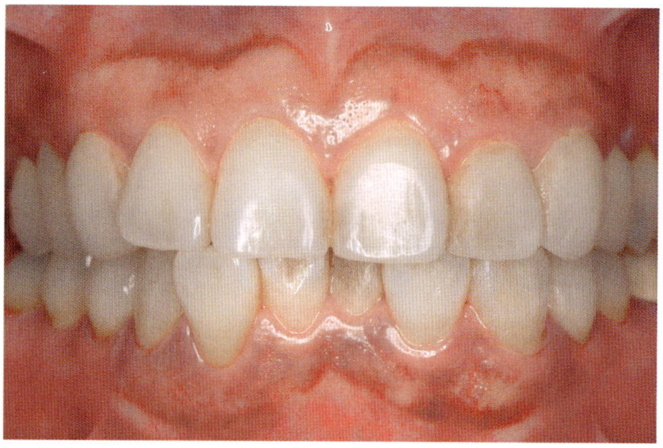

Fig. 7-5 Advanced bleaching case.

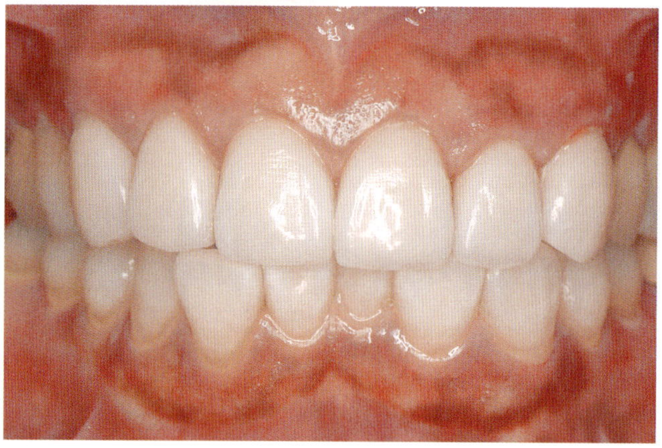

a. Generalized yellow discoloration with former direct resin veneers on the upper anterior teeth and crowding of the lower incisors.

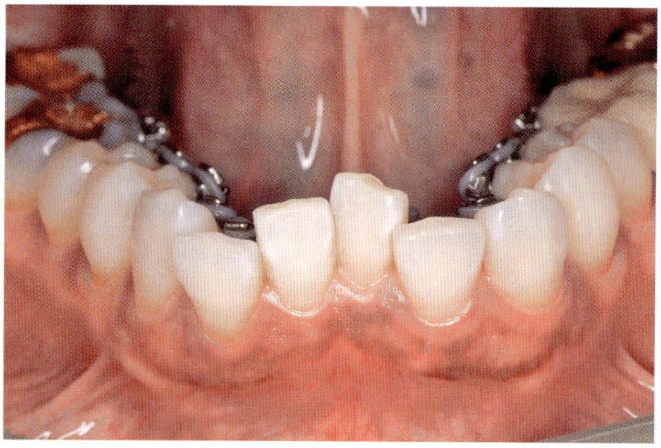

b. Home and power whitening were followed by placement of six porcelain laminate veneers on the upper incisors.

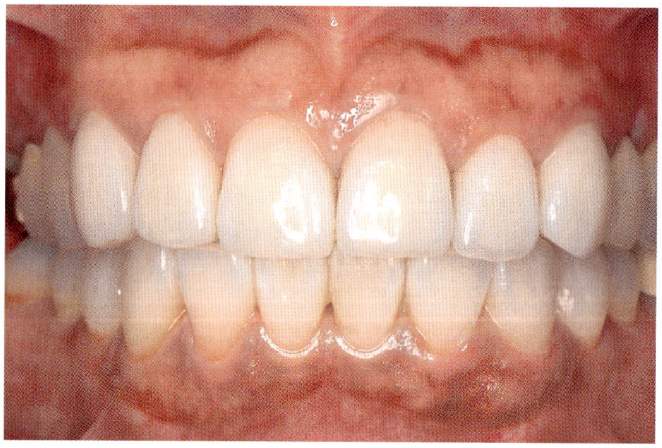

c. Following improvement of esthetics after whitening and veneer placement, the patient desired lingual orthodontics to improve the alignment of the lower teeth.

d. Smile after completion of treatment 10 months later.

Fig. 7-6 Advanced bleaching case.

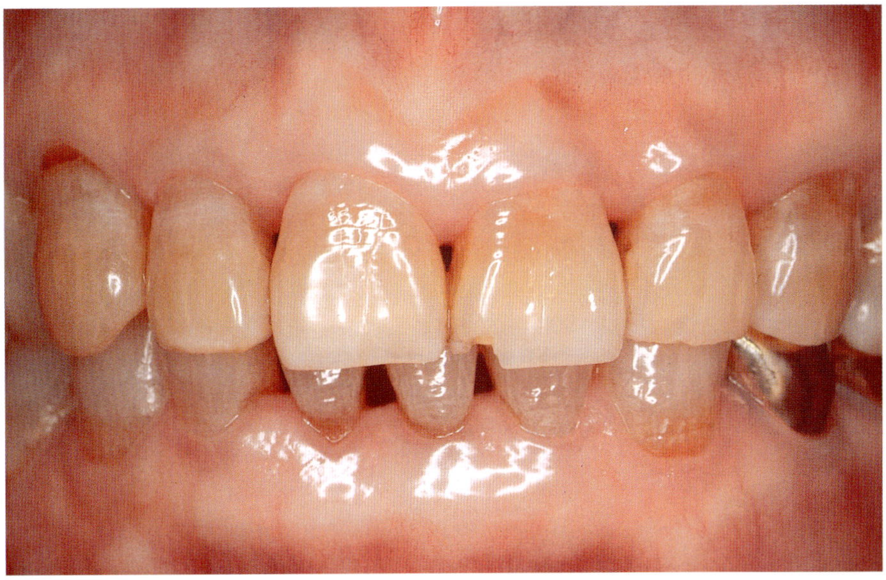

a. The patient desired to replace her lower removable partial denture with implant restorations. Whitening was recommended to treat the generalized yellow to brown discoloration.

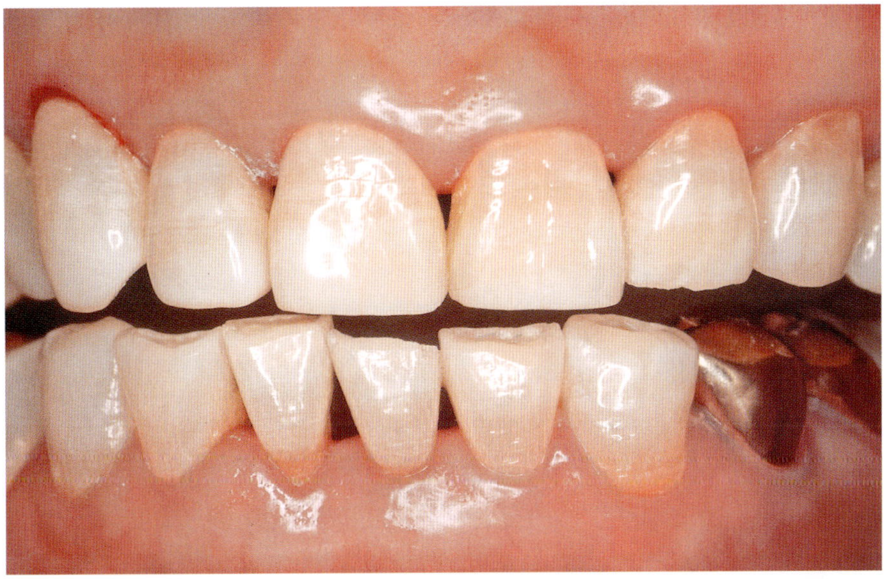

b. Home and power whitening were combined during the healing phase after implant surgery.

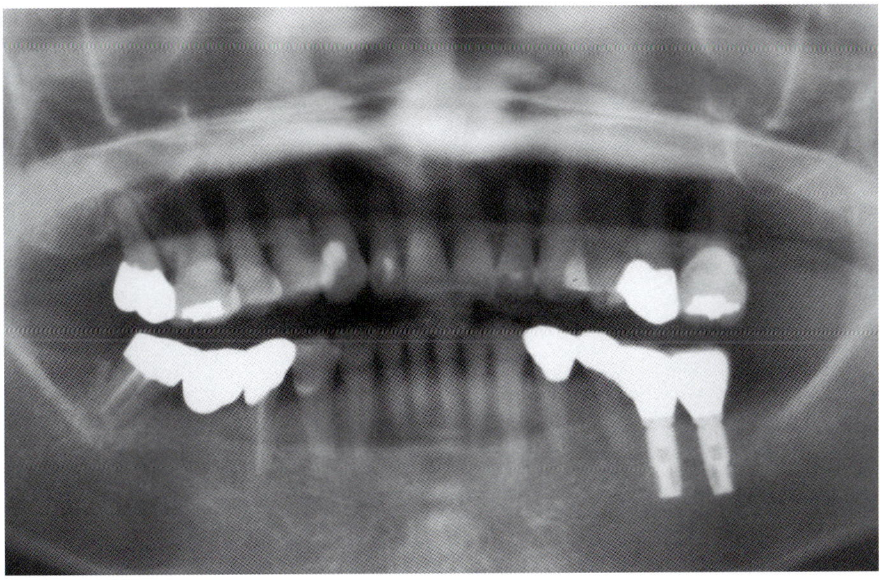

c. Panoramic radiograph after completion of treatment 4 months later.

Tetracycline discolorations

Tetracycline is a broad-spectrum antibiotic used to treat various infections. Tetracycline not only affects the tooth shade, but also causes enamel hypoplasia and deposits in bone. Therefore, tetracycline should be taken with caution from the second trimester of pregnancy on, as this is when tooth development starts, and it should also be used with caution by children up to the age of 8 years. During the tooth mineralization stage, tetracycline seems to penetrate into the dentine and form orthophosphate. As the tooth is exposed to sunlight, the discoloration becomes even more severe (Fig. 7-7). Therefore, the labial side of the anterior teeth is usually darker than the posterior teeth. The shade varies from yellow-brown to purple, and the discoloration is permanent because, unlike bone, there is no remodeling of tooth structure.

Classification of tetracycline discolorations

Tetracycline discolorations may be classified according to the severity of discoloration, shade, and presence of banding (Table 7-2). According to the classification by Jordan and Boksman, mild to moderate tetracycline discoloration with uniformly distributed yellow-grey to yellow-brown discolorations can be treated with tooth whitening. Whitening can be attempted in cases with severe discoloration with marked banding, but the prognosis is questionable. In dark discolorations with surface defects, it is recommended to restore rather than whiten the teeth.

Minocycline is a synthetic derivative of tetracycline that is used to treat acne or various systemic infections. Minocycline is absorbed through the digestive tract and forms an insoluble compound with iron, causing tooth discoloration, even in adults with completed tooth development. Discolorations caused by minocycline are generally mild and possible to treat with tooth whitening.

Table 7-2 Classification of tetracycline discolorations.

	Degree according to Jordan & Boksman, 1984	
1	Mild discoloration	Uniformly distributed yellow-grey discoloration
2	Moderate discoloration	Uniformly distributed yellow-brown discoloration
3	Severe discoloration	Blue-grey or black discoloration with marked banding
4	Untreatable discoloration	Dark discoloration with surface defects

Treatment options for tetracycline discolorations

The various treatment options available for the treatment of tetracycline discolorations range from conservative approaches with no tooth reduction to more aggressive approaches including intentional endodontics and tooth reduction for esthetic restorations (Figs. 7-8 to 7-10). The treatment should be based on the severity of the discoloration and the patient's expectations and desires. In 1982, Abou-Rass reported that intra coronal bleaching of tetracycline-stained teeth has been shown to be predictable and to improve tooth shade without significant clinical complications. In 1997, Haywood reported that good results can be achieved in cooperative patients after 6 months of home whitening and that there was no damage to the enamel surface as determined by scanning electron microscopy.

Treatment options for tetracycline discolorations

- Treatment without tooth reduction
  - Home whitening
  - Power whitening
  - Combination of home and power whitening
- Treatment with tooth reduction
  - Laminate veneers or full-coverage restorations
  - Combination of whitening and restorative treatments
  - Intentional root canal treatment and internal bleaching

••• Since patients asking for esthetic treatment usually have high expectations of treatment outcome, tooth whitening should always be included in the treatment plan.

Fig. 7-7 The color of tetracycline discoloration changed, probably due to exposure to sunlight, as the patient grew up.

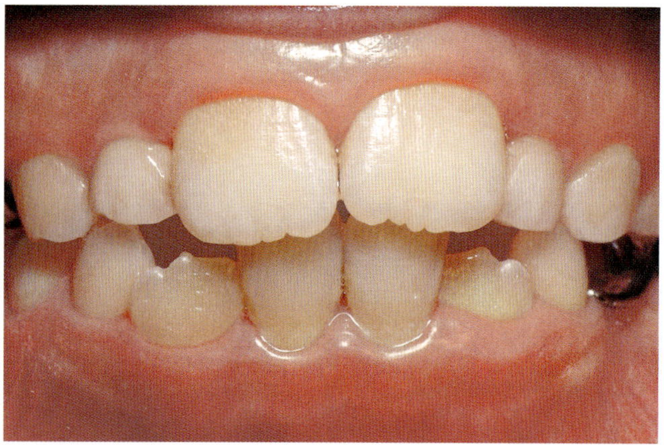

a. On eruption of the central incisors, mild tetracycline discoloration was suspected.

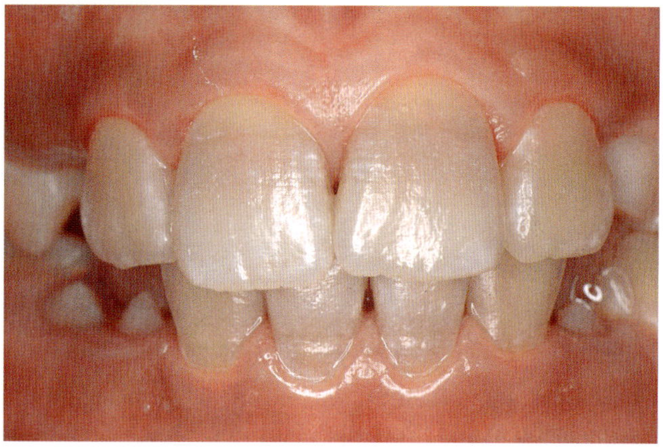

b. Darkening of the tetracycline discoloration could be observed.

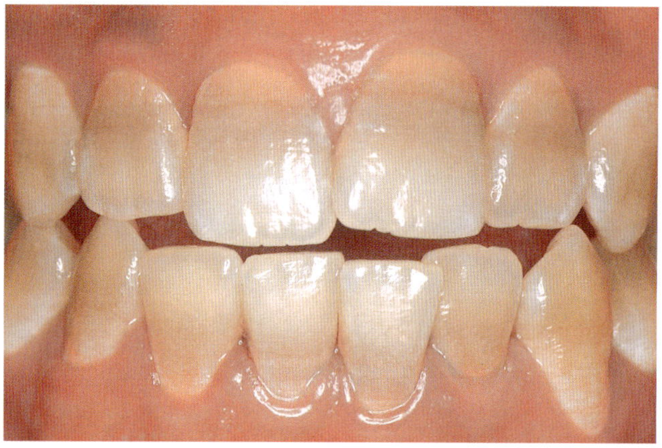

c. The patient and the parents realized the need for treatment as the dark banded areas in the cervical area got worse.

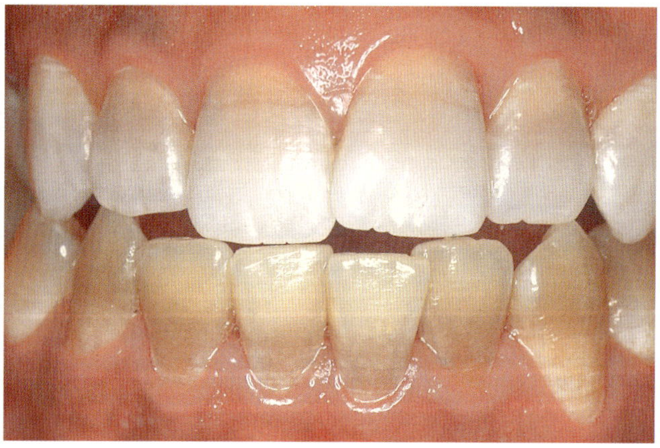

d. Combined home and power whitening was performed on the upper arch for 2 months. Treatment was continued on the lower arch after the patient was satisfied with the color of the upper teeth.

Fig. 7-8 Treatment of tetracycline discoloration without tooth reduction.

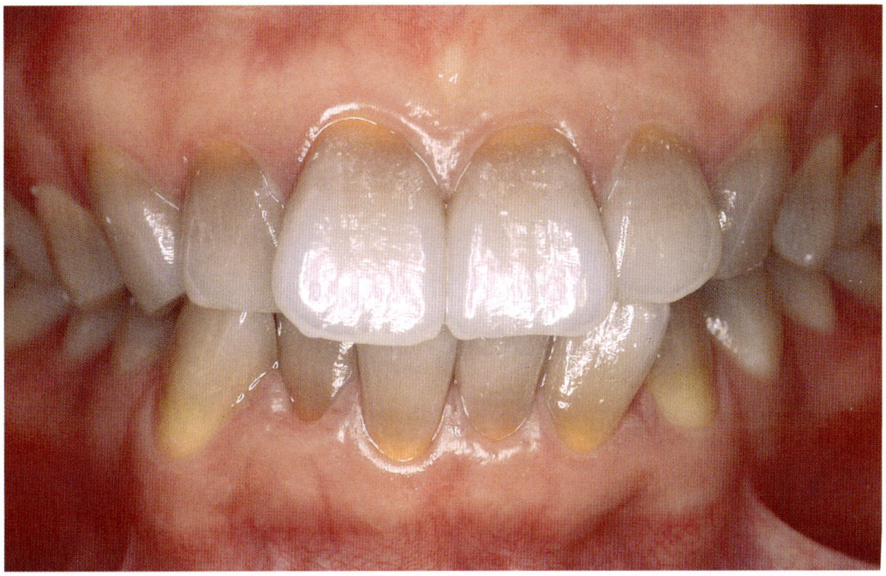

a. Uniformly distributed grey tetracycline discoloration with brown cervical bands.

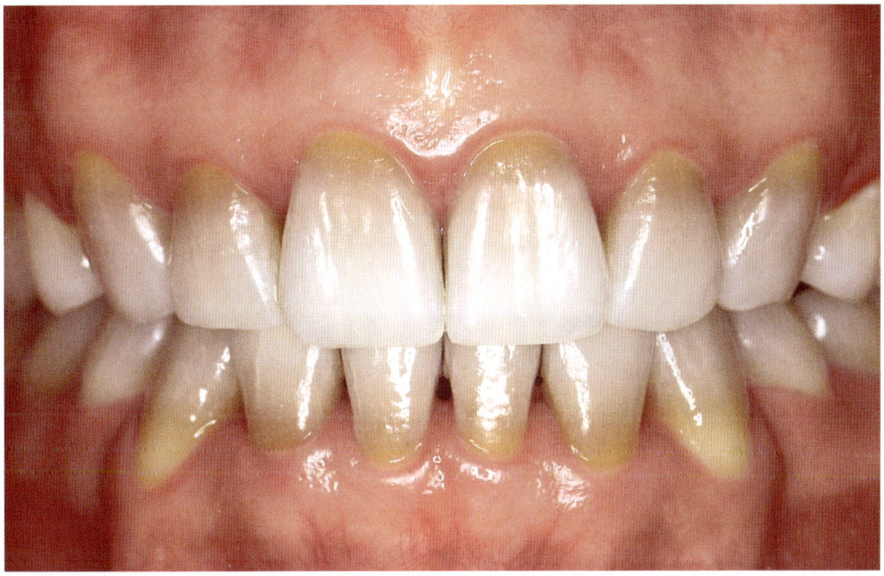

b. Home and power whitening combined was performed for 4 months, followed by orthodontic treatment.

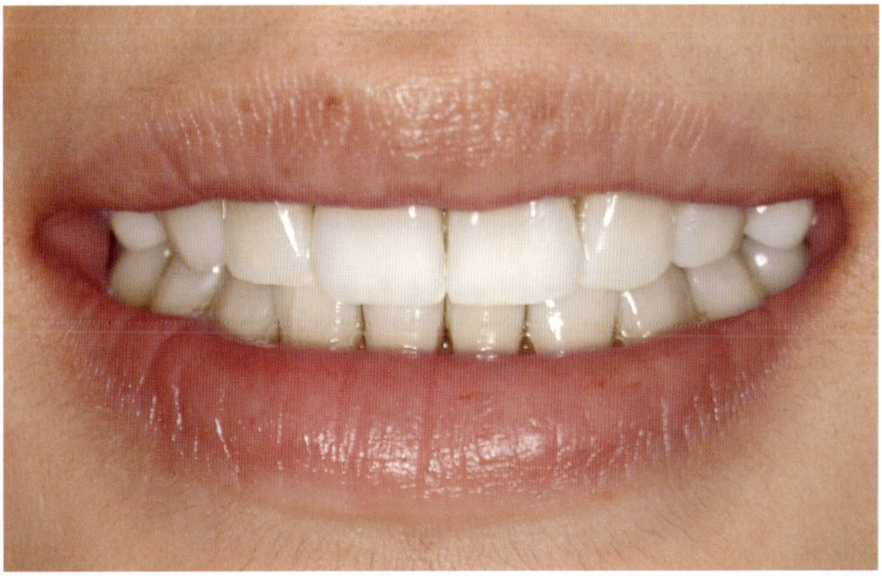

c. Happy smile after treatment.

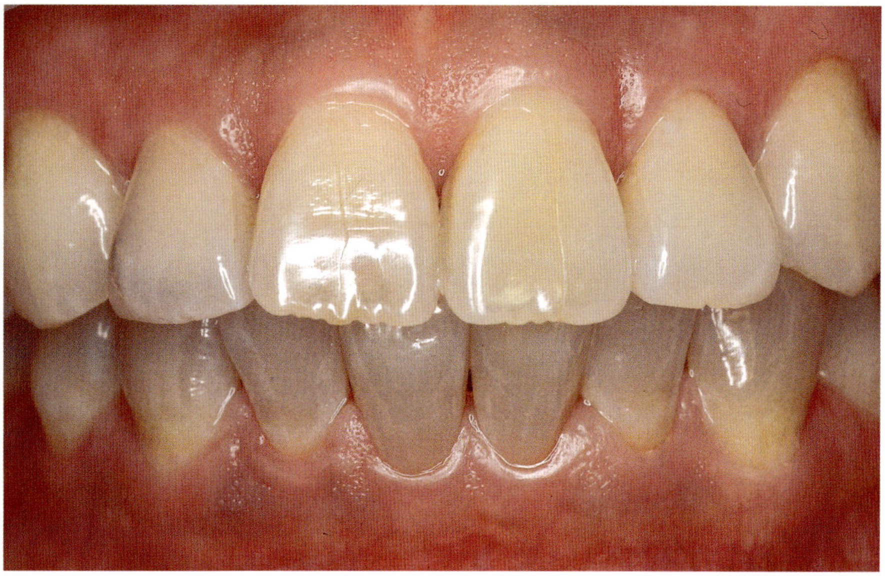

Fig. 7-9 Treatment of tetracycline discoloration with combinations of whitening and restorative treatment.

a. Uniformly distributed brown to grey discoloration. The patient desired improvement of the color and shape of the upper incisors.

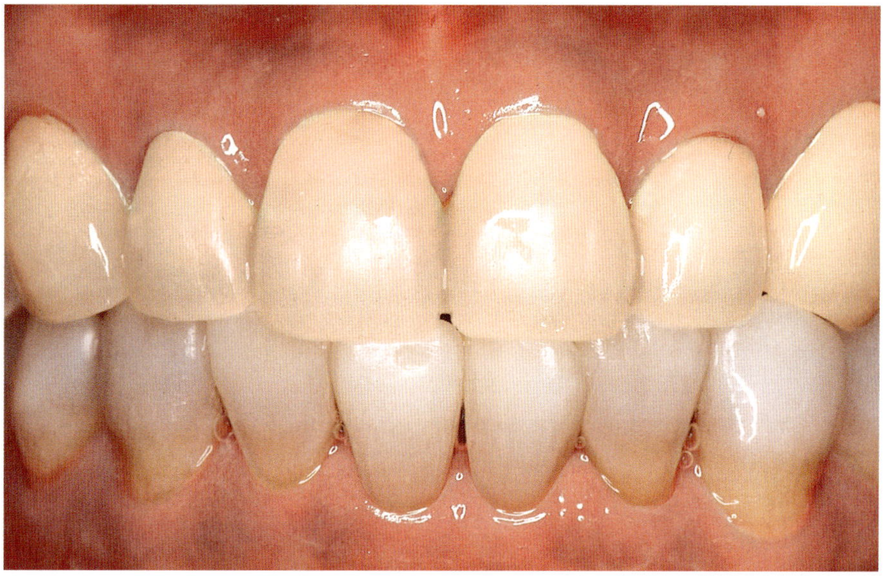

b. Color difference of the upper temporary restoration and the whitened lower teeth can be observed.

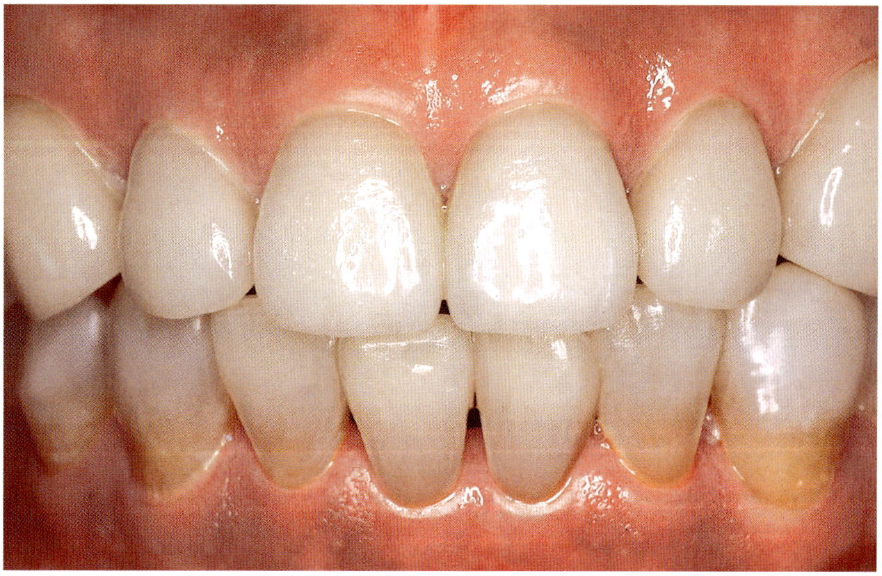

c. Home and power whitening combined was performed for 3 months, followed by placement of six upper anterior Empress crowns. Remaining yellowish discoloration in the cervical area can be noticed.

Fig. 7-10 Treatment of tetracycline discoloration with intentional root canal treatment and internal bleaching.

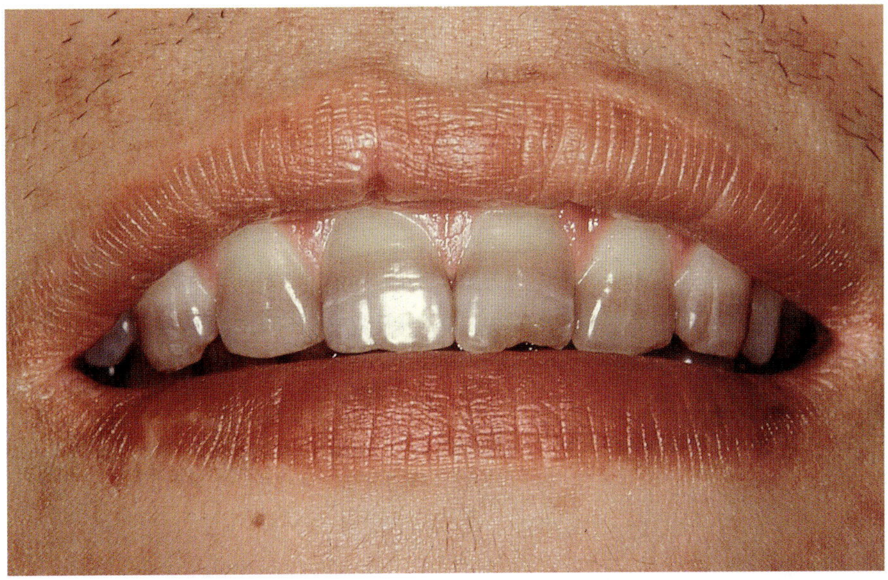

a. Brown to grey tetracycline discoloration with visible bands.

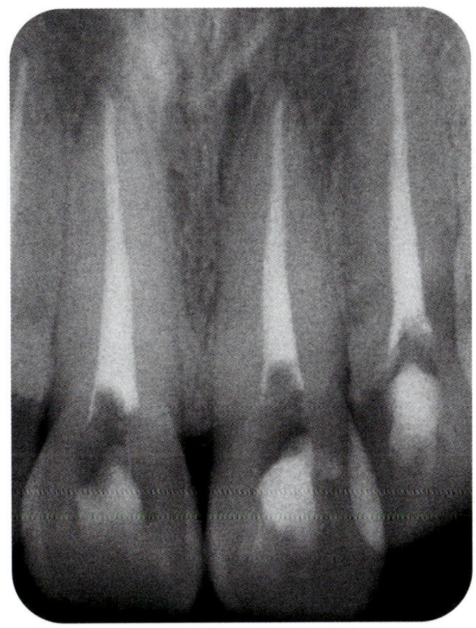

b. Periapical radiograph showing intentional root canal filling state.

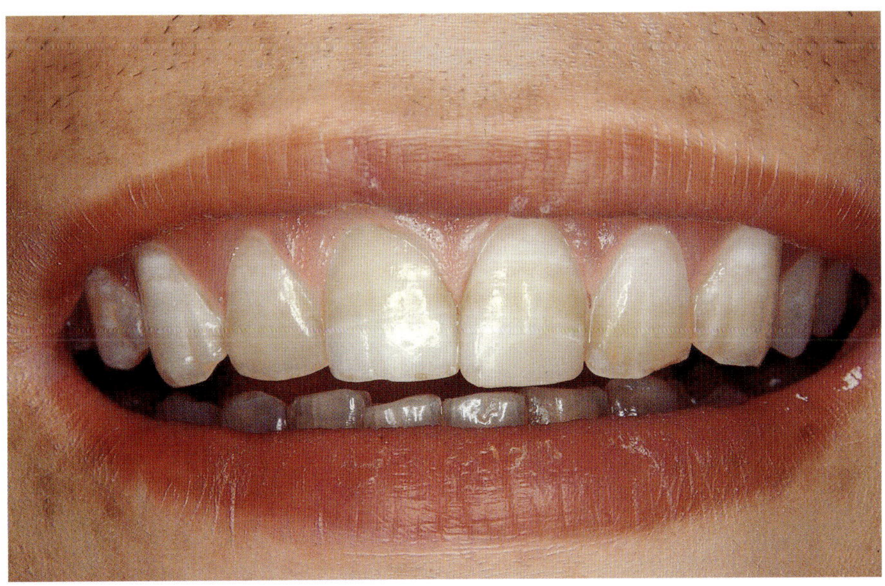

c. Esthetic result after 8 sessions of walking bleaching.

Q&A

Question 1. Is it possible to place bonded restorations immediately after tooth whitening?

Answer: If bonding treatments such as composite resin fillings, laminate or all-ceramic crown restorations are required after tooth whitening, it is best to wait 2weeks for shade stabilization and recovery of enamel bond strength.

Question 2. Can I selectively whiten dark, banded areas during power whitening?

Answer: The highly concentrated whitening gel can be placed selectively on the banded areas of tetracycline-stained teeth, but uniform placement of the gel on the tooth usually produces an overall better result.

Question 3. Does the dark shade of tetracycline-stained teeth show through all-ceramic restorations?

Answer: Esthetic results can be achieved with all-ceramic restorations when proper selection of the core shade is made.

Question 4. How do you usually treat tetracycline discoloration?

Answer: Proper treatment depends on the severity of the discoloration and the patient's wishes. If the patient prefers conservative treatment without any tooth reduction, a combination of home and power whitening for 3 to 6 months is recommended. If the patient agrees to tooth reduction, all-ceramic or full veneer restorations can be placed.

References

Abou-Rass M. The elimination of tetracycline discoloration by intentional endodontics and internal bleaching. J Endodont 1982; 8:101.

Arens DE. A practical method of bleaching tetracycline-stained teeth. School of Dent, Indiana Univ. 1972; 34:812-817.

Carolyn F.G. Color change following vital bleaching tetracycline-stained teeth. Pediatric Dent. 1985; 7(3):205-208.

Cohen S. Bleaching tetracycline-stained vital teeth. Oral Surg. 1970.

Davies AK. Photo-oxidation of Tetracycline Adsorbd on Hydroxyapatite in Relation to the Light-induced Staining of Teeth. J Dent Res 1985; 64(6):936-939.

Deliperi S. Integration of Composite and Ceramic Restorations in Tetracycline-Bleached Teeth: A Case Report. J Esthet Restor Dent 2006; 18:126-134.

Fiedler RS. Combined professional and home care nightguard bleaching of tetracycline-stained teeth. General Dent 2000.

Goldstein RE, Garber DA. Complete Dental Bleaching, Quintessence Publishing Co, Inc, 1995.

Haywood VB, Caughman WF. At-Home Whitening and Selective Bonding of Tetracycline-stained Teeth. Contemporary Esthetics and Restorative Practice 2001; 5(10):20-26.Haywood VB. Tooth Whitening: Indications and Outcomes of Nightguard Vital Bleaching, Quintessence Publishing Co, Inc, 2007.

Haywood VB, Leonard RH, Dickinson GL. Efficacy of six-months nightguard vital bleaching of tetracycline-stained teeth. J Esthet Dent 1997; 9(1):13-19.Haywood VB. Extended Bleaching of Tetracycline-stained teeth: a case report. Contemporary Esthetics and Restorative Practice 1997; 1(1):14-21.

Hisamitsu H, Toko T. Tooth Whitening basics and clinical techniques. Quintessence Japan, 2004.

Kwon S. Tooth Whitening State of the Art, Dental Publishing Co, Inc, 2004.

Leonard RH, Haywood VB, Caplan DJ, Tart ND. Nightguard Vital Bleaching of Tetracycline-Stained teeth: 90 months Post Treatment. J Esthet Restor Dent 2003; 15(3):142-154.

Leonard RH, Haywood VB, Eagle JC, Garland GE, Caplan DJ, Matthews KP, Tart ND. Nightguard vital bleaching of Tetracycline-stained teeth: 54 months Post Treatment. J Esthet Dent 1999, 11:265-277.

Matis BA. Extended Bleaching of Tetracycline-Stained Teeth: A 5-Year Study. Oper Dent 2006; 31-6:643-651.

Moffitt JM. Prediction of tetracycline-induced tooth discoloration. JADA 1974; 88:547-552.

Ritter AV. Tetracycline Dental Staining. J Esthet Restor Dent 2005.

chapter

8

Safety and sensitivity

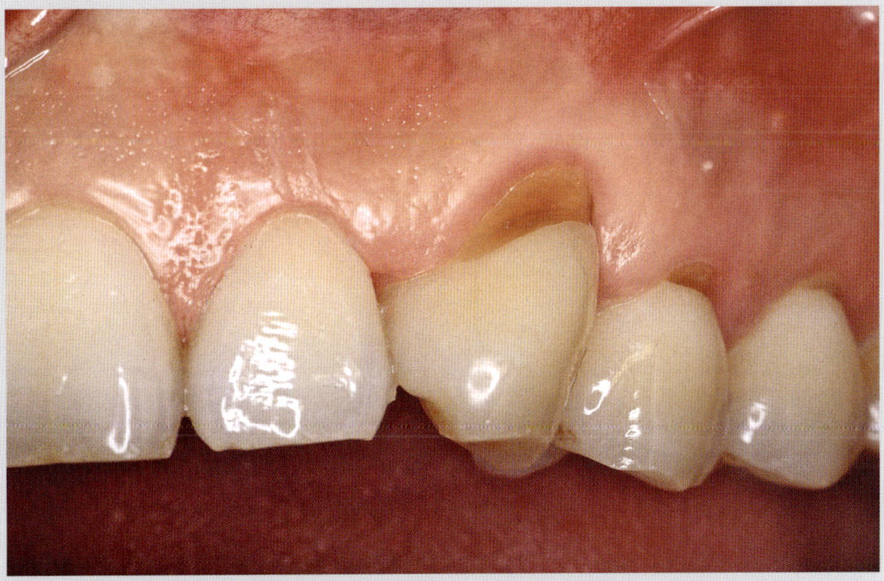

Peroxides have been used for tooth whitening with minimal risks for many years. In a retrospective review of the literature, Yarborough concluded that "the safety and efficacy of hydrogen peroxide is well established". However, adverse effects due to the use of inappropriate materials or the abuse of the materials have been reported. In order to minimize the risks associated with tooth whitening, the whole procedure should be performed under the supervision of a dentist.

Side effects of tooth whitening

Tooth sensitivity

Tooth sensitivity is a common side effect of tooth whitening. Data from various studies of 10% carbamide peroxide indicate that from 15 to 65% of the patients reported sensitivity (Haywood et al., 1994; Schulte et al., 1994; Leonard et al., 1997; Tam 1999a). A higher incidence of sensitivity, ranging from 67 to 78%, was reported after in-office bleaching with hydrogen peroxide in combination with heat (Cohen and Chase, 1979; Nathanson and Parra, 1987). The mechanism of sensitivity after tooth whitening has not been fully established. Studies have shown that hydrogen peroxide, whether applied directly or derived from carbamide peroxide, readily penetrates the tooth and enters the pulp chamber (Cooper et al., 1992). This may cause sensitivity in the form of reversible pulpits. Sensitivity during tooth whitening can be controlled by either passive or active methods, according to the severity experienced.

- **Passive methods:** If the sensitivity related to tooth whitening is mild or moderate, sensitivity can be reduced by modifying the treatment time, frequency and concentration of the whitening material.
- **Active methods:** If the sensitivity related to tooth whitening is severe, sensitivity can be treated with desensitizing agents. Fluoride acts as a tubular blocking agent and can be placed in the whitening tray and worn for 10 to 20 minutes. Potassium nitrate has a direct calming effect on nerve transmission and acts as a strong desensitizing agent. Desensitizing gels containing 3 to 5% potassium nitrate are available and can be worn in the tray for 10 to 30 minutes.
  Pastes containing amorphous calcium phosphate, which fill in the microporosity of the teeth, can be used for 10 to 20 minutes in the whitening tray (Fig. 8-1).
- **Treatment modalities for patients with pre-existing sensitivity:** Patients with pre-existing sensitivity should use a toothpaste for sensitive teeth for 2 weeks or wear a tray with neutral sodium fluoride for 2 weeks prior to starting tooth whitening. If the sensitivity is localized, the sensitive lesions should be either filled temporarily or restored with composite resin of a lighter shade (Fig. 8-2).

Gingival irritation

High concentrations of hydrogen peroxide can be very caustic to mucous membranes. Contact should therefore be avoided by carefully isolating the gingiva during the power whitening procedure to avoid burns and bleaching of the gingiva. The lower concentrations of hydrogen peroxide or carbamide peroxide used during home whitening can cause mild irritation to the gingiva, but mechanical irritation due to ill-fitting trays is more frequently the cause of the gingival irritation.

Tooth surface morphology

Numerous studies have indicated little changes in enamel surface texture (Fig. 8-3) associated with peroxide bleaching (McGuckin et al., 1992). Alterations observed include shallow depressions, increased porosity and slight erosions, which can be expected to normalize through salivary remineralization.

Effects on restorations

- **Amalgam restorations:** Increased release of mercury from dental amalgams exposed to carbamide peroxide for extended periods has been reported (Hummert et al., 1993, Rotstein et al., 1997). The amount of mercury released varies with type of amalgam and type of bleaching agent.
- **Composite resin restorations:** The surface hardness, texture and color of composite resin restorations is largely unaffected by tooth whitening.
- **Glass-ionomer and other cements:** Tooth whitening may increase the solubility of glass-ionomer and other cements (Swift and Perdiago, 1998).
- **Others:** Porcelain or other ceramic restorations as well as dental gold appear to be generally unaffected by tooth whitening procedures.

Genotoxicity and carcinogenicity

Hydrogen peroxide seems to have a weak local carcinogenic potential, but a genotoxic action cannot be ruled-out since free radicals formed from hydrogen peroxide may attack the DNA (Dahl, 2003).

Toxicity

The acute effects of hydrogen peroxide ingestion are dependent on the amount ingested and the concentration of the hydrogen peroxide solution. Since power whitening is performed in the office with meticulous protection, there is little risk of swallowing the whitening material. During home whitening, the amount of whitening material in two trays is only 3.5mg. Therefore, there is little concern about the effects of swallowing the material.

••• In order to minimize the risks associated with tooth whitening, the whole procedure should be performed under the supervision of a dentist.

Fig. 8-1 Use of desensitizing agents.

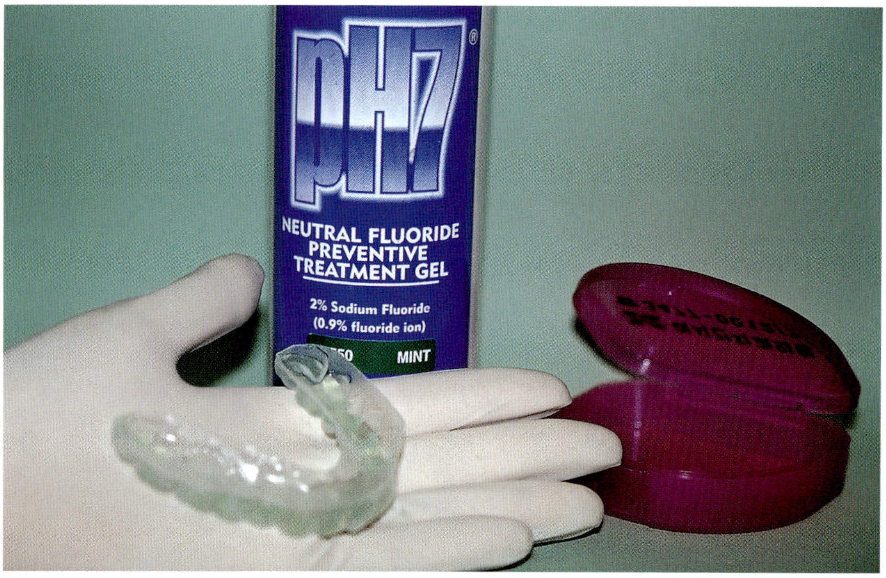

a. Desensitization with neutral sodium fluoride (pH 7, Pascal, USA).

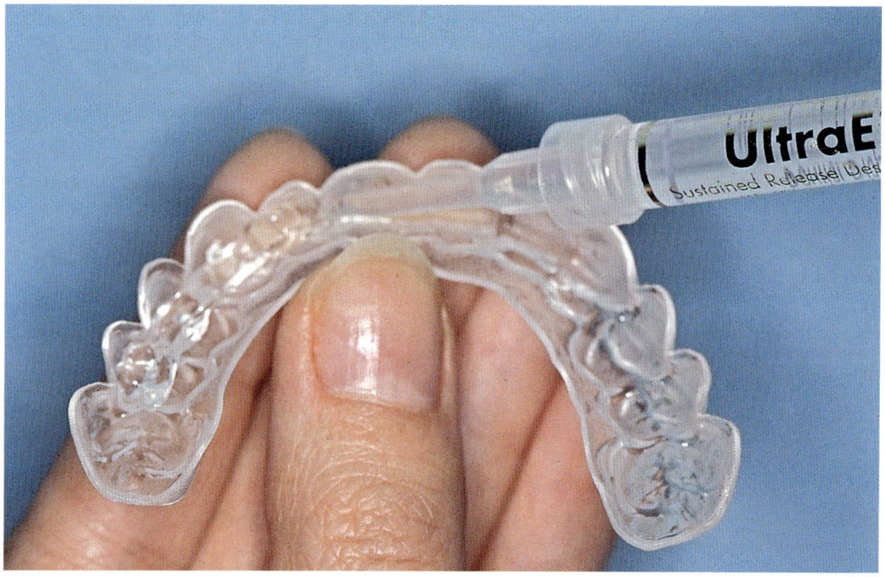

b. Desensitization with a 3% potassium nitrate gel (UltraEZ, Ultradent Products, Inc. USA).

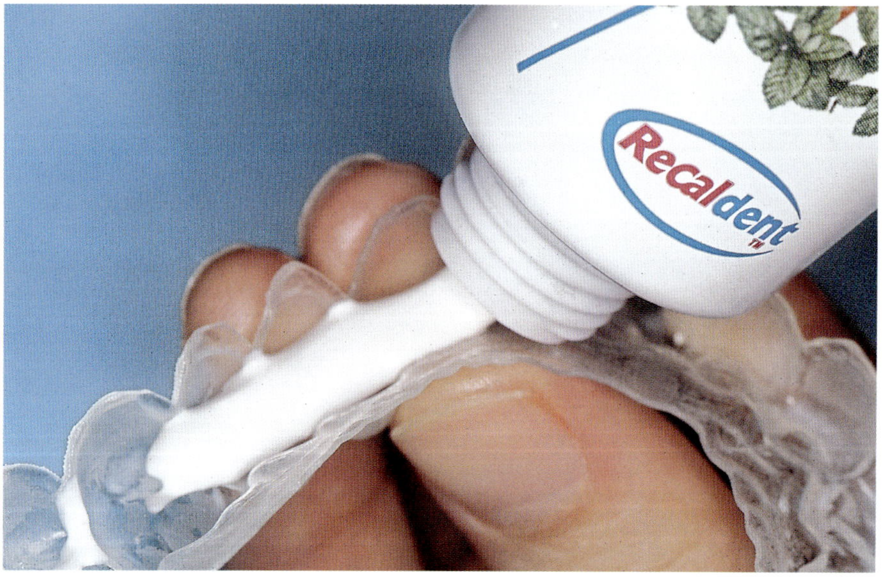

c. Desensitization with a paste containing amorphous calcium phosphate (MI Paste with Recaldent, GC America).

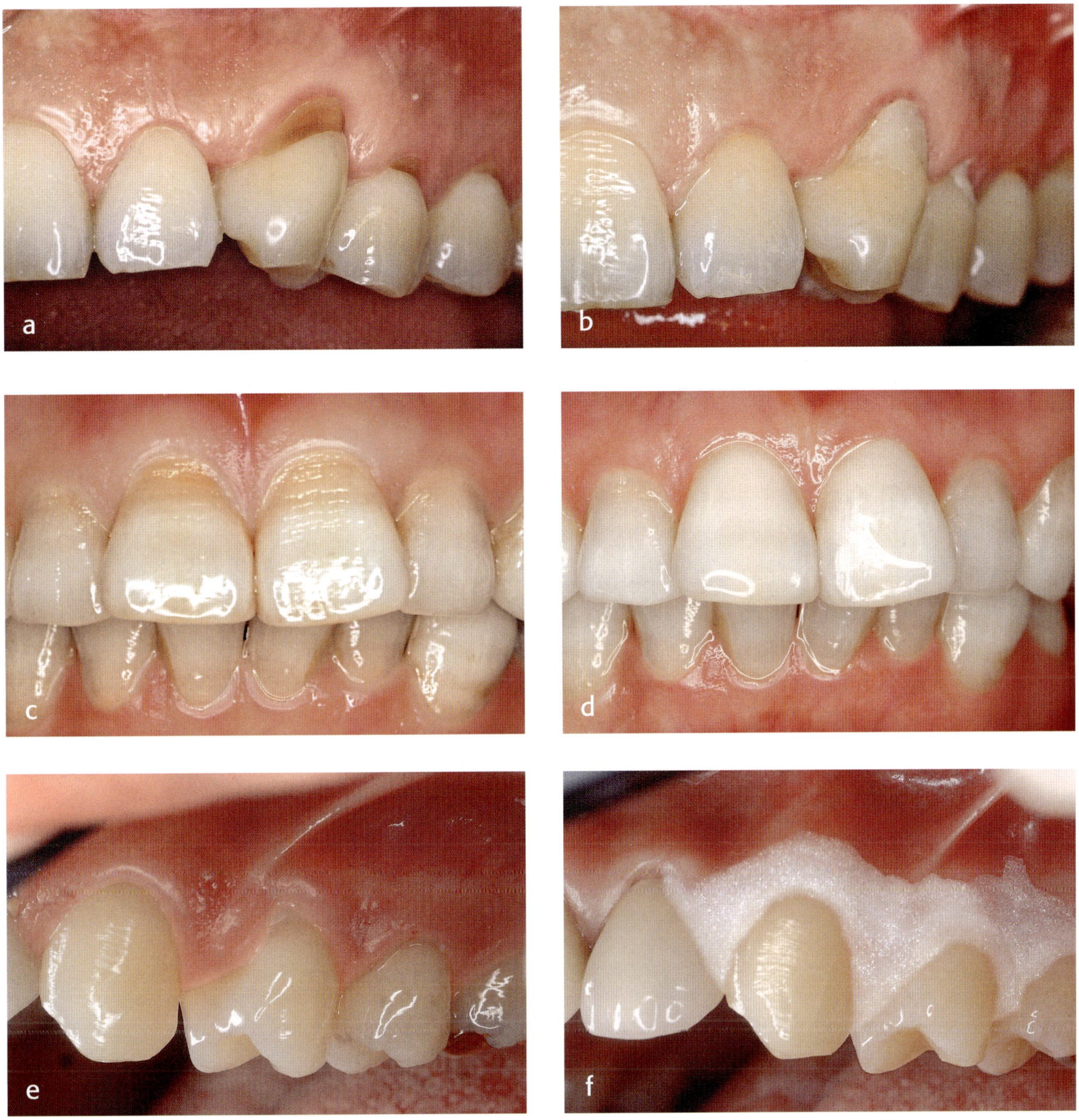

Fig. 8-2 Treatment modalities for patients with pre-existing sensitivity.

a,b. The sensitive cervical area is temporarily restored with resin reinforced glass ionomer. After tooth whitening, the area can be finally replaced with composite resin.

c,d. The sensitive cervical area is restored with composite resin of a lighter shade before tooth whitening.

e,f. During power whitening, the sensitive cervical area is protected by a resin barrier and restored after whitening.

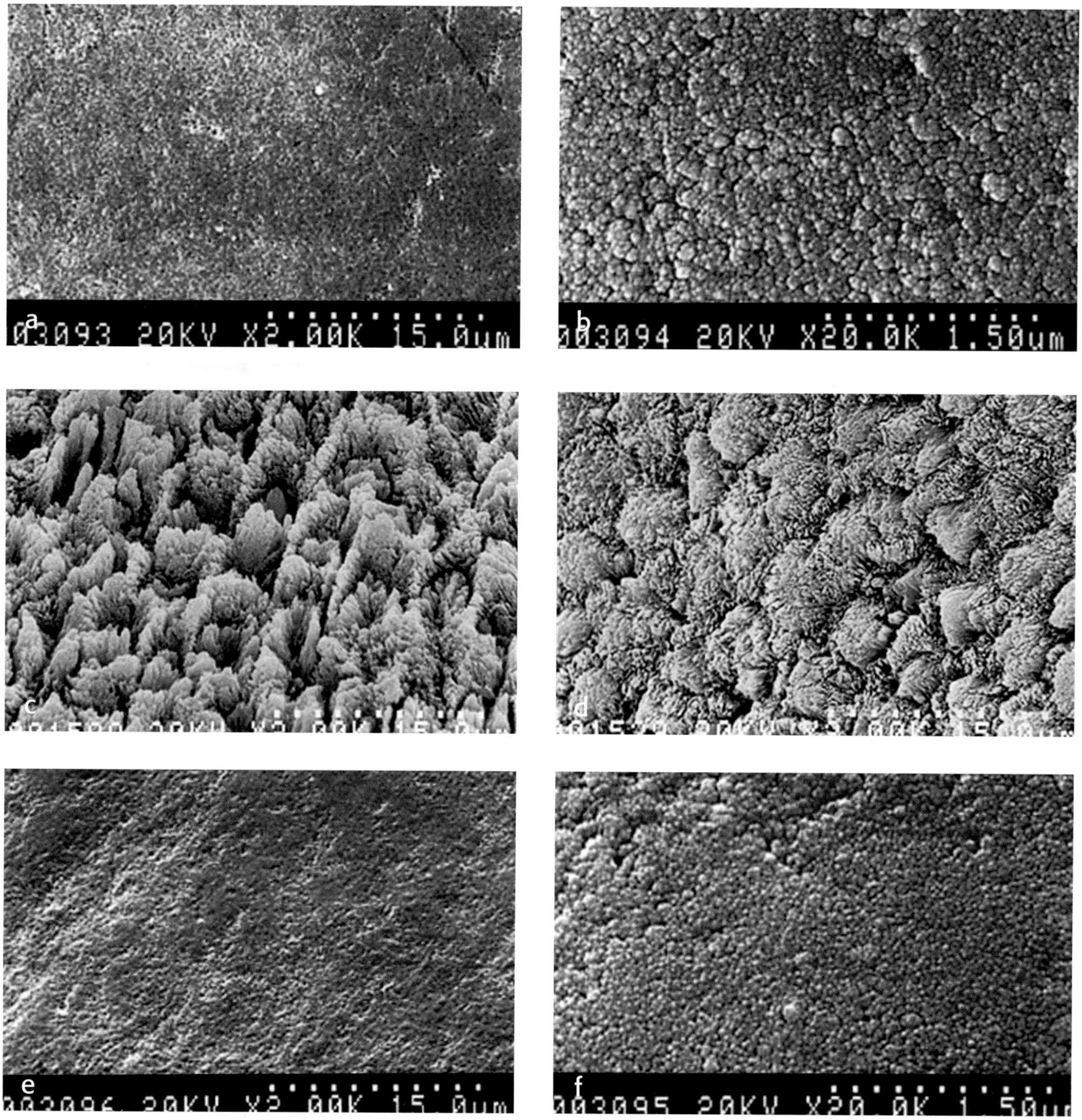

Fig. 8-3 Effect of 10% carbamide peroxide on tooth surface morphology.

a,b. Untreated enamel. Rough and amorphous morphology can be observed.

c,d. Surface morphology after acid etching with 35% phosphoric acid for 30 seconds. Honeycomb and cobblestone patterns can be observed.

e,f. Surface morphology after application of 10% carbamide peroxide for 40 hours. Note that 10% carbamide peroxide had little effect on surface morphology.

Q&A

Question 1. What do you do when there are posterior amalgam fillings?

Answer: When prolonged whitening is required, multiple amalgam restorations can be replaced by composite restorations prior to starting whitening treatment (Fig. 8-4).

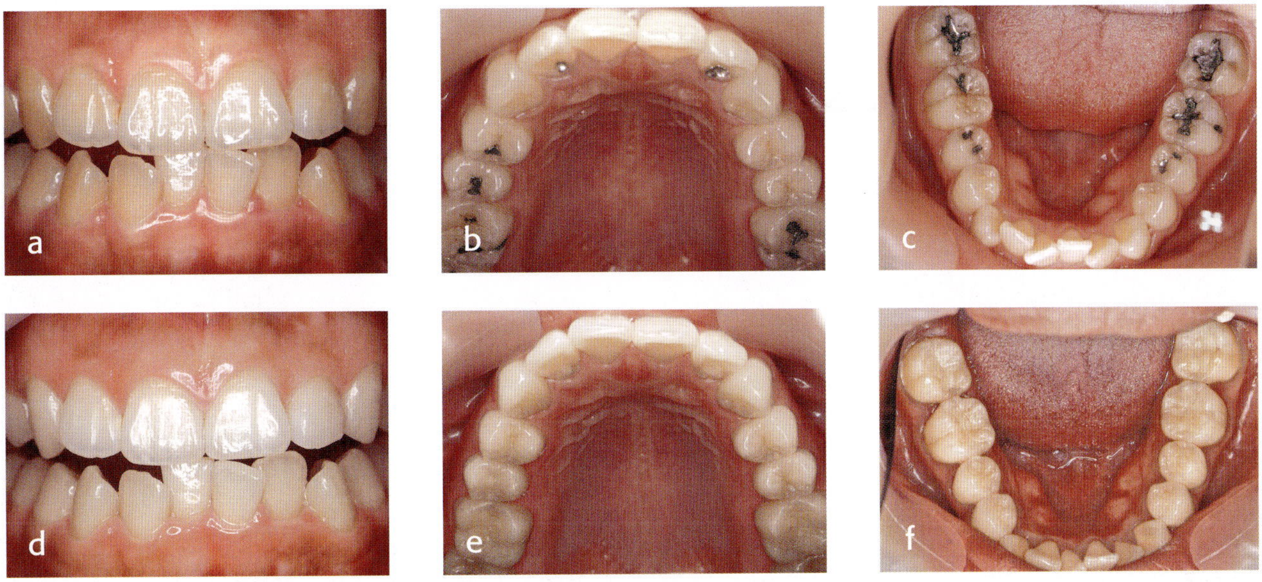

Fig. 8-4 Replacement of amalgam restorations prior to tooth whitening.
a,b,c. Generalized yellow discoloration with multiple amalgam restorations.
d,e,f. The old amalgam restorations were replaced with composite resin fillings prior to tooth whitening at the patient's request.

Question 2. Will whitening damage my crowns or fillings?

Answer: Tooth whitening will not damage your crowns or fillings. Anterior composite resin restorations will probably need replacement after tooth whitening because the color will not match anymore.

Question 3. Is pregnancy a contraindication to whitening?

Answer: There has been no report that tooth whitening is harmful to pregnant women, but care should be taken during pregnancy. It would be best to delay the treatment until after delivery and completion of nursing.

References

Bitter NC. A scanning electron microscope study of the long-term effect of bleaching agents on the enamel surface in vivo. Gen Dent 1998;46:84-88.

Cohen SC, Chase C. Human pulpal response to bleaching procedures on vital teeth. J Endod 1979;5:134-138.

Cooper J, Bokmeyer TJ, Bowles WH. Penetration of the pulp chamber by carbamide peroxide bleaching agents. J Endodont 1992;18(7):315-317.

Dahl JE. Tooth Bleaching – A critical Review of the Biological Aspects. Crit Rev Oral Biol Med 2003; 14(4):292-304.

Dickson KF, Caravati EM. Hydrogen peroxide exposure-325 exposures reported to a regional poison control center. Clin Toxicol 1994;32:705-714.

Dishmann MV, Covey DA, Baughan LW. The effects of peroxide bleaching on composite to enamel bond strength. Dent Mater 1994;9:33-36.

European commission, Scientific Committee on Consumer Products. Opinion on hydrogen peroxide in tooth whitening products [sccp/0844/04]. Available at: http://ec.europa.eu.

Goldstein RE, Garber DA. Complete Dental Bleaching, Quintessence Publishing Co, Inc, 1995.

Goldstein RE. In-office bleaching: where we came from, where are we today? J Am Dent Assoc Suppl 1997; 128:11S-15S.

Haywood VB, Leonard RH, Neilson CF, Brunson WD. Effectiveness, side effects and long term status of Nightguard Vital Bleaching. J Am Dent Assoc 1994; 125:1219-26.

Haywood VB. History, safety and effectiveness of current bleaching techniques and applications of the Nightguard Vital Bleaching technique. Quintessence Int 1992; 23:471-88.

Hisamitsu H, Toko T. Tooth Whitening basics and clinical techniques. Quintessence Japan, 2004.

Hummert TW, Osborne JW, Norling BK, Cardenas HL. Mercury in solution following exposure of various amalgams to carbamide peroxides. Am J Dent 1993;6:305-309.

Ito A, Wanatabe H, Naito M, Naito Y. Induction of duodenal tumors in mice by oral administration of hydrogen peroxide. Gann 1981; 72:174-5.

Ito A, Wanatabe H, Naito M, Naito Y. Kawashima K. Correlation between induction of duodenal tumor by hydrogen peroxide and catalase activity in mice. Gann 1984; 75:17-21.

JADA Guidelines for the acceptance of peroxide containing oral hygiene. J Am Dent Assoc 1994; 125:1140-2.

Kwon S. Tooth Whitening State of the Art, Dental Publishing Co, Inc, 2004.

Leonard RH. Efficacy, longevity, side effects, and patient perceptions of nightguard vital bleaching. Compend Contin Educ Dent 1998;19:766-774.

Leonard RH, Haywood VB, Phillips C. Risk factors for developing tooth sensitivity and gingival irritation associated with nightguard vital bleaching. Quintessence Int 1997;28:527-534.

Li Y. Biological properties of peroxide-containing tooth whiteners. Food Chem Toxicol 1996;34:887-904.

Li Y. Peroxide-containing tooth whiteners: an update on safety. Compend Cont Educ Dent 2000; 21(Suppl 28):S4-S9.

Li Y. Tooth bleaching using peroxide-containing agents: current status of safety issues. Compend Contin Educ Dent 1998; 19(8):783-94.

McCaslin AJ. Haywood VB, Potter BJ, Dickinson GL, Russel CM. Assessing dentin colour changes from Nightguard Vital Bleaching. J Am Dent Assoc 1999; 130:1485-1490.

Nathanson D, Parra C. Bleaching vital teeth - a review of clinical study. Compend Contin Educ Dent 1987;8:490-498.

Nathanson D. Vital tooth bleaching: sensitivity and pulpal considerations. J Am Dent Assoc 1997; 128:41s-44s.

Ritter AV, Leonard RH, St Georges AJ, Caplan DJ, Haywood VB. Safety and stability of nightguard vital bleaching: 9 to 12 years post-treatment. J Esthet Rest Dent 2002;14:275-285.

Rotstein I. In vitro determination and quantification of 30% hydrogen peroxide penetration through dentin and cementum during bleaching. Oral Surg Oral Med Oral Pathol 1991;72:602-606.

Rotstein I, Mor C, Arwaz JR. Changes in surface levels of mercury, silver, tin, and copper of dental amalgam treated with carbamide peroxide and hydrogen peroxide in vitro. Oral Surg Oral Med Oral Pathol Oral Radiol 1997;83:506-509.

Schulte JR, Morrissette DB, Gasior EJ, Czajewski MV. The effects of bleaching application time on the dental pulp. J Am Dent Assoc 1994;125:1330-1335.

Swift EJ Jr, Perdigão J. Effects of bleaching on teeth and restorations. Compend Contin Educ Dent 1998;19:815-820.

Swift EJ Jr, May KN Jr, Wilder AD Jr, Heymann HO, Bayne SC. Two-year clinical evaluation of tooth whitening using an at-home bleaching system. J Esthet Dent 1999;11:36-42.

Tam L. Clinical trial of three 10% carbamide peroxide bleaching products. J Can Dent Assoc 1999a; 65:201-205.

Tam L. The safety of home bleaching techniques. J Can Dent Assoc 1999b; 65:453-455.

Thitinanthapan W, Satamanont P, Vongsavan N. In vitro penetration of the pulp chamber by three brands of Carbamide peroxide. J Esthet Dent 1999; 11(5):244-259.

Titley KC, Torneck CD, Smith DC, Chernecky R, Adibfar A. Scanning electron microscopy observations on the penetration and structure on the resin tags in bleached and unbleached bovine enamel. J Endodont 1991;17(2):72-75.

Zalkind M. Arwaz JR. Goldman A, Rotstein I. Surface morphology changes in human enamel, dentin and cementum following bleaching: a scanning electron microscope study. Endodont Dent Traumatol 1996; 12(2):82-84.

chapter

9

Maintenance

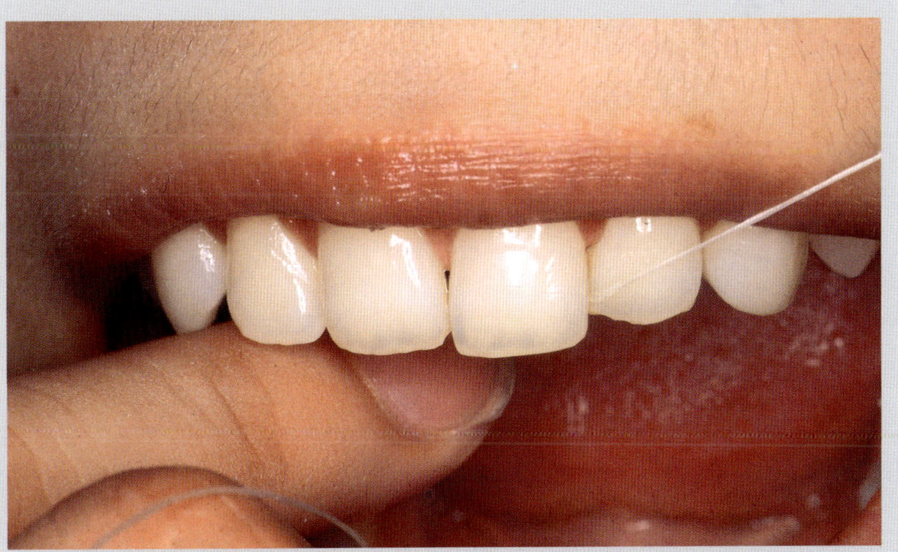

Parameters of success and failure

It is difficult to determine the success and failure of a whitening treatment since the patient's opinion may differ from that of the dentist. The three parameters of success and failure may provide an objective guideline for the evaluation of a whitening treatment.

Parameters of success and failure
- Patient's satisfaction
- Shade change
- Completion of tooth whitening

Patient satisfaction

There are many factors that affect the satisfaction of the patient (Table 9-1). Among those, a shade change that is dramatically noticeable to the patient may be the most important factor. Since accurate shade changes are difficult to assess, various shade measuring methods should be used during tooth whitening. In addition to shade change, a systematic approach with well-trained dental staff members will establish a positive relationship between the patient and the staff, resulting in an increased satisfaction rate.

In 2001, the CRA Newsletter reported that 95% of the respondents were satisfied or very satisfied with home whitening, whereas 42% of the respondents were satisfied or very satisfied with in-office whitening. Recently, the busy lifestyle of modern society has resulted in an increased demand for power whitening, and with the improvement of new power whitening systems, increased satisfaction can be expected.

Table 9-1 Factors that affect patient satisfaction with tooth whitening.

- Visible shade change
- Variety of whitening programs offered
- Good service
- Consultation and performance by well-trained dental staff members
- No discomfort during whitening
- Speedy treatment
- No or little relapse
- Easy touch-up whitening
- Reasonable treatment fee

Shade change

The change in shade (ΔE) as defined by the Commission Internationale de l' Éclairage(CIE) L*a*b* color system is commonly used to evaluate shade changes objectively. ΔE is calculated using the equation

$$\Delta E = (\Delta L^{*2} + \Delta a^{*2} + \Delta b^{*2})^{1/2}$$

where L* represents lightness, a* corresponds to the red-green axis (positive value indicates red; negative indicates green), and b* corresponds to the yellow-blue axis (a positive value indicates yellow; negative value indicates blue). In order to be distinguished by human perception, ΔL must be larger than 2.0 and ΔE must be larger than 4.0. After tooth whitening, ΔE should therefore be at least greater than 4.0.

In the ADA Seal Program, which evaluates the effectiveness and safety of tooth whitening materials, the effectiveness of the tooth whitening material is evaluated based on shade change. The shade change is assessed using a colorimeter, spectrophotometer or a value-oriented shade guide. The shade change is evaluated immediately after bleaching as well as 3 and 6 months later. The results must meet the standards specified as follows.

Shade change for ADA seal

	Δeu*
Immediately after tooth whitening	95% ≥ 1eu
Three months after tooth whitening	85% ≥ 1eu
Six months after tooth whitening	75% ≥ 1eu

* 1eu ≥ 2 sgu, 2 units in a value oriented shade guide (sgu: Shade Guide Unit)
≥ 4.0 ΔE units L*a*b*

Therefore, at least 2 units improvement in a value-oriented shade guide or a ΔE of 4 or more in the L*a*b* color system is required for ADA approval.

The CIE color system used by many researchers is not commonly used in the clinical practice. Clinically, the best way to demonstrate the color change is to whiten the upper and lower arch separately. Once the upper arch is completed, the dentist and the patient can assess the shade difference. If the patient is satisfied with the color of the upper arch, the lower teeth can be whitened to match the shade of the upper teeth. Shade changes can be determined by visual inspection with shade tabs and recorded as a shade map in the patient's chart, or they can be determined by taking a photograph of the teeth along with the baseline shade tabs as a reference.

Completion of tooth whitening

Tooth whitening is considered to be successful when it is completed. According to Miller, the drop-out rate of home bleaching reaches 50%, and one of the reasons patients are recalled repeatedly during home bleaching is to continuously motivate patients towards completing the treatment. Combining home and power whitening may be the best way to motivate the patient to complete the treatment.

Longevity of tooth whitening

Haywood stated that the tooth shade tends to get darker during the initial 2 weeks after bleaching, but then stabilizes and maintains the shade for 1 to 3 years. He reported that, in some cases, the shade is maintained permanently. The longevity of whitening should not be compared to that of restorative treatments like composite resin fillings or full-coverage restorations. Without regular touch-ups, long-term success cannot be guaranteed for tooth whitening treatments. Similar to professional oral hygiene care, tooth whitening should be performed with regular touch-ups to maintain the whitened color for a long time.

Maintenance care

Home care

It is always interesting to note that, as the color of the teeth improves, the patient's interest in oral hygiene care improves as well. Home care includes proper tooth brushing and control of diet to avoid highly staining food. Whitening tooth paste, whitening floss or over-the-counter strip-type whitening materials may be used for maintenance of the whitened teeth (Fig. 9-1). Written instructions should always be provided to inform the patient about proper maintenance care (Fig. 9-2).

Professional care

Regular visits to the dental office and professional mechanical tooth cleaning for removal of calculus and stains are required. Through these monitoring visits, it is possible to evaluate whether the shade is being maintained, and proper timing of touch-ups can be determined.

Touch-up

The tooth shade is reportedly maintained for 1 to 3 years after tooth whitening. However, the shade does not actually relapse to the original shade. It may darken by a few shade units. In order to maintain the lightened shade permanently, simple touch-ups are required once every 1 to 2 years. If tooth whitening is performed by home whitening, the whitening tray may be kept by the patient and be used for touch-ups. The patient may purchase a refill kit to do one week of touch-up whitening. Patients who had power whitening may require retreatment periodically. Most patients tend to lose their whitening tray. In these cases, one to two sessions of power whitening may be performed as a touch-up treatment (Fig. 9-3).

••• After the whitening treatment has been successfully completed, proper maintenance care should be provided for long-term success.

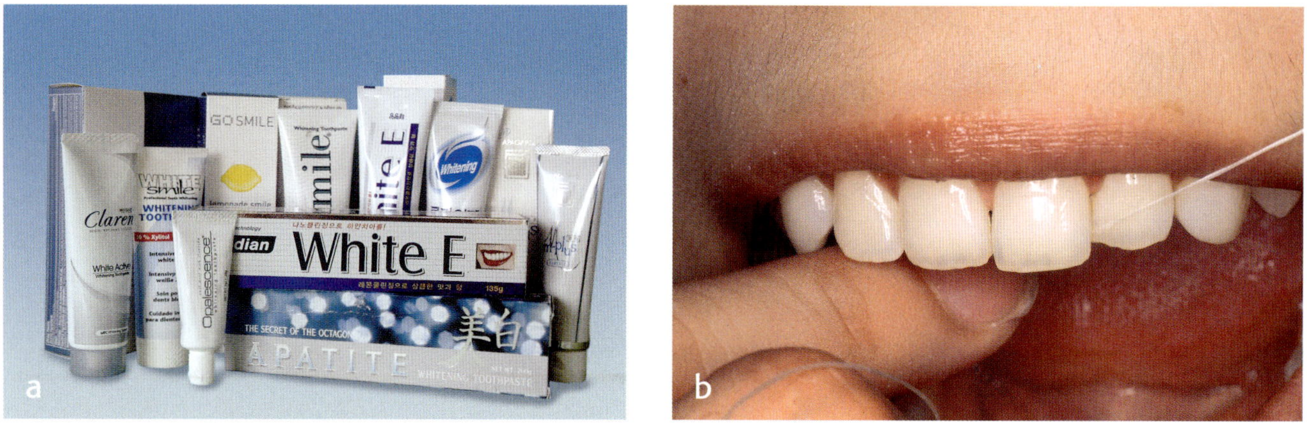

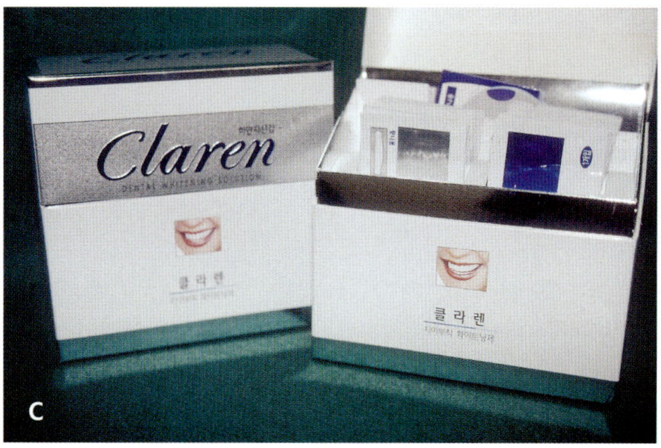

Fig. 9-1 Home care.

a. Various whitening toothpastes are available on the market.

b. Whitening floss.

c. Whitening strips for easy touch-ups.

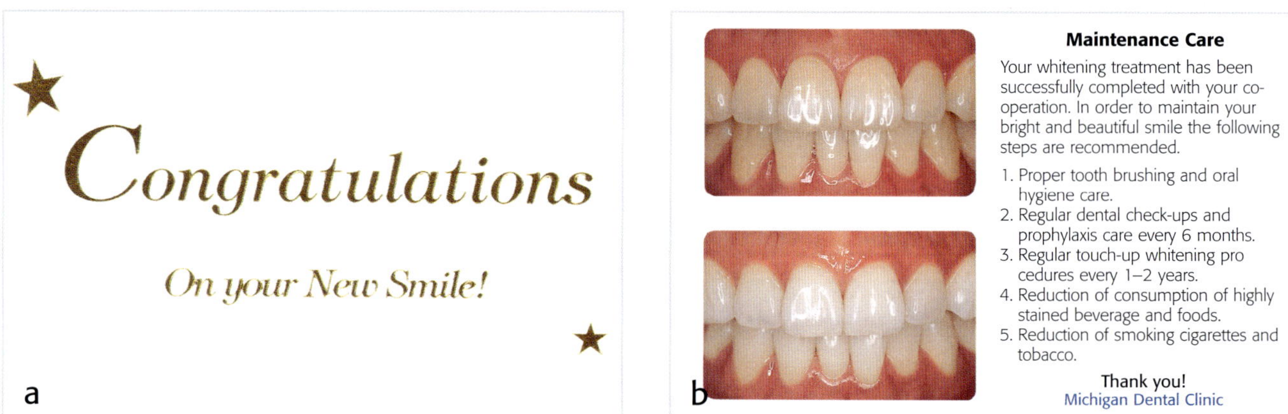

Fig. 9-2 Written maintenance care instructions.

a. Front of maintenance card.

b. Before and after pictures with maintenance care instructions.

Fig. 9-3 Touch-up whitening.

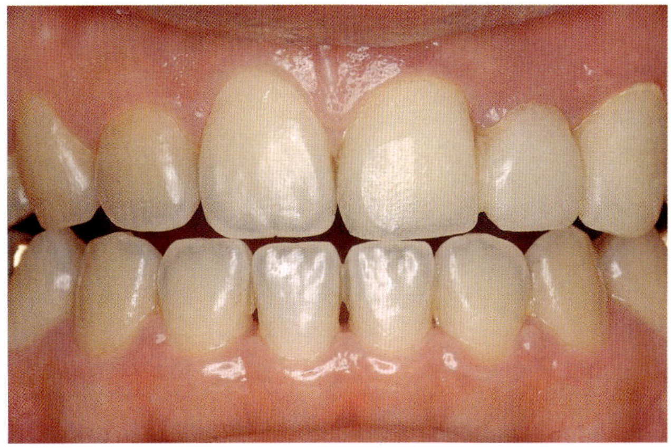

a. Patient with generalized yellow discoloration during prosthodontic treatment of the upper left anterior teeth.

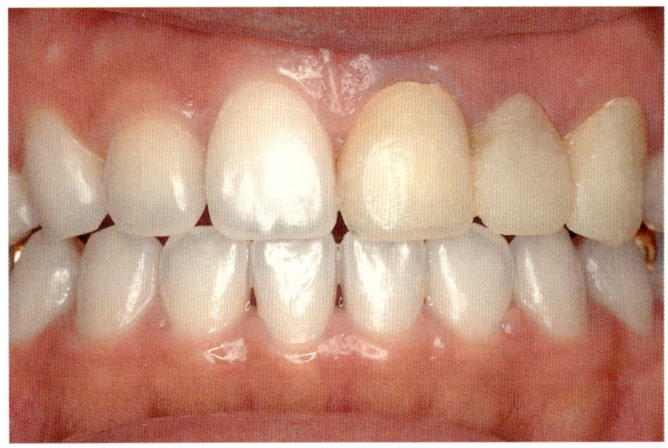

b. Prior to placement of the final restoration, 5 sessions of power whitening were performed. Note the color difference compared to the temporary bridge.

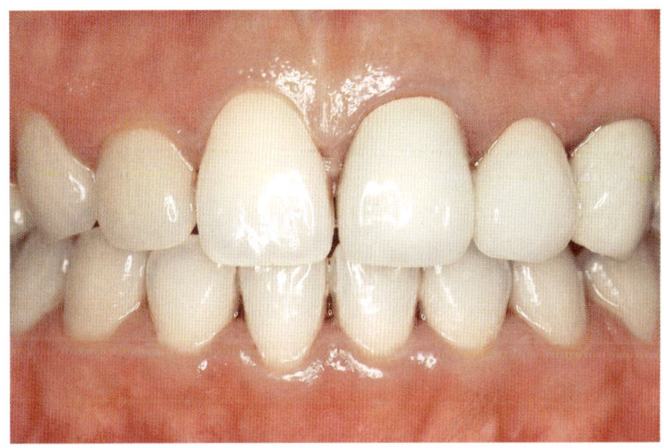

c. The patient returned after six years for a scaling procedure and touch-up whitening. Note that the color has been maintained quite well even without any touch-up.

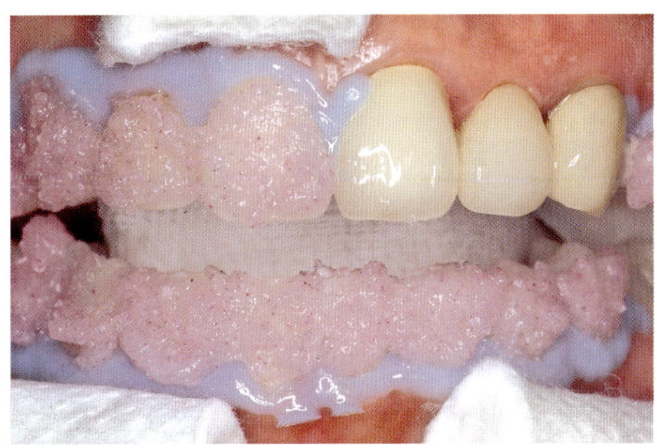

d. Touch-up power whitening.

Q&A

Question 1.	What is the best way to assess the shade change clinically?
Answer:	Clinically, the best way to demonstrate the color change is to whiten the upper and lower arch separately in order to show the color difference.
Question 2.	How long does the lightness from whitening last?
Answer:	It usually lasts one to three years. In some patients, there is no reversal.
Question 3.	How often is it necessary to undertake touch-up maintenance treatments?
Answer:	Regular touch-up whitening procedures may be required every 1 to 2 years.

References

American Dental Association Council on Dental Therapeutics: Guidelines for the acceptance of peroxide-containing oral hygiene products, J Am Dent Assoc 1994; 125:1140.

CRA Newsletter 25:2;2001.

Haywood VB, Heymann HO: Nightguard vital bleaching, Quintessence Int 1989; 20:173.

Leonard RH: Efficacy, longevity, side effects, and patient perceptions of nightguard vital bleaching, Compend Contin Educ Dent 1998; 19:766.

Miller M. Reality: Information source for esthetic dentistry 2000; Vol. 14. Reality Publishing Company: Houston

Sherer JL: Whiteners-bleaching, AGD Impact 1992; 20:14.

chapter

10

History of tooth whitening

(Linda H. Greenwall)

Tooth discoloration has been a problem for patients for many centuries. There have been numerous attempts to whiten teeth over this time with various medicaments being used. In fact, during Roman times, uric acid (Rotstein, 1999) was used to lighten teeth as well as compounds called nitrum, which contained potassium carbonate and/or sodium carbonate rubbed onto the surface of teeth to restore their color (Ring, 1985). Many of the earlier attempts to whiten teeth, although highly innovative, were not successful, and bleaching techniques were considered to be experimental and unpredictable (Greenwall, 2001). Developments in technology and research continue to this day as further alternative methods are sought to continue the quest to whiten teeth in a faster, safer and more predictable way.

Chapple stated in 1877 that the oldest medicament used for bleaching teeth was probably oxalic acid (Bogue, 1872). These early attempts, though revolutionary at the time, were unsuccessful and were considered to be experimental and unpredictable. As hydrogen peroxide proved to be useful as a bleaching agent (Fisher, 1911) capable of penetrating into the enamel and dentin to remove the internal cause of discoloration (Sulieman, 2004), further attempts to whiten teeth progressed. In-office power bleaching is the oldest form of tooth whitening. It was attempted as a convenient way to whiten teeth using strong chemicals, heat and light to encourage tooth whitening at the chairside. Many methods to stimulate the penetration and absorption of hydrogen peroxide were developed, and the high-intensity light unit developed by Abbot in 1918 is a basic unit that is still in use today.

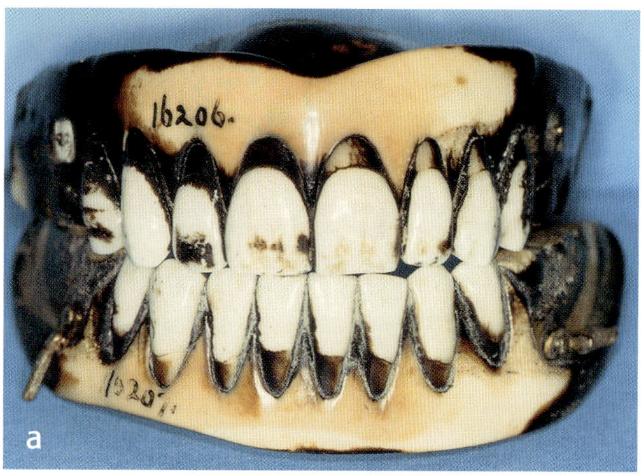

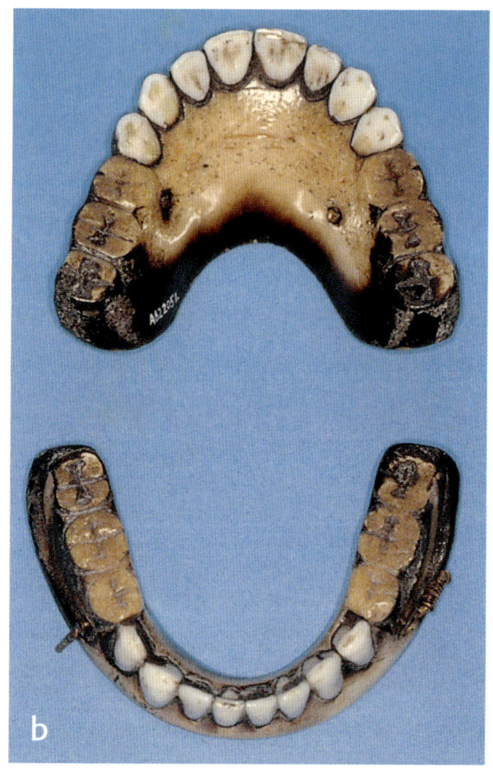

Fig. 10-1 Old spring hinge dentures.
a. Even in the old days, white porcelain teeth were used to emphasize esthetics in the anterior region.
b. It is interesting to note the dark discoloration due to excessive smoking.
(Historical slides are reproduced with kind permission from the archives of the Science Museum in South Kensington, London, UK.)

The patient's pain threshold was used as an indicator of the level of intensity of heat and light and to identify areas of tissue burning (Haywood, 1997). Generally between 3 and 6 appointments were required to achieve a satisfactory outcome. Even in the early years, there were problems associated with postoperative tooth sensitivity. The need for isolation, either with a full arch rubber dam or a light cured dam, has been a problem as only the upper 6 or 8 teeth are normally treated. There was no reliable way of predicting success. Color regression was a particular problem and still is to this day (Matis et al., 2007).

In 1989, Haywood and Heymann introduced the concept and associated research of nightguard vital bleaching, in which a tray was made for the upper and lower teeth and the bleaching gel (normally 10% carbamide peroxide) was placed in the tray for use overnight. The initial materials were quite runny, and the trays had to be designed to better retain these gels (Darnell and Moore, 1990). Newer materials contained carbopol, which allows for the slow release of oxygen, remaining effective overnight (Matis et al., 1999). The next generation of materials contained desensitizers such as fluoride, potassium nitrate and amorphous calcium phosphate. This technique had great effectiveness, predictability and safety. Sensitivity still occurred but was reduced and better managed.

Over-the-counter tooth whitening materials were first introduced onto the market in 1990 as manufacturers realized that they could reach a wider uptake amongst the general public for these products. The early over-the-counter kits were three-stage products. Patients bought these new kits, and they were often overused and misused, resulting in damage to the enamel (Cubbon and Ore, 1991). A variety of new materials, such as preformed transparent tooth strips (Gerlach, 2000) loaded with 5.3%-10% hydrogen peroxide worn for 30-60 minutes and wrapped over the front teeth (Gerlach et al., 2000) and paint-on gels containing 18% carbamide peroxide and bleaching maintenance top-up applicators have since been introduced. These bleaching strips and wraps are more effective and have achieved a significant improvement of tooth whiteness (Matis et al., 2005). They are especially effective in patients who have evenly shaped teeth and an already light shade of teeth.

The quest for more efficient whitening eventually led to introduction of dental lasers and advanced light technology, including halogen and LED lights. The ozone machine has also been utilized in attempts at tooth whitening with reasonable success (Lynch, 2006, Baysan and Lynch, 2005).

Through a continuous process of development that has improved the effectiveness and convenience of bleaching agents and the associated catalyzing lights, tooth whitening has evolved from its humble beginnings (Ciesara et al., 2002) into the most requested service from patients amongst all forms of dentistry.

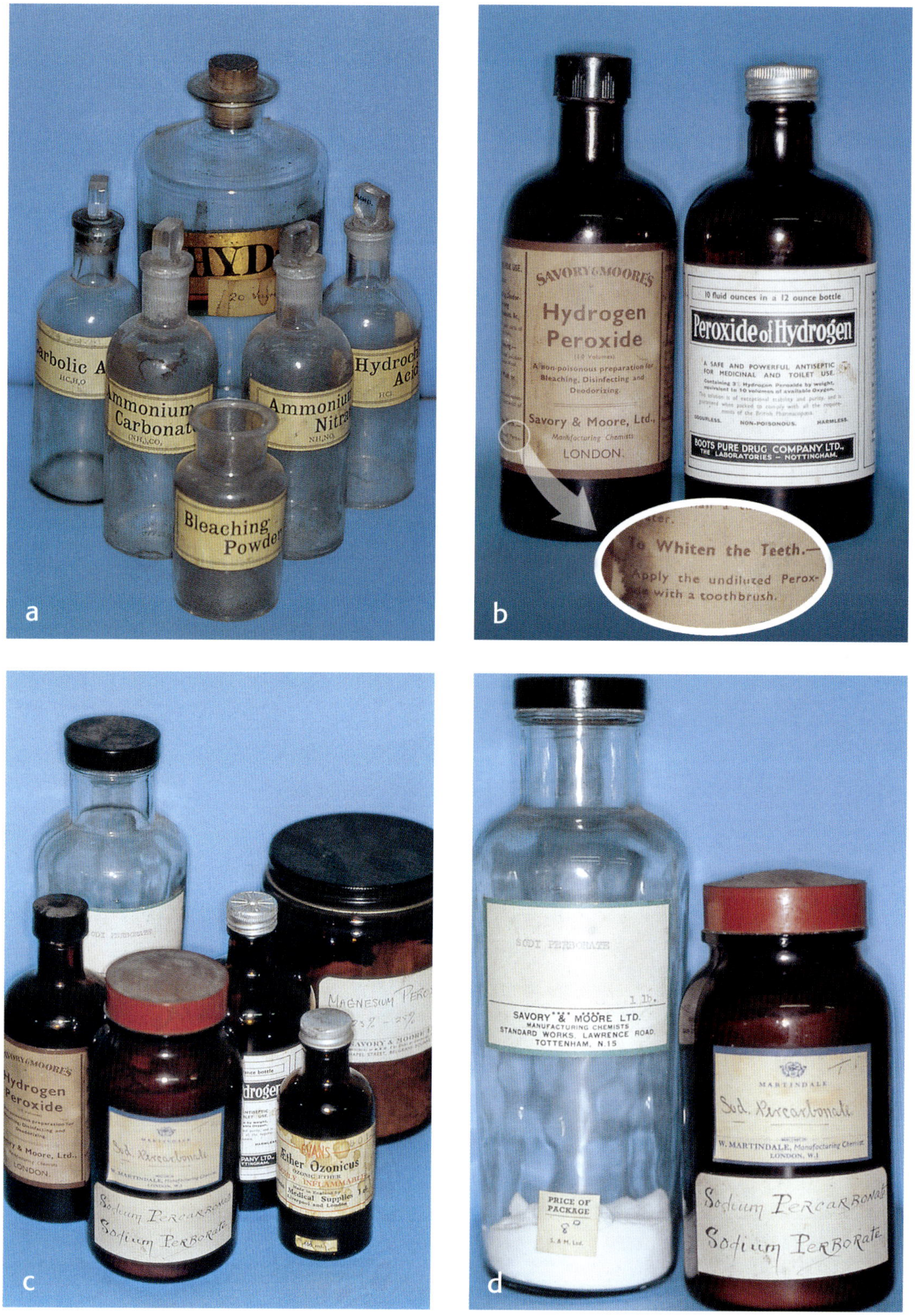

Fig. 10-2 Tooth whitening materials used in the past.

a. Tooth whitening materials used in 1820. Various concentrations of hydrogen peroxide, hydrochloric acid and ammonium compounds were employed.

b. Hydrogen peroxide used in 1860.

c,d. Various whitening materials used from 1860 to 1920.

Table 10-1 History of tooth bleaching (adapted from data in Haywood 1992).

Date	Name	Material used	Discoloration
1799	Macintosh	Invented chloride of lime, or bleaching powder	
1848	Dwinelle	Chloride of lime	Non-vital teeth
1860	Truman	Chloride and acetic acid Labarraque's solution (liquid chloride of soda)	Non-vital teeth
1861	Woodnut	Advised placing the bleaching medicament and changing it at subsequent appointments	
1868	Latimer	Oxalic acid	Vital teeth
1877	Chapple	Hydrochloric acid, oxalic acid	All discolorations
1878	Taft	Oxalic acid and calcium hypochlorite	
1884	Harlan	Used the first hydrogen peroxide (called hydrogen dioxide)	All discolorations
1893	Atkinson	Used 3% pyrozone as a mouthwash, which also lightened teeth 25% pyrozone was the most effective	
1895	Garretson	Applied chlorine to the tooth surface	Non-vital teeth
1910	Prins	Applied 30% hydrogen peroxide to teeth	Non-vital and vital
1916	Kaine	18% hydrochloric acid (muriatic acid) and heat lamp	Fluorosed teeth
1918	Abbot	Discovered a high-intensity light that produces a rapid temperature rise in the hydrogen peroxide to accelerate chemical tooth bleaching	Vital teeth
1924	Prinz	First recorded use of a solution of perborate in hydrogen peroxide activated by a light source	Vital teeth
1942	Younger	5 parts of 30% hydrogen peroxide heat lamp anesthetic	
1958	Pearson	Used 35% hydrogen peroxide inside tooth and also suggested 25% hydrogen peroxide and 75% ether, which was activated by a lamp, producing light and heat to release solvent qualities of ether	Non-vital teeth
1961	Spasser	Walking bleach technique Sodium perborate and water is sealed into the pulp chamber	Non-vital teeth
1965	Bouschar	5 parts 30% hydrogen peroxide, 5 parts 36% hydrochloric acid, 1 part diethyl ether	Orange colored fluorosis stains
1965	Stewart	Thermocatalytic technique Pellet saturated with superoxyl is inserted into the pulp chamber and heated with hot instrument	Non-vital teeth

Table 10-1 History of tooth bleaching (adapted from data in Haywood 1992), continued.

Date	Name	Material used	Discoloration
1966	McInnes	Repeats Bouschar's technique using controlled hydrochloric acid-pumice abrasion technique	Predictable?
1967	Cohen & Parkins	35% hydrogen peroxide and a heating instrument	Tetracycline stains
1967	Nutting and Poe	Combination walking bleach technique Superoxyl in pulp chamber (30% hydrogen peroxide)	Non-vital teeth
1968	Klusmier	Home bleaching concept started as an incidental finding; Gly-Oxide, which contains 10% carbamide peroxide, is placed in a custom-fitted orthodontic positioner	Vital teeth
1972	Klusmier	Used the same technique with Proxigel as it was thicker and stayed in the tray longer	Vital teeth
1975	Chandra & Chawla	30% hydrogen peroxide 18% hydrochloric acid flour of Paris	Fluorosis stains
1977	Falkenstein	1-minute etch with 30% hydrogen peroxide 10% hydrochloric acid 100 watt(104 °F) light gun	Tetracycline stains
1979	Compton	30% hydrogen peroxide heat element(130–145 °F)	Tetracycline stains
1979	Harrington and Natkin	Reported on external resorption associated with bleaching pulpless teeth	Non-vital teeth
1982	Abou-Rass	Recommended intentional endodontic treatment with internal bleaching	Tetracycline stains
1984	Zaragoza	70% hydrogen peroxide + heat for both arches	Vital teeth
1986	Munro	Used Gly-Oxide to control bacterial growth after periodontal root planning. Noticed tooth lightening	Vital teeth
1987	Feinman	In-office bleaching using 30% H_2O_2 and heat from bleaching light	Vital teeth
1988	Coastal Dental Study Club	Mouth guard bleaching technique	Vital teeth
1988	Munro	Presented findings to manufacturer, resulting in first commercial bleaching product: White + Brite (Omnii Int.)	Vital teeth
1989	Croll	Microabrasion technique 10% hydrochloric acid and pumice in a paste	Vital teeth, Superficial enamel discoloration, hypocalcification extrinsic stains
1989	Haywood & Heymann	Nightguard vital bleaching, 10% carbamide peroxide in a tray	All stains, vital and non-vital teeth

Table 10-1 History of tooth bleaching (adapted from data in Haywood 1992), continued.

Date	Name	Material used	Discoloration
1990		Introduction of commercial over-the-counter bleaching vital teeth products	Vital teeth
1991	Numerous authors	Power bleaching 30% hydrogen peroxide using a light to activate bleach.	All stains, vital teeth
1991	Garber and Goldstein	Combination of bleaching power and home bleaching	Vital teeth
1991	Hall	Recommended no etching teeth before vital bleaching procedures	Vital teeth
1994	American Dental Association	Safety and efficacy established for tooth bleaching agents under the ADA seal of approval	
1996	Food and Drug Administration	ADA-approved ion laser technology: argon and CO_2 lasers for tooth whitening with patented chemicals	
1996	Reyto	Laser tooth whitening	Vital teeth
1997	Settembrini et al	Inside/outside bleaching	Non-vital and vital teeth
1998	Carrillo et al	Open pulp chamber 10% carbamide peroxide in custom tray	Vital
2000	Miara	Compressed bleaching technique in patient's own bleaching tray	Vital teeth
2000	Kugel	5.3% hydrogen peroxide OTC tooth whitening strips	Vital teeth
2000	Gerlach	5–10% hydrogen peroxide OTC tooth whitening strips	Vital teeth
2004	Kurthy	Deep bleaching technique	Vital teeth
2005	Lynch*	Ozone whitening using ozone machine	Vital teeth
2006	Kwon	Sealed bleaching for power whitening; Prevents evaporation of active agent by placing a wrap onto the power whitening gel.	Vital teeth
2006		Various whitening applications; Use brush applications, pen and varnish	Vital teeth
Present Day		■ Plasma arc, halogen, UV, LED and light-activated bleaching techniques ■ Reduction in time with power gels for in-office bleaching ■ Laser-activated bleaching ■ Home bleaching available in different concentrations and with new desensitizers	Vital teeth

(With permission from Martin Dunitz Ltd.)

References

Baysan A and Lynch E: The use of ozone in dentistry and medicine. Prim Dent Care 2005 Apr:12 (2) 47-52.

Bogue EA. Bleaching Teeth. Dental Cosmos 1872;14 (1):1-3.

Chapple JA. Restoring discoloured teeth to normal. Dental Cosmos 1877;19:499.

Ciesara E, Dayan AD, Dushner H, Maier H and White D. The Safety of Tooth Whitening. Blackwell Munksgaard. Oxford. United Kingdom. First Edition. 2002.

Cubbon T and Ore D. Hard tissue and home tooth whiteners. CDS Review 1991;85:32-35.

Darnell DH and Moore WV. Vital tooth bleaching with the white and bright technique. Compend Continuing Education in Dentistry. 1990;11:86-94.

Fischer G. The bleaching of discoloured teeth with H_2O_2 Dent Cosmos 1911;53:246-247.

Gerlach RW. Shifting paradigms in whitening.: introduction of a novel system for vital tooth bleaching. Compend of Continuing Education in Dentistry. 2000; 21:4-9.

Gerlach RW Gibb RD and Sagel PA. A randomized clinical trial comparing a novel 5.3% hydrogen peroxide whitening strip to 10%, 15% and 20% carbamide peroxide tray-based bleaching systems. Compend Continuing Education in Dentistry 2000;21:22-8.

Greenwall LH. Chapter 2, page 24. Bleaching Techniques in Restorative Dentistry. Martin Dunitz. First Edition. London UK. 2001.

Haywood VB. History, safety and effectiveness of current bleaching techniques and applications of the nightguard bleaching technique. Quintessence Int 92 Jul 23(7) 1992;471-88.

Haywood VB. Historical development of whiteners: clinical safety and efficacy. Dental Update 24 (3) 1997;98-105.

Haywood VB and Heymann H. Nightguard vital bleaching. Quintessence Int 1989;20: 173-176.

Hall DA. Should etching be performed as part of a vital bleaching technique? Quintessence Int. 1991;22: 679-686.

Lee, Y. The Effectiveness of Sealing Technique on in-office Bleaching. Department of Dentistry, Yonsei University. Master of Science. 2007.

Matis BA, Cochran M, Wang G, Franco M, Eckert GJ, Carlotti RJ, Bryan C. A clinical evaluation using whitening wraps and strips. Oper Dent 2005 Sep- Oct: 30(5):588-92.

Matis BA, Cochran MA Franco M, Al Ammer W, Eckert GJ, Stropes M. Eight in-office tooth whitening systems evaluated in vivo: a pilot study. Operative Dent Jul-Aug 2007;32(4):322-7.

Matis BA, Gaiao U, Blackman D, Scultz FA, Eckert GJ. In vivo degradation of bleaching gel used in whitening teeth. J Am Dent Assoc. 1999;130 (2): 227-35.

Ring ME. Dentistry, an Illustrated History. Mosby Year Book Inc St Louis USA. 1985.

Rotstein I. Personal Communication 1999.

Sulieman M. An overview of bleaching techniques:1: History, chemistry, safety and legal aspects. Dental Update Dec 31(10) 2004;608-10, 612-4,616.

Index